CLEVELAND CLINIC HEART BOOK

CLEVELAND
CLINIC
HEART BOOK

ERIC J. TOPOL, M.D.

Editor-in-Chief

A CMD Publishing Book

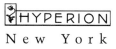

New York

The *Cleveland Clinic Heart Book* is the definitive book on heart disease, covering all areas from prevention to treatment presented by the nation's #1 heart center. To stay current with diagnostic and treatment advancements, consult the *Cleveland Clinic Heart Advisor* newsletter, which provides the latest up-to-date information from the same trusted source that has brought this book to you. For information on how to receive the newsletter, call 1-800-829-2506.

Founded in 1921, the Cleveland Clinic is one of the nation's largest medical group practices with more than 1,000 physicians and scientists on staff. Within the Cleveland Clinic is the nation's top heart center, as ranked by *U.S. News & World Report.* The Cleveland Clinic Heart Center's top cardiologists and cardiac surgeons have provided the knowledge for the content of this book. For further information, write to the Cleveland Clinic Heart Center, 9500 Euclid Ave., Cleveland, OH 44195, or visit the Web site at www.clevelandclinic.org/heartcenter.

As with any medical literature or advice, we recommend that you always consult with your physician before embarking on any changes to your current treatment or if you have any questions regarding your care. The *Cleveland Clinic Heart Book* is not intended to substitute for your physician's care nor does this book support or endorse any product or company.

Library of Congress Cataloging-in-Publication Data

Cleveland Clinic heart book: the definitive guide for the entire family from the nation's leading heart center / Cleveland Clinic ; foreword by Michael D. Eisner ; introduction by Eric J. Topol–1st ed.
    p. cm.
    Includes index.
    ISBN 0-7868-6495-8
    1.Heart–Diseases–Popular works. I. Title: Heart Book. II. Cleveland Clinic Foundation.

RC672.C55 2000
616.1'2–dc21   99-059778

Cover design by Paul Perlow Design.
Text design by Blake Logan.

ISBN: 0-7868-6495-8

FIRST EDITION

10 9 8 7 6 5 4 3 2 1

Dedicated to Our Patients

Foreword

In 1994, at the age of 52, I learned the hard way that it's a mistake to take one's heart for granted.

Unfortunately, it's easy to lure ourselves into thinking that this all-important muscle is somehow self-sufficient. After all, from the moment we're born, when most of the other muscles in our body are just flailing about, the heart is already dutifully doing its job. Other muscles may get tired or sore or strained, but the heart quietly goes about beating. Even when we sleep and all of our other muscles rest and rejuvenate, the heart keeps on working, relentlessly pulsing deep within the chest, as if some sort of perpetual motion machine.

Then, as happened to me, we abruptly learn otherwise. I was in Sun Valley, curiously feeling pain in my arms. I decided to fly home the next day and that night found myself on an operating table, having healthy vessels from my legs patched in to replace the clogged ones that led into my heart.

I was lucky and received the care I needed in time. I got a second chance. I decided to make the most of it.

And so I came to be aware of the Cleveland Clinic, where incredible advances in coronary care have become almost routine. I learned how, though proper diet, exercise, and lifestyle, I can help keep my heart healthy. I was amazed how simple and effective the Clinic's advice was and how filled with common sense. I only wished I had followed this kind of guidance before that trip to Sun Valley.

Because of the importance of making these heart health options more widely known, I suggested the creation of this book. I discussed the idea with the Cleveland Clinic and with Bob Miller of Hyperion. It seemed that a book would be a way to make the Clinic's guidance and wisdom available to anyone who is coping with a heart problem and, even more important, to anyone whose heart is still completely healthy.

Unlike other muscles in the body, our heart does not come in a matched set. We only get one. It should never be taken for granted. So, you might think of this book as a step-by-step user's manual on how to take good care of your heart—so your heart can take good care of you.

Michael D. Eisner
Chairman and Chief Executive Officer
The Walt Disney Company

Acknowledgments

CLEVELAND CLINIC HEART CENTER

CHAIRMEN

Delos M. Cosgrove, M.D.
Chairman of Thoracic & Cardiovascular Surgery

Norman J. Starr, M.D.
Chairman of Cardiothoracic Anesthesiology

Eric J. Topol, M.D.
Chairman of Cardiology

CARDIOLOGISTS
(by Section)

CARDIAC CATHETERIZATION
Frederick A. Heupler, Jr., M.D.
John R. Kramer, M.D.
Mehdi Razavi, M.D.

CARDIOVASCULAR IMAGING
Imran Afridi, M.D.
Craig Asher, M.D.
Fetnat Fouad, M.D.
Mario J. Garcia, M.D.
Brian P. Griffin, M.D.
Richard A. Grimm, D.O.
Loretta R. Isada, M.D.
Allan L. Klein, M.D.
Harry M. Lever, M.D.
Leonardo Rodriguez, M.D
Ellen Mayer Sabik, M.D.
William J. Stewart, M.D.
James D. Thomas, M.D.

CLINICAL CARDIOLOGY
Matthew G. Deedy, M.D.
Sasan Ghaffari, M.D.
Fuad Y. Jubran, M.D.
Donald F. Hammer, M.D.
Roger. M. Mills, M.D.
Steven Nissen, M.D.
Curtis M. Rimmerman, M.D.
Killian C. Robinson, M.D.
Donald A. Underwood, M.D.

HEART FAILURE AND TRANSPLANTATION
Corinne Bott-Silverman, M.D.
Gary S. Francis, M.D.
Garrie J. Haas, M.D.
Robert E. Hobbs, M.D.
Karen P. James, M.D.
Michael S. Lauer, M.D.
Suzanne R. Lutton, M.D.
Gustavo Rincon, M.D.
Randall C. Starling, M.D.
Hilal Yamani, M.D.
James B. Young, M.D.

INTERVENTIONAL CARDIOLOGY
Sorin J. Brener, M.D.
Khosrow Dorosti, M.D.
Stephen G. Ellis, M.D.
Irving Franco, M.D.
A. Michael Lincoff, M.D.
David J. Moliterno, M.D.
Russell E. Raymond, D.O.
Mitchell J. Silver, D.O.
Conrad C. Simpfendorfer, M.D.
E. Murat Tuzcu, M.D.
Patrick L. Whitlow, M.D.
Sanjay S. Yadav, M.D.

PACEMAKER/ELECTROPHYSIOLOGY
Lon W. Castle, M.D.
Mina K. Chung, M.D.
Frederick J. Jaeger, D.O.
Andrea Natale, M.D.
Mark J. Niebauer, M.D.
Walid Saliba, M.D.
Patrick J. Tchou, M.D.
Bruce L. Wilkoff, M.D.

PREVENTIVE CARDIOLOGY
Gordon G. Blackburn, Ph.D.
JoAnne Foody, M.D.
Joseph P. Frolkis, M.D., Ph.D.
Dennis L. Sprecher, M.D.

SURGEONS
Michael K. Banbury, M.D.
Eugene H. Blackstone, M.D.

Malcolm M. DeCamp, Jr., M.D.
A. Marc Gillinov, M.D.
Bruce W. Lytle, M.D.
Patrick M. McCarthy, M.D.
Sudish Murthy, M.D.
Jose Luis Navia, M.D.
B. Gosta Pettersson, M.D., Ph.D.
Thomas W. Rice, M.D.
Joseph F. Sabik III, M.D.
Nicholas G. Smedira, M.D.

ANESTHESIOLOGISTS
John T. Apostolakis, M.D.
Darryl M. Atwell, M.D.
C. Alan Bashour, M.D.
Paula M. Bokesch, M.D.
M. Gregory Bourdakis, M.D.
Randall Correia, M.D.
Pierre deVilliers, M.D.
E. George Estafanous, M.D.
Charles J. Hearn, D.O.
Steven R. Insler, D.O.
Eric F. Kaiser, M.D.
Colleen Gorman Koch, M.D.
Erik J. Kraenzler, M.D.
Michael G. Licina, M.D.
Emad B. Mossad, M.D.
Michael S. O'Conner, D.O.
John H. Petre, Ph.D.
Dominique Prud'homme, M.D.
Robert M. Savage, M.D.
Lee K. Wallace, M.D.
Jean-Pierre Yared, M.D.

IMAGING SPECIALISTS
Richard C. Brunken, M.D.
Sebastian A. Cook, M.D.
Scott D. Flamm, M.D.
Raymundo T. Go, M.D.
Donald R. Neumann, M.D., Ph.D.
Richard D. White, M.D.

PEDIATRIC CARDIOLOGISTS
Maryanne Kichuk, M.D.
Larry A. Latson, M.D.
Douglas S. Moodie, M.D., M.S.
Daniel J. Murphy, Jr., M.D.

Lourdes R. Prieto, M.D.
Richard Sterba, M.D.

PEDIATRIC AND CONGENITAL HEART SURGEONS
Jonathon Drummond-Webb, M.B., CH.B.
Roger Mee, M.B., CH.B.

PUBLISHING AND PRODUCTION ACKNOWLEDGMENTS

CLEVELAND CLINIC HEART CENTER
Holli Birrer
Jon Catanese
John Clough, M.D.
Nancy Heim
Mary Heisler, R.N.
Jeffrey Loerch
Phyllis Marino
Linda Noble
Betsy Stovsky, R.N.

HYPERION
Anne Cole
Wendy Lefkon
Linda Prather

CMD PUBLISHING
a division of
Current Medical Directions, Inc./
Three V Health, Inc.
Greg Annussek
Donna Balopole
Andrea Lins
Jennifer Mitchell
Kim Pohl

WRITERS
Kristine Napier, R.D., L.D.
Lyn Yonack

HERMITAGE PUBLISHING SERVICES
Page Composition

FETTERS INFOMANAGEMENT
Indexing

Introduction

The human desire not only to live but also to improve the quality of life has accelerated the pace of heart disease research. It has pushed forward the frontiers of therapies for malformed, sick, weakened, clogged, and failing hearts of all ages and sizes at a startling rate. As a result, people with nearly every form of heart disease today have options—viable and excellent options to return them to a more functional lifestyle, if not a full recovery.

The *Cleveland Clinic Heart Book* describes these options and guides the reader to making them a reality.

One of the greatest challenges we face in cardiology is preventing death and disability from coronary artery disease (CAD). According to the American Heart Association (AHA), nearly 14 million Americans have CAD, which is responsible for half of all heart-related deaths.

In this era of seemingly boundless technology, we scarcely acknowledge a time when CAD could not be diagnosed until it narrowed blood vessels so severely as to cause myocardial infarction (heart attack) or instant death. Today, the tools of a cardiologist's trade are many and magical—thanks in large part to the legendary F. Mason Sones, Jr., M.D., a Cleveland Clinic cardiologist regarded as one of the most important contributors to modern cardiology. His pioneering work linked catheterization, x-ray studies, and cinematography, lighting the previously dark world of CAD and revolutionizing the course of cardiology and cardiovascular surgery.

A Magical Beginning

His story is fascinating. Opening a window into the heart happened quite by accident four decades ago. Conventional medical wisdom of the day held that invading the coronary arteries with a catheter and dye to identify blockages would be fatal, as had been shown in dog experiments. Instead, Sones' plan was to inject contrast material just near the opening of diseased vessels in an attempt to photograph them. But in a basement laboratory late one night in 1958, Sones was retracting the catheter across the aortic valve when what he thought was certain disaster struck. "I hit the switch to rev up the x-ray generator so I could see," recalled Dr. Sones in accepting the 1983 prestigious Albert Lasker Clinical Medical Research Award for pioneering coronary angiography. "As the picture came on, I could see that the catheter was in the guy's right coronary artery. And there I was down in the hole," he continued, describing the cardiologist's usual compromised position in the antiquated catheterization laboratory. "I yelled, 'Pull it out! Pull it out.' By that time, about 30 ccs of the dye had gone into the coronary artery... I thought that his heart would fibrillate, as the dogs' hearts had in our animal studies, and I would have to open his chest and shock his heart to bring it out of fibrillation."

The next agonizing 8 seconds proved fortuitous, revealing a new world of possibilities in selective coronary arteriography. The patient's heart did not fibrillate as Sones had expected—it stopped. "I knew that if we could get him to cough, it would produce a pulse pressure inside the arteries that would drive out the dye." Miraculously, the patient coughed three times—restoring his heart beat. "I knew at once that if the human heart could tolerate 30 ccs of dye, we would be able to safely inject small amounts directly into the coronary artery."

That late night accident granted heart specialists the view of CAD they needed to advance treatment options. At once, angiography and the arteriograms it produced became the blueprints cardiovascular surgeons used to identify coronary artery lesions requiring bypass surgery. Two decades later, arteriograms provided a clear picture for interventional cardiologists pioneering percutaneous (through the skin) revascularization, or nonsurgical procedures to restore blood flow to the heart.

Today, angioplasty plus stenting has replaced angioplasty as state-of-the-art therapy, representing more than 80 percent of percutaneous revascularizations in the United States, for a total of 600,000 procedures annually.

Fortunately, angiography can diagnose narrowing arteries before they cause serious trouble, and the images it produces aid heart specialists in recommending the most appropriate therapy: either coronary artery bypass graft (CABG) surgery or a catheter intervention by an interventional cardiologist. Each year about a million people undergo bypass surgery or percutaneous revascularization to restore blood flow to the heart and in so doing receive the gift of new life.

Cardiac specialists continue to advance their skills and technologies, never settling for the current technology and always asking questions—the answers to which improve the chance of success and ultimately quality of life. They now know, for example, that balloon angioplasty augmented by stenting is superior to balloon angioplasty alone, once the gold standard of nonsurgical revascularization. Thanks to a large, 63-center study conducted in the United States and Canada, EPISTENT, cardiologists recently learned that angioplasty plus stenting produces superior results when given with a potent drug that inhibits blood clotting.

Preventing Myocardial Infarctions

A main goal of treatments for heart disease is to prevent heart attacks (myocardial infarctions). In groundbreaking research, we now understand that the popular view of myocardial infarction is incorrect. Exciting research spilling forth at this very time has opened the next frontier in cardiology. At one time, we thought that most myocardial infarctions occur when one major artery is severely obstructed—closed off by 80 percent or more—by atherosclerosis. Today, we are just realizing that instead, 70 percent of myocardial infarctions are caused by much smaller obstructions, which narrow the artery by perhaps only a third or so. Such obstructions are too small to cause symptoms or to be detected by an angiogram, a special x-ray of the heart. It is in our newly evolving understanding of why this happens that we are now approaching CAD from a new angle, and seeking new therapies that we hope will prevent the majority of myocardial infarctions.

We are learning, for example, that the body's immune system—its defense mechanism—is one of the instigators in causing myocardial infarctions. We are just beginning to appreciate that the inflammatory processes produced by the body's immune system are a key culprit in the CAD process. Now understanding these processes, we better understand why plaque—the atherosclerotic patches inside the blood vessels—rupture and cause a myocardial infarction, even though they barely block an artery. In the next generation of heart disease research, we will determine how to combine the many and varied therapies to stop all the processes that damage blood vessels and lead to myocardial infarctions. We are exploring, for example, the possibility of using the new arthritis anti-inflammatory drugs such as COX-2 and tumor necrosis factor (TNF) inhibitors in people with CAD.

Stopping Restenosis

We must be multifocused in our approach to heart disease. Not only must we seek to prevent and treat CAD, but we must also look after the people that have been treated. An issue we continually tackle is restenosis, or the renarrowing of heart vessels after angioplasty, the bane of the interventional cardiologist's existence. Even with the added help of stents, the restenosis rate is still 10 to 20 percent within 6 months of treatment. Investigators have been working on reducing this rate by implanting irradiated stents.

The concept of using radiation to reduce cell growth—and restenosis is simply one form of cell growth—is not a new one. The benefits of radiation are well-described in stopping cancer cell proliferation and also in reducing scar size by limiting cell overgrowth in people with a tendency to form bulky scars called keloid tissue. In the case of stents, the hope is that radiation will lessen cell growth inside the stent, thereby reducing the chance of restenosis. Cardiologists also theorize that the radiation may be sufficient to penetrate plaque all the way down to the artery wall, further limiting cell growth.

Carotid Artery Involvement

The heart is not the only organ affected by atherosclerosis. One-half million Americans suffer strokes each year, which often result in death or considerable disability. Minimizing risk factors is key to preventing stroke, and a main risk factor is carotid artery stenosis, or blocked carotid arteries, which accounts for approximately 20 to 30 percent of all strokes. The carotid arteries are the pipelines carrying precious oxygen-rich blood to the brain. When one or both carotid arteries becomes blocked by atherosclerosis—the same condition that blocks heart vessels, causing angina (chest pain) and myocardial infarction—surgeons can sometimes scrape them clean in a procedure called endarterectomy. This is major and tricky surgery, however, and alternatives are needed for several types of high-risk patients. Some people with carotid artery stenosis, for example, are too sick with heart disease, lung disease, or neurologic instability or simply too weak from advancing age to have the procedure done. Others have already undergone endarterectomy and suffer from restenosis. Another group of people have both blocked carotid and coronary arteries, and performing both carotid endarterectomy and CABG surgery in them is quite risky. In addition, an alternative procedure is needed for people who develop restenosis after carotid endarterectomy and whose other carotid artery is also blocked.

Now, there is an option for these high-risk people: balloon angioplasty and stenting. In this treatment, cardiologists advance the treating catheter through a vein in the groin all the way up to the blocked neck arteries. This technique reduces complication rates significantly by eliminating the need for major surgery and allowing monitoring of the patient's neurologic status during the intervention. In addition, radiologists use ultrasound imaging and angiograms to check that blood flow to the brain is adequate during the procedure.

CAD Prevention

Expanding the options for people with CAD is important, and stepping up preventive efforts is just as critical.

At the Cleveland Clinic Heart Center, prevention is divided into two efforts. Primary prevention is aimed at preventing arterial blockage in people not yet diagnosed with artery-clogging heart disease but who have one or more risk factors. In secondary prevention, cardiologists take a more aggressive approach with people who have already suffered the consequences of CAD: angina, myocardial infarction, stroke, or the need for a procedure to bypass blocked vessels.

Utilizing a sophisticated, multidisciplinary approach, preventive cardiologists review all risk factors, including genetic markers. Preventive cardiologists at the Cleveland Clinic have made important global contributions in the roles that genetic markers such as lipoprotein(a), homocysteine, Apo(E), and fibrinogen play in instigating or worsening heart disease. Their nationally recognized research has recently revealed that lipoprotein(a) significantly increases the risk of CAD in women of all ages and also in younger men. Related research found that lipoprotein(a) predicts cardiovascular disease in women independently of low-density lipoprotein (LDL, or "bad") cholesterol levels. Ultimately, such findings will translate into an earlier diagnosis that can prevent heart disease from developing, which means decreased health care costs and greatly improved quality of life.

Heart Failure

Heart failure is the only form of heart disease increasing in prevalence, owing largely to an incidence that doubles every decade after age 45 and an increasing lifespan. Four million Americans now have this condition; at the current rate of increase, 6 million Americans will have heart failure by the year 2030. A devastating disease, heart failure is the leading and most expensive cause of hospitalization after age 45, accounting for $10 to $40 million of direct health care costs yearly. In a medical milieu where people leave the hospital 2 to 3 days after major surgery, heart failure patients remain hospitalized an average of 9 days at a time and usually several times yearly.

Today, heart failure specialists realize a goal more enthusiastic than improving life and lifespan of people with heart failure: to diagnose heart failure early and treat it aggressively before the heart literally works itself to death. Early treatment is aimed at preventing unfavorable "ventricular remodeling," or the dangerous stretching and thinning that renders heart muscles useless. How? By monitoring people at high risk of heart failure, and watching for its earliest signs (swollen ankles, shortness of breath on limited exertion, and decreasing ability to exercise) and then acting on these signs promptly. Such early signs signal the need for more sophisticated testing, such as echocardiography and the institution of aggressive drug therapy. Heart failure specialists such as those at the Cleveland Clinic Heart Center, one of the largest heart failure treatment centers in the world, are experienced in using classes of medications both more aggressively and in new but more effective combinations. Simultaneously, advances are being made in mechanical assist devices that keep the heart beating as heart failure patients await surgical reconstruction of their hearts or a new heart. The choices are many and excellent, as described in this book.

Congenital Heart Defects

Congenital heart defects—the most common type of birth defect—affect 8 to 10 of every 1,000 newborns. Heart defects are diagnosed at several junctures: before birth, at birth, and sometimes not until later in life, even into adulthood, when the defect becomes severe enough to cause symptoms. Although difficult to fathom, pediatric heart surgeons now operate on the tiniest of hearts, including those of 1- or 2-pound infants.

While any heart defect is serious and can be frightening for new parents, some defects are particularly worrisome. Not only are they complex—a complexity complicated by their ever so minute size—but they are rare. That means that few pediatric heart surgeons have had extensive experience in repairing these defects. It remains essential for parents to know all their treatment options and seek the best care available.

About This Book

In this comprehensive book, medical and surgical heart specialists from the Cleveland Clinic Heart Center have summarized the very latest understanding of the heart muscle itself, as well as the advances and options available in diagnosing and treating CAD, valvular problems, arrhythmias, heart failure, blood vessel diseases, and congenital anomalies. Concerned with each patient's everyday ability to live well, Cleveland Clinic cardiologists have included information about the practical aspects of living with heart disease.

The advice in this book emanates from a medical center that is considered a leading authority on heart disease. For the fifth consecutive year, the Cleveland Clinic Heart Center was ranked first in the country for treating heart disease. The Clinic's track record is excellent in all matters of the heart, from balloon angioplasty to heart transplant. Among other things, the sheer volume of patients seen—Cleveland Clinic heart surgeons, for example, perform over 4,500 open-heart operations annually—grants the Clinic the expertise that only experience can bring.

We hope this book gives you the information you need to help improve your cardiovascular health today, and for many years to come.

Eric J. Topol, M.D.
Chairman and Professor
Department of Cardiology
Cleveland Clinic

Co-Chairman
Cleveland Clinic Heart Center

Director
The Joseph J. Jacobs Center for Thrombosis and Vascular Biology
Cleveland Clinic Heart Center

Contents

CHAPTER 1

How the Heart and Circulatory System Work

The heart, consequently, is the beginning of life...it is the household divinity which, discharging its function, nourishes, cherishes, quickens the whole body, and is indeed the foundation of life, the source of all action.
—*William Harvey*, English physician

What stronger breastplate than a heart untainted!
—*Shakespeare*, Henry VI

Introduction

The heart. Speak the word and poetic images may well come to mind. From playing cards to Valentine's Day cards, from romantic poetry to musical lyrics, the use of the term and of the image offers up a range of sentiments and associations. The heart is at the fiery core of existence, and it is the source of strength and emotions. Yet, abruptly the heart can grow cold or be broken.

How is it that one word is able to embrace such complicated, often contradictory notions of the human experience?

The answer may well lie in the biologic heart itself. Like its metaphoric counterpart, this organ lies at the center—at the heart—of the circulatory system. It is the source of physical strength and vitality. A person with a vigorous heart typically feels animated, full of energy, rosy from the top of the head to the tips of the toes. Excitement, fear, exhilaration, or the push toward physical excellence can make palpable the heart's rhythmic power in the center of the chest.

However, the heart can also be fragile. When the heart is not functioning well, it can likely be felt—if not in actual discomfort—in an inability to engage vigorously in ordinary activities and in a widespread, often vague sense of being tired, spent, or ill. And when the heart stops, life stops.

Nevertheless, when stripped of its symbolic and romantic associations, the plain fact is that the heart is a pump. It is the driving force by which the blood delivers nutrients, oxygen, and other substances to nourish the various parts of the body. The heart is also the means by which the body's waste products are pumped away from the cells so that they can be removed from the body. The heart may sound rather mechanical—and so it is. But the fact that the heart is a pump does not alter its complexity or its wonder.

Today's doctors and researchers, much like the poets and philosophers of earlier centuries, have turned a keen eye and a driving curiosity to understand the complex workings of the human heart. Cardiology, the study of the heart, has applied intense scientific scrutiny and made tremendous strides during the past few decades not only in understanding how the heart works, but also in what happens to undermine it. Perhaps even more exciting, cardiologists are learning how to prevent, reverse, and correct heart problems and heart disease.

None of this increased medical and scientific knowledge has diminished our romantic notions of the heart. The more we learn about the human heart, the more wondrous it seems.

The Location and Structure of the Heart

The heart nestles in the area of the thorax (chest) between the lungs and behind the sternum (breastbone) called the mediastinum of the thoracic cavity. Although the heart lies between the lungs in the center of the chest, its base balloons out from the breastbone toward the front of the chest. This slight tilt is why the heart appears to be on the left side of the body. Because the bottom part of this cone-shaped organ lies so close to the surface, you can readily feel—and often hear—the heart's pulsating beat. At its bottom, the heart is attached to the diaphragm, the muscular membrane that separates the thoracic cavity from the abdominal cavity. At its front, the heart is attached to the sternum, on the sides to the pleura (the membranes that enclose the lungs), and at the back to the esophagus, trachea, and principal bronchi, the lung's larger air passages.

The heart's structure is relatively simple. The walls of the heart have three layers of tissue. The outer surface is made up of a thin membrane called the epicardium. The middle layer is the muscular wall, called the myocardium, or cardiac muscle. Unlike the body's other muscles, the myocardium is capable of contracting rhythmically, which allows it to respond to the heart's electrical impulses.

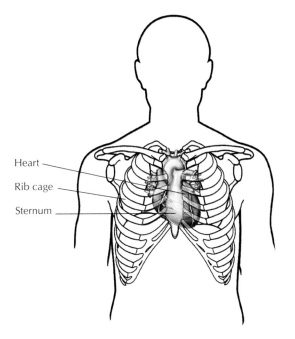

Heart
Rib cage
Sternum

The heart is a fist-sized muscular organ located in the chest cavity under the rib cage to the left of the sternum (breastbone) and between the lungs. At its bottom, the heart is extended to the body's left.

The heart's smooth inner lining is called the endocardium. A silky, fibrous sac, the pericardium, encloses the heart. Within the innermost layer of the pericardium, between the epicardium and the parietal pericardium, its fibrous outer layer, is the pericardial cavity. This space is normally filled with a small amount of clear fluid that reduces friction between the two membranes.

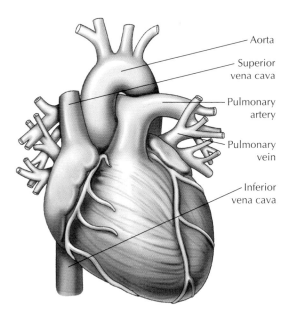

Aorta
Superior vena cava
Pulmonary artery
Pulmonary vein
Inferior vena cava

The major blood vessels that enter the heart: the aorta, the pulmonary arteries and veins, and the superior and inferior venae cavae.

The great blood vessels are the large vessels that enter the heart:

- The aorta, the body's main artery, which sends oxygenated blood from the heart out to the body

- The pulmonary arteries and veins, which bring blood to and from the lungs

- The superior and inferior venae cavae, the body's principal veins, which return deoxygenated blood to the heart from the upper and lower sections of the body respectively

Each of the heart's two sides is responsible for separate but related tasks. The right side receives the oxygen-depleted blood on its journey back from the body and passes it to the lungs, where it is oxygenated. The left side pumps oxygen-replenished blood out to the body.

The heart contains an atrium and a ventricle, an upper and lower chamber, on each side. The atria are small filling pockets that also serve as low-pressure pumps. Their walls are thin; a thicker muscular wall, the atrial septum, divides the right and left atria and prevents blood from flowing directly between the two chambers.

Below the atria are the right and left ventricles, which are separated by the ventricular septum. Because the ventricles act as major pumping stations, they have thicker, more muscular walls than do the atria.

The atria and ventricles work in concert to create the cardiac cycle. The atrium supplies blood to the ventricle, which then pumps the blood out. By feeding a steady flow of blood to the ventricle, the atrium serves as a reservoir, ensuring that the pump never runs dry. That way, when-

The heart's left and right sides are divided by the septum. The heart is divided into four chambers—the right and left atria on top, the right and left ventricles beneath them. The left ventricle is the heart's major pumping chamber. The four heart valves, tricuspid, aortic, pulmonic, and mitral, control the flow of blood through the chambers.

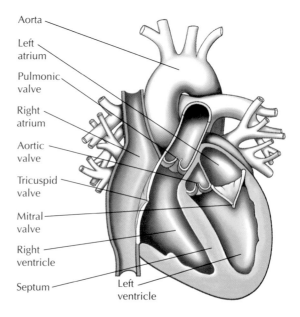

Aorta
Left atrium
Pulmonic valve
Right atrium
Aortic valve
Tricuspid valve
Mitral valve
Right ventricle
Septum
Left ventricle

ever you sit up quickly or disengage abruptly from some type of strenuous activity, your body continues to receive just the right supply of blood.

Four valves—delicate, billowing flaps attached to the chamber wall—ensure that blood flows in only one direction between chambers of the heart and into the major blood vessels. The tricuspid valve operates between the right atrium and right ventricle. The pulmonic (or pulmonary) valve is located between the right ventricle and the pulmonary artery. The mitral valve, so named because it resembles a bishop's headdress, is also called the bicuspid valve; it is located between the left atrium and left ventricle. The aortic valve leads from the left ventricle to the aorta.

Each valve has a set of flaps, called leaflets or cusps. The mitral valve has two cusps; the others have three. The tricuspid and mitral valves are larger and more fragile than the other valves and depend on fibrous cords called chordae tendineae for support. These supporting structures are attached to fingerlike projections called papillary muscles.

Whenever there is a difference in pressure across the valves, these petal-shaped leaflets undulate gently to allow the blood free passage. The flaps then fold down over themselves to enclose the opening. The valves do not seal the passageway completely, however. Instead, a steady trickle of blood is allowed to seep through. All four valves operate on a one-way basis so that blood cannot flow backwards through them.

For more information on valves, see Chapter 6, Diseases of the Heart Valves.

The Mechanics of the Heart

A little larger than a fist, the human heart is a strong, hollow, four-chambered muscular pump. It weighs little more than a pound and yet is able to move more than 5 quarts of blood each minute—approximately 2,000 gallons of blood each day—throughout the body. While it may be customary to talk about the heart as though it were a distinct object—something to hold in your hand (or to wear on your sleeve)—the heart actually occupies the center of an elaborate, extensive cardiovascular system.

Working together with the lungs and vascular system (blood vessels), the heart provides the propulsion behind the blood's circulation. Other parts of the body—the kidneys, liver, brain, and nervous system—contribute to the smooth functioning of the cardiovascular system by regulating the tempo, adjusting the pace, and making corrections in the rhythm as needed.

With each beat, the heart muscle expands and contracts, sending 2 to 3 ounces of blood through the vascular system, an elaborate network of elastic veins, arteries, and smaller vessels, to the body's tissues and organs. The typical heart rate—the pace at which the heart pumps—is 72 beats per minute, or more than a beat per second. Each day, the heart beats faithfully, on average, 100,000 times. In a 70-year lifetime, an average human heart beats more than 2.5 billion times.

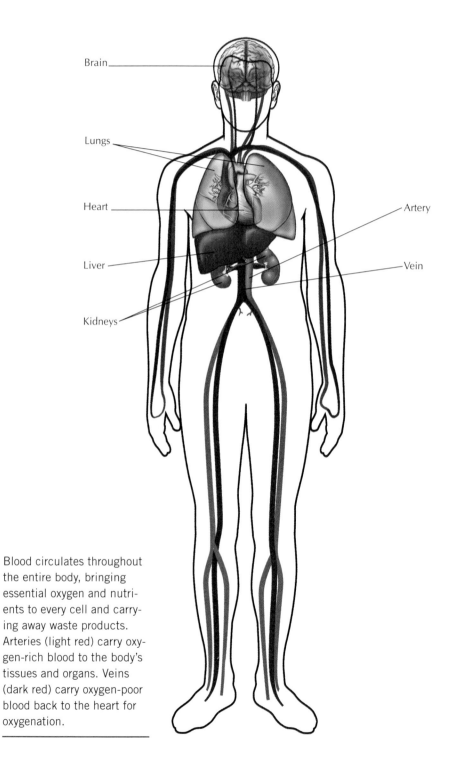

Brain

Lungs

Heart

Artery

Liver

Vein

Kidneys

Blood circulates throughout the entire body, bringing essential oxygen and nutrients to every cell and carrying away waste products. Arteries (light red) carry oxygen-rich blood to the body's tissues and organs. Veins (dark red) carry oxygen-poor blood back to the heart for oxygenation.

Moreover, this steadfast instrument responds to and accommodates a variety of factors. The heart's rate and rhythm vary from person to person and from activity to activity. The heart naturally pulses more slowly when a person is at rest and hastens its pace during exercise or strenuous activity, thus decreasing or increasing the amount of oxygen transported to muscles and tissues in accordance with the body's needs. Other factors, including pain, emotional stress, and hormonal changes, also affect the heart's rate and rhythm.

The Dynamics of the Heart

The Heart's Electrical System

The structure of the heart muscle accounts for the precise sequence of coordinated movements that propels the blood throughout the cardiovascular system. A natural pacemaker, the sinoatrial node (SA node or sinus node) is located within a small bundle of highly specialized cells at the juncture of the right atrium and the superior vena cava. Considered the starting point of the heartbeat, the SA node generates the

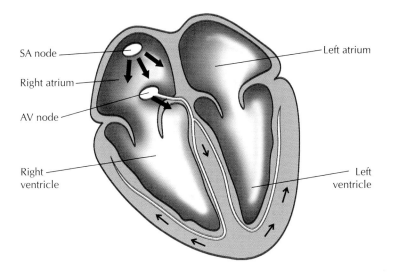

The heartbeat—the heart's pumping action—is controlled by electrical impulses that signal the myocardium to expand and contract. The impulses are generated at the sinus node (sinoatrial or SA node), located in the right atrium. This cluster of nerve cells functions as the body's natural pacemaker, the system that keeps the heart pacing in an even rhythm. Impulses travel through predetermined electrical pathways to reach the atrioventricular (AV) node, an electrical relay station near the border of the right atrium and right ventricle.

rhythmic electrical impulses that guide the chambers of the heart in their contractions.

The heart's electrical system generates a wavelike movement within the myocardium. As they pass through the heart, electrical ripples stimulate the smooth sections of the myocardium, causing rhythmic contractions to progress from the top to the bottom. This is the heartbeat, or pulse. It is this electrical activity that an electrocardiogram (ECG or EKG) measures (see page 67).

The SA node builds up electrical energy and then discharges it, causing a slight twitch that prompts the atria to contract. The electrical pulse travels down the right atrium and passes through the atrioventricular or AV node, a group of nerve cells located where the atria and ventricle meet—almost at the center of the heart. The AV node checks the electrical current as it crosses the heart.

As the pulse moves to the ventricle, it is slowed and distributed to the muscular network that is engineered to handle the more strenuous work of this chamber. After the ventricle contracts, the cycle begins again. The exact pace of this cycle—just how fast or slowly a person's heart beats—is cued by messages from the brain (see page 16), and is subject to conditions such as outside temperature, level of activity, pain, and emotional stress.

For more information on the heart's electrical system, see Chapter 7, Rhythm Disorders.

The Cardiac Cycle

The heartbeat has two phases.

- *Diastole:* The phase of the heart cycle during which the heart relaxes and the muscle fibers lengthen. As the heart dilates, the cavities fill with blood. As a rule, diastole of the atria occurs before diastole of the ventricles.

- *Systole:* The phase of the heart cycle during which a given part is in contraction. During the systolic phase the myocardial fibers contract, that is, they tighten and shorten. Blood surges through the aorta and the pulmonary artery.

This cardiac cycle directs blood through the heart, to the lungs, and throughout the body. Blood is transported to the body's organs and tissues by means of a highly orchestrated sequence of contractions within the heart's chambers. Between contractions, during the diastolic, or filling, phase of the pumping cycle, the heart muscle relaxes and blood enters the right atrium from the superior and inferior venae cavae, the two large veins that collect blood returning from the upper and lower body, respectively.

Dark bluish in color, this blood is depleted of oxygen and rich in carbon dioxide. The right atrium contracts, moving the blood through the tricuspid valve into the right ventricle. Once the right ventricle is filled, the right atrium relaxes at the same time that the ventricle con-

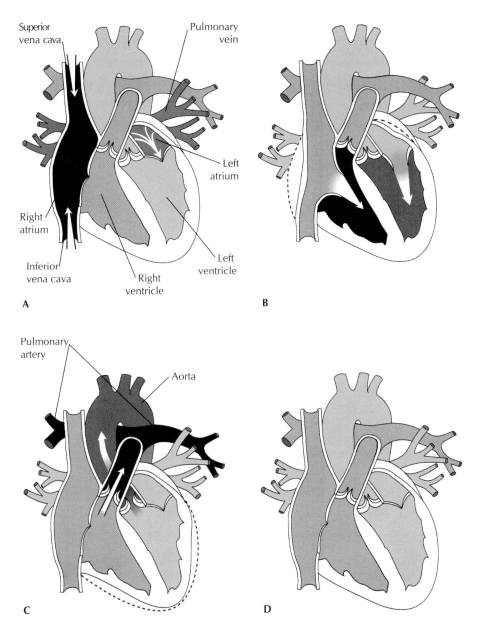

Blood flow in the heart: (A) Atrial filling. Oxygen-deprived blood enters the right atrium from the superior and inferior venae cavae; the pulmonary vein empties oxygen-rich blood into the left atrium. (B) Atrial contraction. Blood flows from the right atrium to the right ventricle and from the left atrium to the left ventricle. (C) Ventricular contraction. The right ventricle contracts and pumps blood through the pulmonary artery to the lungs, where it picks up oxygen; the left ventricle contracts and pumps blood through the aorta to the entire body. (D) Ventricular relaxation. As the ventricles relax, valves snap shut to prevent blood from flowing back. This process is repeated continuously. Dashed line indicates contraction.

tracts. The tricuspid valve closes, stopping blood from flowing back into the atrium.

The cardiac cycle is continuous, not sequential. Both the right and left atria fill and empty at the same time. Simultaneously, the right side of the heart fills with oxygen-poor blood and circulates it to the lungs (pulmonary circulation), while the left side fills with oxygen-rich blood and circulates it throughout the body (systemic arterial circulation).

Pulmonary Circulation

As the tricuspid valve closes, the blood enters a part of the circulatory system called pulmonary circulation. From the right ventricle, the blood passes through the pulmonary arteries to the lungs, where it is purified and oxygenated. In the lungs, the blood streams through smaller arteries and then into capillaries.

The capillary walls are sufficiently permeable to allow gases to filter through. Oxygen crosses from the tiny air sacs in the lungs through capillary walls into the blood. At the same time, carbon dioxide, a waste product generated by cellular metabolism, passes from the blood into the air sacs. Carbon dioxide is expelled from the body when a person exhales.

Once oxygenated, the blood is transported back to the left atrium through the pulmonary veins. Between heartbeats, the atrium contracts, pushing the blood through the mitral valve into the left ventricle. As pressure increases during heart contractions, the mitral valve closes. The muscular left ventricle wields its powerful pumping action, forcing the oxygen-rich blood out through the aortic valve into the aorta, the body's principal artery, and on through the rest of the circulatory system.

Coronary Circulation

The oxygen-rich blood that leaves the heart via the aorta to circulate to the organs and tissues of the body must also reach the heart muscle itself. The heart is outfitted with its own specialized vascular system, called coronary circulation. At the base of the aorta, where it diverges from the heart, a pair of blood vessels called the coronary arteries branch off. These specialized arteries send branches downward that encircle and spread out over the surface of the heart, so that blood also nourishes the heart muscle.

The right coronary artery provides blood principally to the right side of the heart, which is smaller, as it pumps blood only to the lungs. The left coronary artery divides into two large vessels: the left anterior descending artery and the circumflex coronary artery. Together, they thread through the front surface of the heart and supply blood to the more muscular left side of the heart, which pumps blood to the rest of the body. The rest of the right coronary artery and its main branch, the pos-

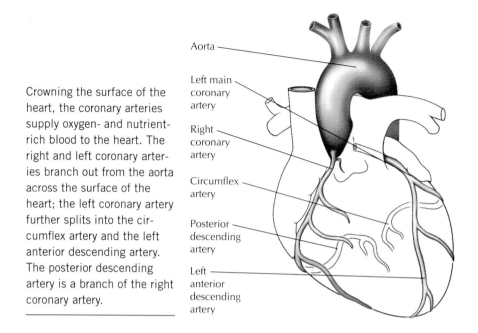

Crowning the surface of the heart, the coronary arteries supply oxygen- and nutrient-rich blood to the heart. The right and left coronary arteries branch out from the aorta across the surface of the heart; the left coronary artery further splits into the circumflex artery and the left anterior descending artery. The posterior descending artery is a branch of the right coronary artery.

Aorta

Left main coronary artery

Right coronary artery

Circumflex artery

Posterior descending artery

Left anterior descending artery

terior descending artery, together with branches of the circumflex artery, run across the surface of the heart's underside.

Collateral Circulation

The collateral circulation system is a distinct vascular network that overlaps the coronary network. It is composed of blood vessels that are microscopic and, under normal conditions, not open. When the coronary arteries narrow to the point that blood flow to the heart muscle is blocked (coronary artery disease, CAD), collateral vessels may enlarge and become active, making it possible for two sources of blood to be available to a portion of the heart.

When a collateral vessel enlarges, blood flows around the blockage either to another artery nearby or to the same artery past the blockage. Open collateral vessels thus provide additional protection from tissue death if the blood supply to the heart muscle is blocked.

The Propulsion of the Heart

Rich in oxygen and nutrients, the blood now continues its travels to the body's tissues and organs through the vascular system. This elaborate network of elastic tubes or blood vessels, if laid end-to-end, would stretch for about 60,000 miles—a length that would encircle the earth more than twice. As they stretch away from the heart, the blood vessels become smaller; as they near the heart, they become larger. The three main types of blood vessels are arteries, veins, and capillaries.

The *arteries* carry oxygenated blood to all of the body's organs and tissues, and the veins carry oxygen-depleted and carbon-dioxide-rich blood back from the organs and tissues to the right side of the heart. In pulmonary circulation, the roles are reversed: The arteries bring oxygen-poor blood to the lungs and the pulmonary veins transport oxygen-rich blood back to the heart. Because the arterial network works harder and blood in the arteries is under greater pressure than blood in the veins, arterial walls tend to be more muscular and elastic than venous ones.

Arterial circulation begins with the aorta, the body's major artery and the main trunk of the arterial system. A tube about 3 centimeters in diameter, the aorta originates in the upper surface of the left ventricle. Three shorter tubes protrude from it. As the aorta leads away from the left ventricle, it divides into large arteries that, in turn, branch into smaller vessels called arterioles.

Tiny *capillaries* with thin permeable walls connect arteries and veins and branch out into the farthest extremities, providing oxygen and nutrients to the tissues and absorbing carbon dioxide from them. The oxygen-depleted blood is then transported by the venous system away from the tissues.

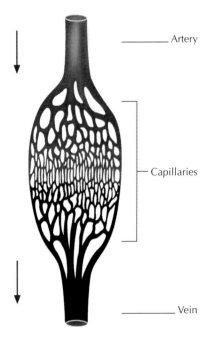

The body has three kinds of blood vessels—arteries, capillaries, and veins. Blood flows away from the heart through the arteries, which become smaller until they become capillaries. Capillaries are thin enough to permit oxygen, nutrients, carbon dioxide, and waste products to pass to and from the body's tissues. They connect the arteries to the veins; blood flows through the veins back to the heart.

Artery

Capillaries

Vein

The *veins* differ from the arteries in a number of ways. There are more veins than arteries in the vascular system. Compared to arteries, veins have a larger capacity and thinner walls; the muscles are less smooth and the tissues less elastic. They depend on the action of surrounding muscles to move the blood along. Valves in the veins prevent blood from flowing backward.

The inferior vena cava is the principal vein in the lower part of the body. It brings blood from the abdomen and legs into the right atrium. The superior vena cava, the upper body's principal vein, returns blood from the head and arms into the right atrium.

Most veins empty their blood into either the superior or the inferior vena cava. The veins from the stomach, spleen, pancreas, and small intestine link up to form the portal vein, which runs into the liver, where some cellular waste is filtered and potentially harmful waste products are either neutralized or excreted. The blood then drains through the hepatic veins into the inferior vena cava.

The combined blood from the superior and inferior venae cavae and the coronary veins enters the right atrium, passes through the right ventricle, and is forced through the pulmonary artery to the lungs, where carbon dioxide is removed and expelled and oxygen is picked up. The bright red oxygenated blood circles back to the left side of the heart, and the cycle begins again as the blood is pumped out through the aorta to be distributed by smaller arteries to all parts of the body. By the time people reach their seventieth birthdays, the blood in their bodies will have made this journey more than 110 million times.

Blood

The heart's structure and dynamics are superbly suited to moving blood throughout the body; every organ, every tissue, every cell in the body needs blood, with the oxygen and nutrients it provides, in order to live.

Blood is not merely a red fluid. It is a tissue—a group of cells acting together to perform highly specialized functions. It is thick because it contains a concentration of millions of cells, each laboring according to its particular task. Blood is approximately 78 percent water and 22 percent solids.

Most of the blood is plasma, a colorless or pale yellow fluid consisting mainly of water. Suspended within the plasma are the three types of blood cells—erythrocytes (red blood cells), leukocytes (white blood cells), and thrombocytes (platelets). Blood also contains fat globules as well as carbohydrates, proteins, hormones, and gases, including oxygen, carbon dioxide, and nitrogen. These elements sustain life and promote the health of all the body's tissues and organs.

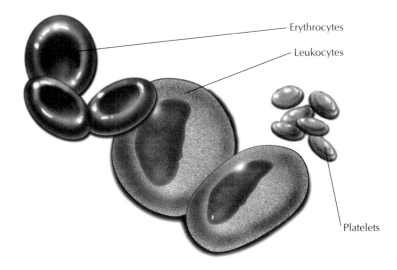

Erythrocytes

Leukocytes

Platelets

Plasma, a fluid consisting mainly of water, is the main component of blood. Suspended within the plasma are the three types of blood cells—erythrocytes, or red blood cells, which carry oxygen; leukocytes, or white blood cells, which fight infections; and thrombocytes, or platelets, which play an important role in blood clotting.

On average, the volume of blood in a man's body is between 10 and 12 pints; in a woman's body, it is 8 to 9 pints. Generally, the total blood volume circulating within the body makes up approximately 8 percent of the total body weight.

Oxygen-rich arterial blood that leaves the heart is bright red. Typically, it pulsates as it issues from a cut artery. Oxygen-deprived venous blood that returns to the heart is usually dark red and flows steadily from a cut vein. As a rule, blood moves in the aorta at an average speed of 30 centimeters per second; the entire trip around the vascular system takes about 20 seconds.

The blood transports oxygen from the lungs and nutrients from the gastrointestinal system to the body's tissues and carries away carbon dioxide and other waste products that would poison the system. It also regulates body temperature, distributes hormones and other agents to manage cell function, and delivers antibodies, which help the body guard against infectious foreign substances, and clotting factors, which help the body's tissues heal when injured.

Blood Pressure

Blood pressure is the result of two forces—the force that the heart's pumping action exerts on the artery walls as blood circulates and the force of the arteries as they resist that flow. Their elasticity, shape, and size largely determine the degree to which the arteries (including the arterioles) dilate or constrict. The presence of impediments to blood flow along the artery wall—especially plaque—can also affect blood pressure.

Because the heart cycle involves both contracting and relaxing, blood pressure is measured in two values, expressed as a fraction—the systolic value over the diastolic value. The systolic value reflects the pressure exerted on the artery wall when the heart contracts; the diastolic value represents the pressure when the heart rests between beats.

Since force is needed to move blood from the heart throughout the circulatory system, blood pressure reaches its highest values in the left ventricle during systole. It decreases in the arterial system as blood moves away from the heart. It is lowest in the capillaries.

Blood pressure is expressed in millimeters of mercury (mm Hg), which refers to how high the pressure in the arteries can raise a column of mercury in a sphygmomanometer, a device for measuring blood pressure. In a healthy, relaxed adult, systolic pressure ranges from 100 to 130 mm Hg, and diastolic pressure normally measures around 80 mm Hg.

Central blood pressure is the pressure in the heart chambers, in a great vein, or in an artery surrounding the heart muscle. Blood pressure measured in the aorta or surrounding arteries is called central arterial blood pressure. Blood pressure measured in a vein is called venous blood pressure.

Blood pressure varies with activity. It is lower during sleep and rest because the heart slows and blood vessels relax, and it is higher during exercise. Whenever more oxygen is needed by working muscles and other tissue, the heart pumps faster to push more blood through the blood vessels. At the same time, the blood vessels constrict. As a result, blood pressure rises.

Generally, the body makes immediate adjustments as demand changes. When you rise from a prone position, for example, the blood vessels in your legs and stomach quickly constrict to ensure that enough blood returns to the heart and brain. You may feel dizzy or lightheaded for a minute, because there may be a slight delay in your body's ability to make the adjustment. Since the body's ability to adjust may slow a bit with age, older people may feel dizzy when they change position or level of activity.

Kidneys

The kidneys, a pair of large organs at the back of the abdomen, serve as filters for the blood. They also regulate the amount of water in the body and control the blood's acid-base balance.

As blood passes through the kidneys, any excess water, electrolytes, sodium, and potassium are removed and sent to the bladder to be excreted. Should blood pressure begin to fall, the kidneys release renin, an enzyme that generates a cascade of events that results in a rise in blood pressure. When blood pressure rises, renin production ceases.

If a person becomes dehydrated—a condition that occurs when there is too little fluid in the blood—the kidneys work to preserve fluid. Whenever sodium and fluid volume increase, the kidneys generate more urine in order to flush excess salt out of the body.

Liver

The body's largest solid organ, the liver, weighs about 3 pounds. It is situated on the body's right side at the bottom of the sternum, just below the diaphragm. All the blood from the stomach and the intestines passes through the liver before continuing to the heart and lungs.

The liver aids in the body's ability to metabolize and use the energy in food by regulating the blood level of glucose, the chief source of energy for living organisms. The liver also plays a key role in maintaining the blood level of iron.

The liver also acts as a large filter, screening out potentially toxic waste products from the blood. Once extracted, these harmful substances, including those that come from foods, alcohol, and medications, are either neutralized or excreted. In addition, the liver helps to regulate blood volume, and it produces and regulates clotting factors, thus ensuring that the blood contains the chemicals needed to heal injuries throughout the body.

Whenever alcohol, drugs, or viruses, such as the one that causes hepatitis, damage the liver, it cannot adequately handle the blood that filters through it. When this happens, the blood backs up and seeks alternate routes, thus impeding the smooth flow of blood through the cardiovascular system.

Brain and Nervous System

As poets have written for centuries, a strong and vital link exists between the head and the heart—although perhaps not quite in the way they imagined. The brain and nervous system maintain constant communications with the cardiovascular system by way of chemicals called neurotransmitters. The nervous system regulates heart and blood pressure, keeps the chemical composition of the blood in balance, and helps the cardiovascular system stay responsive to internal and external environments.

For example, when a person is frightened, nervous, or facing physical or emotional threat, the hormones and neurotransmitters norepinephrine and epinephrine (adrenaline) signal the heart to hasten its pace and the blood vessels constrict. Sometimes referred to as the "fight-or-flight" hormone, norepinephrine is produced by the adrenal glands. It prompts

Gender Differences

While structurally the heart is the same in men and women, a woman's heart is generally smaller. An adult woman's heart weighs about 8 ounces whereas an adult man's weighs about 10 ounces. Also, a woman's maximum heart rate tends to be 10 percent greater. Her lung capacity is 10 percent less and her aerobic capacity—the maximum capability to use oxygen during physical exertion—is usually 15 to 20 percent lower than a man's. Women have less blood volume and water than do men, and a woman's blood contains about 5 percent less hemoglobin, the oxygen-carrying pigment of red blood cells, than a man's does.

blood glucose levels and blood pressure to rise and signals the heart to pump harder, forcing more blood to the muscles and priming a person for action. Other neurotransmitters, such as the hormone acetylcholine, reverse the fight-or-flight response when the danger dissipates.

Other neurotransmitters relay signals to the brain about pressure in the vessels, pressure and volume within the heart's chambers, and salt or potassium levels in the blood. Whenever there is a shortage of oxygen— during a workout, for example—the brain's respiratory center sends a message to speed up breathing, so more oxygen is delivered to the lungs and blood.

Understanding the Heart

The intricacies and inner workings of the cardiovascular system are extraordinary. Each day, the healthy heart beats steadfastly, continuously, and vigorously. Indeed, unless something goes wrong, these cyclical events occur automatically.

Whether the heart is viewed as the source of emotions or as an anatomic pump—or both—it is worth the time and effort to become familiar with the way it works. A little heart wisdom can help you improve your heart's health and, by extension, your overall health.

If something does go wrong with your heart, a basic understanding of its workings may increase the chance that you will seek timely medical intervention and participate actively in both the treatment process and aftercare, increasing the likelihood that you and your heart will recover. In many cases, all it takes is a bit of awareness and a lifestyle that embraces that awareness. As Nelson Mandela said, "A good head and a good heart are always a formidable combination."

CHAPTER 2

Keeping the Heart Healthy

Introduction

Imagine a gruel-like sludge coating the inside of your arteries and then hardening to block the flow that keeps your heart beating and you alive. This is what happens in atherosclerosis, which affects about 14 million Americans and can lead to coronary artery disease (CAD). The Greek roots of the word atherosclerosis well describe the process within affected arteries. "Athero" means gruel or paste and "sclerosis" means hardness. Untreated, the atherosclerotic process can completely occlude, or block, arteries. When atherosclerosis causes severe or total occlusion, chest pain called angina or myocardial infarction (heart attack) can occur.

Many of the important risk factors in atherosclerosis are modifiable, or within your control. A smaller number of these factors are outside your control. Reducing—or better yet, eliminating—the risk factors you can control means significantly reducing your risk of atherosclerosis and myocardial infarction. Being aware of the risk factors you cannot change can increase your vigilance for the first signs and symptoms of CAD.

Risk Factors You Cannot Change

While many risk factors are within your control, some are not. There is good reason to be aware of risk factors you cannot change: Knowing your risk can make you more diligent in reducing those risk factors that you can control. For example, if you are a man over the age of 55, you should be especially vigilant in reducing blood cholesterol and controlling hypertension (high blood pressure).

Risk factors that you cannot change include the following:

■ *Age.* Approximately four out of five people who die of CAD are age 65 or older.

■ *Gender.* Men have a greater risk of myocardial infarction than do women, especially early in life. Even after menopause, when women's death rate from heart disease escalates, men are still at

Additional Risk Factors in Women

On average, men suffer myocardial infarctions 10 years earlier in life than do women. As women approach the age of menopause, their risk of heart disease and stroke begins to rise steadily.

■ *Menopause.* As women approach menopause, they start to lose the protective effect of estrogen, the female sex hormone whose manufacture ends with menopause. Studies show that the loss of natural estrogen as women age may contribute to a higher risk of heart disease after menopause. When menopause is artificially induced—through a hysterectomy (the surgical removal of the uterus), for example—the risk of heart disease rises sharply. When menopause occurs naturally, the risk rises more gradually.

    Some women elect to take hormone replacement therapy (HRT), artificial estrogen and progesterone, to combat the uncomfortable side effects of menopause and to prevent diseases such as osteoporosis (degeneration of the bones) and heart disease. The beneficial effects of HRT for the prevention of heart disease are still being studied, and because of the risk of breast cancer associated with HRT, women are advised to consult closely with their doctors to decide if HRT is right for them.

■ *Oral contraceptives.* In the late 1960s, when oral contraceptives were first manufactured, they contained high doses of the hormones estrogen and progestin. Among older women who took these contraceptives and also smoked, the risk of heart disease and stroke rose considerably. Today, lower-dose oral contraceptives appear to carry a lower risk (except for women who smoke or have hypertension).

■ *High triglyceride level.* Research suggests that high levels of blood triglycerides (the most common type of fat in the body) increase the risk of CAD more for women than for men. Triglyceride levels rise in conjunction with higher total cholesterol and LDL cholesterol levels, and with lower HDL cholesterol levels (see Understanding Cholesterol, page 23).

greater risk. However, a woman is more likely to die from a myocardial infarction than a man.

■ *Family history.* Parents who have heart disease are more likely to have children who develop heart disease.

■ *Race.* Because blacks have more severe hypertension than do other racial groups, their risk of heart disease is greater.

■ *Diabetes.* The chance of developing CAD significantly increases for people with diabetes. Even when glucose levels are controlled with insulin and diet, the risk of heart disease is significant. Cardiovascular disease is two to four times more common in people with diabetes. People with diabetes must keep the disease under control, as well as their weight, cholesterol levels, and blood pressure. And smoking must be avoided.

Risk Factors You Can Change

High Blood Cholesterol

Prevention is particularly powerful in the case of blood cholesterol. For every 1 percent reduction in your total blood cholesterol reading, you cut your risk of CAD by 2 percent. For example, if your cholesterol reading is 200 mg/dL (milligrams of cholesterol per deciliter of blood),

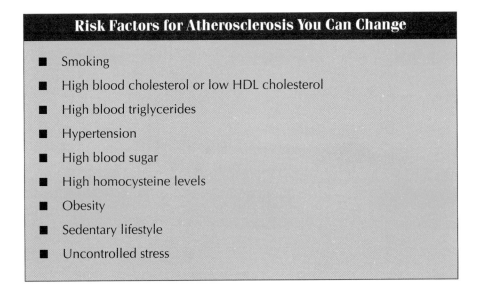

Risk Factors for Atherosclerosis You Can Change

■ Smoking

■ High blood cholesterol or low HDL cholesterol

■ High blood triglycerides

■ Hypertension

■ High blood sugar

■ High homocysteine levels

■ Obesity

■ Sedentary lifestyle

■ Uncontrolled stress

lowering it by 1 percent to 198 mg/dL drops your risk of clogged arteries by 2 percent. Lowering cholesterol 10 percent (from 200 mg/dL to 180 mg/dL, for example) cuts your risk of CAD by 20 percent. Lowering the low-density lipoprotein (LDL) cholesterol reading is even more important than lowering overall cholesterol (see Understanding Cholesterol, page 23).

To reduce the risk of CAD your total cholesterol level should be less than 200 mg/dL, your LDL cholesterol level should be less than 130 mg/dL (less than 100 if you already have CAD), and your level of high-density lipoprotein (HDL) cholesterol should be greater than 45 mg/dL for men and greater than 55 mg/dL for women.

The first way to decrease blood cholesterol levels should always be dietary changes and exercise (see Dietary Guide to Heart Health, page 28 and Exercise, page 39). But if cholesterol levels do not respond to these lifestyle modifications, your doctor may prescribe a cholesterol-lowering medication. Cholesterol-lowering medications include the following:

- The statins (also called HMG-CoA reductase inhibitors) include atorvastatin (Lipitor), cerivastatin (Baycol), fluvastatin (Lescol), lovastatin (Mevacor), pravastatin (Pravachol), and simvastatin (Zocor). The statins are the newest and most powerful of the cholesterol-lowering medications. These drugs work by interfering with the production of cholesterol in the liver. Because the liver still needs some cholesterol, it draws cholesterol out of the bloodstream, and blood cholesterol levels are lowered.

- Niacin (nicotinic acid) works to reduce levels of "bad" cholesterol (LDL) while raising levels of "good" cholesterol (HDL) (see Understanding Cholesterol, page 23).

- Bile-acid binder resins (cholestyramine, colestipol) are another group of medications that lower cholesterol. Cholesterol is a component of bile acids, created in the liver. These medications work by binding to bile acids in the intestines, preventing them from being reabsorbed into the bloodstream. This process creates a greater demand for bile acids and thus, for cholesterol. The additional cholesterol needed is drawn from the bloodstream, lowering blood cholesterol levels.

- Fibrates include clofibrate (Atromid-S), gemfibrozil (Lopid), and fenofibrate (Tricor). The fibrates are generally used to lower levels of triglycerides in the blood (see High Blood Triglycerides, page 23). They work by reducing the amount of triglycerides produced in the liver and by increasing the amount of triglycerides eliminated by the body. The fibrates are usually prescribed for those people who have very high levels of triglycerides, which can cause abdominal pain and pancreatic inflammation.

Understanding Cholesterol

Although cholesterol has a negative image, the truth is that human beings could not live without it. Cholesterol, a waxy fatlike substance called a sterol, is an essential ingredient in many substances the body makes including hormones, skin oils, digestive juices, and vitamin D. The body makes most of the cholesterol it needs in the liver.

Just as oil cannot dissolve in water, cholesterol cannot dissolve in blood. To transport cholesterol where it is needed, the liver manufactures lipoproteins, microscopic ball-shaped fat-protein shells into which it slips cholesterol. Heart problems arise when cholesterol is packaged in these hard-to-get-rid-of bundles.

There are two main types of lipoprotein shells. Shells with less protein are lighter and can hold more cholesterol; they are called low-density lipoproteins (LDLs). Shells with more protein are heavier and can hold less cholesterol; they are called high-density lipoproteins (HDLs).

When there is too much LDL (bad) cholesterol relative to HDL (good) cholesterol, the cholesterol carried in LDLs lodges in the arteries and narrows them, which contributes to CAD. A low level of HDL cholesterol, which removes excess cholesterol from the bloodstream, also increases the risk of CAD.

High Blood Triglycerides

When blood cholesterol levels are checked through a lipid profile test, blood triglyceride levels are also measured. Triglycerides are the form in which fat from food is carried through the bloodstream to be stored. Blood triglycerides become elevated if too many calories of any type are eaten: The body converts excess sugar and alcohol calories into triglycerides for storage as fat. High triglyceride levels can increase a person's chance of developing CAD. An optimal triglyceride level is less than 200 mg/dL.

Hypertension

One in four Americans, some 50 million adults, has hypertension (high blood pressure) although up to half of them do not know it until they suffer a stroke or myocardial infarction. This is why hypertension is called the silent killer. An additional 34 million adults have high normal blood pressure. High normal blood pressure is far more serious than it sounds: At least one-third of all myocardial infarctions and strokes occur in people with high normal blood pressures. Fewer than half of all Americans have optimal blood pressure readings (see Optimal Blood Pressure, page 24).

Optimal Blood Pressure

A blood pressure reading is expressed as two numbers: the systolic (first) number followed by the diastolic (second) number. The systolic number is the pressure of the blood against blood vessel walls when the heart contracts to squeeze out blood. The diastolic is the pressure on the vessel walls between beats when the heart is at rest.

Optimal blood pressure is below 120 systolic and 80 diastolic. High normal blood pressure is defined as pressures between 130/85 mm Hg and 139/89 mm Hg (the measurement "mm Hg" indicates the amount of millimeters of mercury that your blood pressure can raise on a sphygmomanometer; see Taking Your Blood Pressure, page 61). A person has hypertension when blood pressure is over 140/90 mm Hg.

High normal blood pressure is a serious concern because one-third of myocardial infarctions and strokes occur in people with high normal blood pressure.

High Blood Sugar

Uncontrolled diabetes mellitus doubles a man's risk and triples a woman's risk for CAD. Diabetes is a chronic disorder in which the pancreas either cannot produce or adequately utilize insulin, the hormone that breaks down digested sugars. Diabetes can take one of two forms: type 1 diabetes, previously called insulin-dependent diabetes mellitus or juvenile diabetes, and type 2 diabetes, formerly known as noninsulin-dependent diabetes mellitus or adult-onset diabetes.

Some people have a condition called impaired glucose tolerance. While they do not have abnormally high blood sugars, their bodies have to work much harder to keep blood sugars in the normal range by pumping out excessive amounts of insulin. In this process, they suffer some of the same symptoms as do people with diabetes.

Maintaining a lean body weight and exercising regularly reduces the risk of developing type 2 diabetes. Losing weight, exercising, and following a diet planned by a registered dietitian can normalize blood sugars if type 2 diabetes does develop.

Insufficient Vitamins

Low levels of three B vitamins—B_{12}, B_6, and folic acid—can increase CAD risk. Recent evidence suggests that these vitamins can control blood levels of homocysteine, a naturally occurring body amino acid. Studies have found that having high levels of homocysteine in the blood can significantly increase risk of CAD.

Although some people have a genetic tendency to high homocysteine levels, most people can keep levels in check by eating a balanced diet that includes milk products, lean meats, fish, poultry, fruits, green leafy vegetables, and whole grains, foods that contain B vitamins. Your doctor may also advise taking supplemental vitamins. It is nearly impossible to get the daily requirements of folic acid (400 IU) through diet alone.

Obesity

Excess body weight greatly increases a person's risk of developing CAD, largely by increasing hypertension and cholesterol levels and impairing glucose tolerance. Take the example of a lawnmower engine, which is powerful enough to cut grass, but does not have enough energy to propel a car. The one-third of Americans who are seriously overweight place great demands on their hearts every day. Their hearts are continually stressed to meet the physical requirements of excess body weight. The strain can result in high blood pressure, a risk factor for CAD. Heavier people also tend to be sedentary, which further increases the risk of CAD.

Two methods are used to calculate obesity. Central adiposity—the tendency of some people, particularly men, to gain weight around the midsection—increases a person's risk of developing CAD. Excess weight in the midsection triggers metabolic changes that cause significant abnormalities in cholesterol and a higher incidence of impaired glucose tolerance and type 2 diabetes, especially in women. The waist-hip ratio (WHR) is used to measure central adiposity. WHR is the waist circumference divided by the hip circumference. A WHR higher than 1.0 in men and 0.9 in women is considered high risk.

The body mass index, or BMI, also provides a measure of obesity. The National Heart, Lung and Blood Institute's Obesity Education Initiative defines being overweight as having a BMI over 25 and considers people with a BMI greater than 30 as obese (see Calculating Body Mass Index, below).

Calculating Body Mass Index (BMI)

BMI equals body weight in kilograms divided by the square of height in meters (multiply your height in meters by itself to determine the square).

To convert body weight to kilograms, multiply body weight in pounds by 0.45. To convert body height to meters, multiply height in inches by 0.254.

Sedentary Lifestyle

The human body is meant to be active—especially for the heart's sake. Like any other muscle, the heart cannot be as strong as it needs to be without adequate exercise. Exercise confers many other significant benefits to the heart, including fighting the body's tendency to form tiny blood clots in the bloodstream, which can eventually develop into a larger clot that can cause a myocardial infarction. Exercise raises the body's percentage of HDL cholesterol, which protects the heart. Engaging in regular exercise also helps to manage stress and anger.

Uncontrolled Stress or Anger

While stress and anger are a part of life, the reaction to them is what matters—especially as they impact on CAD risk. The cascade of physiologic responses set off by stress and anger is the same emergency response that protected prehistoric people from predators: the fight-or-flight response.

Sensing danger—whether it be a charging woolly mammoth or a screaming boss—the body releases epinephrine (adrenaline) and other hormones that make the heart beat faster and that energize the body. People who are chronically stressed tend to secrete more of a hormone called cortisol, which can raise blood pressure and program the body to retain fluid. These physiologic changes increase the risk of myocardial infarction.

Smoking

Each year, cigarette smoking accounts for nearly 200,000, or one-fifth, of all deaths from heart disease in the United States—90,000 of which are due to atherosclerosis. Smokers have a two- to fourfold greater incidence of CAD and about a 70 percent higher death rate from CAD than do non-smokers.

Inhaling tobacco smoke causes immediate, negative effects on the heart and blood vessels. The impact is cumulative. Some of these ill effects—and reasons to stop smoking—include:

- An increase in heart rate: Within one minute of starting to smoke, heart rate begins to rise; it may increase by as much as 30 percent during the first 10 minutes of smoking.

- An acute increase in blood pressure: Blood vessels constrict, forcing the heart to work harder to deliver oxygen to the rest of the body and to the heart muscle itself. Smoking causes blood pressure variability, which is even more likely to lead to heart damage than high blood pressure alone, and smoking reduces the effectiveness of blood pressure medication.

■ Compromised oxygen supply: One ingredient of tobacco smoke, carbon monoxide, seriously compromises the blood's ability to carry oxygen.

■ In women, smoking is associated with an earlier menopause. The onset of menopause raises heart disease risk because at menopause women nearly stop producing estrogen, the hormone that protects against heart disease. Female smokers who have not yet reached menopause have lower than normal estrogen levels, another means by which smoking increases heart disease risk.

Smoking increases CAD risk by several powerful mechanisms. It increases levels of free fatty acids in the bloodstream and also increases levels of a cholesterol component called very-low-density lipoprotein (VLDL), which raises LDL cholesterol and decreases HDL cholesterol (see Understanding Cholesterol, page 23). Smoking damages the arterial lining, making it an attractive site for blood fats and platelets to accumulate, which either starts or encourages the process of atherosclerosis.

In addition, smoking raises blood pressure, which contributes to heart disease risk. Smoking also causes another abnormality in blood pressure, called blood pressure variability, which is even more damaging. Finally, one ingredient of tobacco smoke, carbon monoxide, exerts a negative effect on the heart by limiting the blood's ability to carry oxygen.

Passive smoking—taking in second-hand smoke—is also a powerful risk factor. Continual exposure to second-hand smoke nearly doubles a person's risk of having a myocardial infarction, and the Environmental Protection Agency calls environmental tobacco smoke a serious and substantial health risk for nonsmokers.

How to Stop Smoking

The highly addictive nature of smoking makes quitting a difficult proposition. Behaviorists point out that having a plan increases the chances of long-term success:

■ Pick a date to stop smoking

■ Record when and why you smoke

■ Record what you do when you smoke

■ As you cut the number of cigarettes you have each day, smoke at different times and different places to help break the connection between smoking and certain activities

■ List your reasons for quitting

■ Find activities to replace smoking

■ Ask your doctor about using nicotine gum, patches, and inhalers

When you first quit smoking, you will likely crave cigarettes, be irritable, feel very hungry, cough often, get headaches, or have difficulty concentrating. These symptoms of withdrawal occur because the body is adjusting to the lack of nicotine, the addictive agent in cigarettes.

Withdrawal symptoms are temporary. They are strongest right after quitting, and generally disappear within 2 weeks. Withdrawal symptoms are far easier to treat than the major diseases that smoking can cause.

A relapse is not a reason to lose hope. Seventy-five percent of people who quit subsequently relapse. Most smokers quit three times before they are successful.

Dietary Guide to Heart Health

Fat Consumption

Managing the amount and type of dietary fat you eat is a key strategy in lowering blood cholesterol levels and reducing CAD risk. Two simple strategies—subtract and substitute—will help in the wise management of dietary fat.

Subtract

The American Heart Association and the National Cholesterol Education Program recommend limiting fat calories to 30 percent of a day's total caloric intake. The Cleveland Clinic Heart Center Preventive Cardiology and Rehabilitation Program recommends holding fat calories to 15 to 25 percent of a day's total calorie intake.

Some evidence suggests that people with diets that contain very low amounts of fat give themselves a great advantage: Not only do they lower serum cholesterol and prevent future development of the plaque that blocks arteries, they also reverse or clear away plaque that already exists. This is called reversing stenosis.

People who have a genetic predisposition to CAD are very sensitive to dietary factors. For them, holding dietary fat to the 15 percent level is especially important. Finally, reducing dietary fat makes weight control easier, because fats are calorically dense: Each gram of fat has two and a half times as many calories as the same amount of proteins and carbohydrates.

Substitute

Choosing heart-healthier fat calories is as important as cutting down on the amount of fat you consume. There are three main types of fatty acids that make up dietary fat: saturated, polyunsaturated, and monounsaturated. Any food that contains fat has all three types of fatty acids, but generally one type predominates; dietary fats are generally called by the name of the predominating fat. For example, olive oil is called a monounsaturated fat because 75 percent of its fatty acids are monounsaturated. However, it also contains some polyunsaturated fat and a little saturated fat.

Fats that are predominantly poly- and monounsaturated fatty acids are liquid at room temperature, and saturated fats are solid. Picture a bottle of liquid olive oil versus the white waxy layer of saturated fat on a slab of roast beef.

As a rule, fats of plant origin, such as vegetable oils, are almost entirely poly- and monounsaturated (the only exceptions are coconut and palm oil, which are primarily saturated fat). Animal fats—those in dairy foods, beef, pork, and chicken—are predominantly saturated.

This clear animal/plant distinction is significant in choosing a healthier fat. Vegetable fats are always better for the heart than are animal fats; mono- and polyunsaturated fats are much healthier choices than are saturated fats.

Saturated fat is the heart's greatest food enemy. It raises blood cholesterol levels, especially of LDL cholesterol. One way that saturated fat is thought to do this is by impairing the liver's ability to remove cholesterol. Normally, LDL receptors at the end of liver cells snag LDL cholesterol as it flows by; the LDL particles are then packaged for removal from the body through the intestinal tract. Saturated fat both reduces the number of LDL receptors and impairs their efficiency.

The best way to limit saturated fat intake is by cutting back on the number of meat and poultry meals and by reducing serving sizes of these foods. Of seven dinner meals, fish can be served for at least two, nonmeat entrees for at least two, and the remaining three meals can be divided between meat and poultry. According to the United States Department of Agriculture (USDA) guidelines, when beef, pork, or chicken is served, a serving should equal 3 ounces—a portion equal to the size and depth of a deck of playing cards.

Vegetable sources of protein—black beans, lentils, tofu (soybean curd), tempeh (a fermented, textured soybean product), and other legumes—can be served for every lunch. It is generally thought that having more plant-based than animal-based meals is one of the healthiest steps to take to reduce CAD risk.

Dairy foods—milk, sour cream, cream cheese, and yogurt—can be enjoyed in their nonfat or low-fat versions. You can also include cheese in your diet in a fat-free or reduced-fat version; if you do not enjoy the taste or texture of fat-free cheese, use a reduced-fat version and limit your serving size to an ounce or two a maximum of three times a week.

Limiting convenience and snack foods also cuts down on saturated fat. Some of these foods are cooked in saturated fats (such as lard), and others are cooked in coconut or palm oil. Even baked varieties are often coated with unhealthy fats.

Monounsaturated fats are the heart-friendliest fats. Substituted for saturated and trans-fats (see Trans-Fatty Acids, page 30) and limited in

Trans-Fatty Acids

Trans-fatty acids are created during hydrogenation, the process by which liquid vegetable oils are converted to solid or semisolid shortening and margarine. Trans-fatty acids give prepared foods a longer shelf life. Although they are created from vegetable oils, trans-fatty acids are more like saturated fats in that they increase total and LDL cholesterol levels and decrease HDL cholesterol levels.

In addition to margarine, many commercially processed convenience foods such as cookies, crackers, chips, frozen dinners, and cake mixes contain trans-fatty acids. Search out alternatives without trans-fatty acids by reading food labels. Although current food labeling laws do not require a listing of trans-fatty acids, a food has them if the list of ingredients includes the words "hydrogenated" or "partially hydrogenated" preceding any type of oil.

Oxidation: Bad Cholesterol Made Worse

The same process that causes rust can wreak havoc in blood vessels. Oxidation ("rusting") in the body is caused by free radicals. As the body uses oxygen, it forms by-products; the main one is oxygen-free radicals. These free radicals are stray, high-energy particles that ricochet wildly, scarring and damaging cells, including LDL cholesterol particles. This turns the LDL particles rancid, and they become swollen. Oxidized and swollen LDL particles are likelier to lodge in and block arteries than are nonoxidized LDL cholesterol. This helps explain why people with normal or even slightly elevated LDL or total cholesterol can have myocardial infarctions.

You can limit LDL cholesterol oxidation with two dietary strategies: When you use added fat, choose monounsaturated fat, which studies indicate limits LDL oxidation. Also, eat 4 to 5 servings of fruits and 4 to 5 servings of vegetables daily—both fruits and vegetables contain generous amounts of antioxidant nutrients. One serving is about $\frac{1}{2}$ cup steamed spinach, 1 orange, 1 cup chopped romaine lettuce, $\frac{3}{4}$ cup fresh strawberries, $\frac{1}{2}$ banana, or $\frac{1}{2}$ cup green peas.

Vitamins E, C and beta carotene (a form of vitamin A) are thought to be antioxidants. Supplemental doses of vitamin E in particular may be recommended for those with heart disease or for those with multiple risk factors for heart disease.

quantity, monounsaturated fats may lower LDL-cholesterol. This is also true for the third type of fat, polyunsaturated fats. Monounsaturated fats, however, offer another advantage over polyunsaturated fats: They seem to protect against LDL oxidation (see Oxidation: Bad Cholesterol Made Worse, page 30). Whenever you use added fat, such as an oil, in baking or cooking, choose a monounsaturated one such as olive or canola. But also remember the first rule about fats: reduce the amount of fat you use in any recipe (see Calorie-and Fat-Reducing Cooking Techniques, page 255).

Calories

How daily calories are consumed may be as important to heart health as the number of calories that are eaten. Designing a diet with the appropriate number of calories is pivotal in losing weight—and slimming down may be the single most important action an overweight person can take to reduce heart disease risk. But how daily calories are divided may also influence CAD risk.

A limited amount of research suggests that people who eat several small meals throughout the day have less significant rises in LDL or cholesterol than do people who eat three or fewer large meals.

As people age, the body loses its fat-burning efficiency. The energy-burning hormones become less competent with age. Insulin, the hormone that allows sugar in the blood to enter cells, becomes less efficient with age. As a result, the body must make more insulin to let the same amount of sugar into cells. Increased circulating insulin causes the body to store sugar as fat.

This does not mean that everyone must grow heavier with age. The body is better able to burn smaller calorie bundles. Hormones, especially insulin, work more efficiently with small amounts of calories at one time, and are less likely to turn calories into fat.

The practical advice is easy: Eat six smaller meals throughout the day rather than three larger meals. An easy way to do this is to plan three meals and then split them into six—this helps to avoid eating junk food at snack times.

How many total calories should you consume in a day? Weight loss can be achieved with no less than 1,500 daily calories. Taking in fewer than 1,500 calories can backfire, leading to overwhelming hunger that can cause bingeing. It is nearly impossible to get all the nutrients the body needs on fewer than 1,500 calories, and such a regime can lead to weakness and fatigue.

The body has a strong ability to preserve itself: Sensing a calorie deprivation, it lowers metabolism. This is why it seems so difficult to lose weight at lower calorie intakes—the body expends less energy and so burns less fat.

Caffeine

The news about caffeine and the heart has been confusing. Caffeine is a stimulant and can cause the heart to beat faster or to skip a beat or two, especially in the presence of heart disease. If you notice this after drinking coffee, discuss it with your doctor, who may advise you to switch to decaffeinated coffee, tea, and soft drinks.

Two issues are relevant in evaluating the effect of coffee on heart health: caffeine and how the coffee is prepared. The long-running debate about caffeine and heart disease was finally settled by researchers at Harvard University, who found that caffeine did not affect heart disease risk in more than 85,000 women between the ages of 34 and 59.

There is some suggestion, however, that coffee prepared without a paper filter may adversely affect blood cholesterol levels. Paper filters trap oils from coffee beans, which are thought to drive up cholesterol levels. Espresso is one type of coffee prepared without a paper filter. If you have CAD and drink coffee prepared without a paper filter, discuss this with your doctor.

While caffeine may not increase the risk of CAD, it may raise both systolic and diastolic blood pressures significantly, especially in people with hypertension. Rises in blood pressure are noted even in people who drink coffee regularly and seem to be more profound with increasing age. People with hypertension should discuss their caffeine intake with their doctors.

Alcohol

You may have heard that red wine is good for the heart. The truth is that the advice about alcohol and heart disease is complicated. Perhaps the most important message is that although a little alcohol may be good for the heart, too much increases cardiovascular problems, including heart rhythm abnormalities and heart failure.

What is too much alcohol? Experts think that anything more than one drink is probably too much. Epidemiological (population-based) data clearly reveal that the benefit of alcohol is more evident among light to moderate drinkers.

A prevalent theory thought to explain alcohol's ability to reduce heart disease focuses on HDL cholesterol. Alcohol seems to raise the level of HDL cholesterol, thereby helping to reduce cholesterol buildup on arterial walls. Another possibility is that alcohol decreases platelet aggregation, or renders platelets less sticky and therefore less likely to clump together. Alcohol also seems to encourage the body to produce greater amounts of tissue plasminogen activator, a chemical that helps break up the tiny clots that continuously form in the bloodstream.

Should alcohol consumption be limited to red wine? Probably not, although red wine may offer benefits beyond its alcohol content. The grapes from which red wine is made are high in flavonoids, a type of phytochemical or health-promoting plant substance. Flavonoids are powerful antioxidants, which protect against heart disease (see Oxidation: Bad Cholesterol Made Worse, page 30). It is not necessary to drink an alcoholic beverage to receive the benefits of flavonoids: A wide variety of fruits and vegetables offer rich amounts. Apples, onions, and green beans are flavonoid-rich choices; green and black tea are also very high in this phytochemical.

The best advice about alcohol:

- If you do not drink now, do not start to decrease your risk of heart disease. There are more powerful ways to reduce risk: adding a 30-minute daily walk, for example, or reducing saturated-fat intake.

- If you drink now, drink in moderation. One drink is an appropriate level. A drink is defined as 12 ounces of beer, 5 ounces of wine, or 1.5 ounces of hard liquor.

Vegetarianism

Adopting a vegetarian diet makes it much easier to achieve the dietary recommendations that reduce CAD risk. It is important to be aware, however, that a vegetarian diet is not necessarily synonymous with a low-fat diet.

Some foods included in a vegetarian diet are high in saturated fats. Cheese and other dairy foods tend to be the worst offenders. Just 3 ounces of cheese, 1 cup of 2 percent cottage cheese, and 3 cups of 2 percent milk tally 886 calories, 47 percent of which are fat (including nearly 30 grams of saturated fat). Substituting low-fat soy cheese, nonfat milk, and nonfat cottage cheese lowers calories to 595 and fat to 16 percent (and less than a gram of saturated fat).

The heart-saving essence of vegetarian diets centers on vegetable sources of protein, which offer advantages over animal protein (beef, chicken, and pork). Vegetable protein is naturally very low in fat—and almost void of saturated fat—and has no cholesterol. The grams of protein in a 2-ounce ground-beef patty come with an unwelcome 12 fat grams, 4 of which are saturated. If the beef is traded for 1 cup of black beans for the same amount of protein, fat is cut to 2 grams and saturated fat to nothing at all; cholesterol drops to 0 from 57 grams. The same serving of black beans is also rich in other nutrients: 14 grams of fiber, lots of folate, and extra calcium.

Fish Oil and Omega-3 Fatty Acids

Inuits (Eskimos) in Greenland revealed to the world that eating fish may decrease CAD risk. Research has consistently uncovered the same association: Death from heart disease is less likely among people who eat at least some fish than among those who do not.

Surprisingly, the fat in fish provides most of the benefit. Fish contain a type of polyunsaturated fatty acid called omega-3. Two omega-3 fatty acids are especially abundant in fish: eicosapentaenoic acid and docosahexaenoic acid.

These fatty acids help fish adapt to the cold water in which they live; they are also thought to confer the health benefits that fish-eaters realize. Omega-3 fatty acids stop the body's immune system from working overtime by slowing the production of prostaglandins, leukotrienes, and thromboxanes.

While the body needs some of these chemicals to function normally, too-high concentrations of them can cause problems: The right amount helps blood vessels contract and relax appropriately to control blood pressure, but too much makes blood vessels contract too forcefully, driving up blood pressure. An overload of these chemicals also encourages platelets to aggregate overzealously, a risk factor for CAD.

Omega-3 fatty acids raise HDL cholesterol, and eating fish may keep HDL cholesterol from dropping, as can occur on a low-fat diet.

The oil in fish may also keep the heart beating in a healthy rhythm. Disruptions in the heart's electrical conducting system, which keeps the heartbeat even and steady, are called arrhythmias (see Chapter 7, Rhythm Disorders). While some arrhythmias are harmless, others are dangerous and can cause the heart to stop beating altogether (cardiac arrest). There is increasing evidence that omega-3 fatty acids may guard against dangerous arrhythmias, fortifying heart muscle against unstable beats. In a recent study, people who ate enough fish to consume 5.5 grams of omega-3 fatty acids in a month—just one 3-ounce serving of salmon weekly—had half the risk of cardiac arrest as people who consumed no omega-3.

Fish may also offer some protection for people who have already suffered one myocardial infarction. Evidence suggests that including two meals of fish (each about 3 ounces) a week may reduce the chances of suffering a second, fatal myocardial infarction. Evidence also suggests that eating fish may keep arteries from closing after angioplasty, a nonsurgical procedure that opens blocked vessels in the heart.

If eating fish is so good for the heart, are fish-oil capsules recommended? Unless a doctor prescribes fish-oil capsules for specific metabolic issues, it is best to rely on eating fish. Fish-oil capsules are a concentrated source of fat calories. While some fish fat is good, too much can cause an elevation in LDL cholesterol and lead to weight gain. Taking fish-oil capsules and then eating a hamburger has no benefit—the negative effects of eating too much red meat and saturated fat cannot be erased with a pill.

If you do not like fish or have a hard time fitting two fish meals into your weekly eating plan, there is an alternative: Flaxseed is high in omega-3 oils. Add flaxseed to bread recipes, sprinkle it on cold and hot cereals, or stir it into juice. Use ground or milled flaxseed, as the body cannot digest the whole seed—it passes through the body unabsorbed. However, avoid flaxseed oil, a concentrated source of calories that can negate the benefits of a nutritious meal. Arugula, a peppery-tasting salad green, is also high in omega-3 fatty acids.

Weight Management

To manage your weight effectively, stop dieting and start thinking long-term good health—weight management rather than weight loss or dieting. Dieting is a short-term proposition; when the diet ends, many people return to the eating habits that helped them accumulate the extra pounds.

Setting the stage for weight management by assessing your readiness and attitude is the first step toward success. There are several factors to think through when making the commitment to weight loss:

- Is the timing correct to make the lifelong changes necessary to achieve success?

- Can you eat different foods—and amounts—than what you eat now? Are you ready to do this over the long haul, rather than temporarily?

- Are you ready to learn about lifelong good nutrition and about the foods (and the correct serving sizes) the body needs on a daily basis for good health? (The foods the body needs to manage weight are the same foods it needs for a healthier heart.)

- Will you exercise regularly?

If you are ready, a slow and steady process is recommended. The following guidelines will help you lay a solid foundation for a new, lifelong eating style that will help achieve permanent weight control.

- Learn about food and nutrition first. Before you begin changing your dietary habits, it is important to consult with your doctor or a registered dietitian. A dietitian can teach you how to choose the food you need for good nutrition as well as weight management. Although some people may call themselves nutritionists, only professionals with the appropriate education and clinical experience can have the initials R.D., for registered dietitian, after their name.

- Always have a list when grocery shopping, and purchase only the foods your body needs for long-term good health. Omit cookies, chips, and other snack foods you often purchase for other family members. The family shopper has an opportunity to shape eating habits.

- Do eat what you enjoy, but eat less. Too much deprivation may cause you to abandon your new eating style or to eat more than usual to make up for lack of taste.

Food Log

Name: _____

Date: _____ / _____ / _____

	Time	M	S	Foods Eaten	Quantity	How Prepared
Morning						
Afternoon						
Evening						
Nighttime						

Use this sample page from a food diary to keep track of the foods you eat. You may also want to record your activities or feelings at the times you eat to give you a better idea of your eating habits. (M, meal; S, snack)

- Track what you eat. Keep a daily log of what, how much, and when you eat. Food diaries are a proven method to help you control what you eat and how often you eat. You will also identify problem areas, such as those times of the day when you turn to food more often. Identifying these problems will help in solving them.

- Understand what is meant by a serving size. Avoid guesswork: Use a measuring cup or spoon to measure the amount indicated.

- Take the time to exercise daily (see Exercise, page 39). People who exercise have an easier time managing weight; exercise increases metabolism, which burns off extra calories. An exercise physiologist can help you design a realistic exercise program.

- Forgive yourself for the occasional setback. People who immediately forgive their dietary regressions have fewer of them, because negative self-talk can lead to overeating to heal the pain of guilt.

- Do not be tempted by weight-loss aids. Most pills and powders do not work and may be dangerous, especially if they contain stimulants. In some cases of extreme obesity, when the risks of severe obesity outweigh the risks associated with taking a medication, a doctor may prescribe a weight-loss medication. These medications are just an adjunct to weight loss, and they cannot replace the other efforts needed to achieve lifelong weight control.

- Treats are a normal part of life. Plan one favorite dessert each week. To control the portion size of treats, purchase one serving of one item and savor every bite.

Blood Pressure

Salt and Blood Pressure

Cutting back on sodium, one ingredient of table salt, can help lower blood pressure. But this is just one strategy to control high blood pressure. Adding certain foods to a regular eating plan is at least as important as reducing sodium intake in controlling blood pressure.

Food labels list the amount of sodium per serving in milligrams. Most people with hypertension should stop at a total of 2,400 milligrams daily; your doctor will indicate an ideal daily sodium intake for you. People with heart failure may have to limit sodium more strictly than people with hypertension who do not have heart failure. The "% of Daily Value" for sodium pertains to the average American, not to anyone with heart disease.

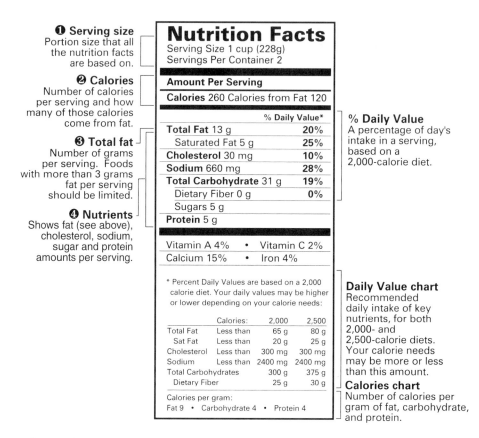

❶ **Serving size**
Portion size that all the nutrition facts are based on.

❷ **Calories**
Number of calories per serving and how many of those calories come from fat.

❸ **Total fat**
Number of grams per serving. Foods with more than 3 grams fat per serving should be limited.

❹ **Nutrients**
Shows fat (see above), cholesterol, sodium, sugar and protein amounts per serving.

Nutrition Facts
Serving Size 1 cup (228g)
Servings Per Container 2

Amount Per Serving

Calories 260 Calories from Fat 120

	% Daily Value*
Total Fat 13 g	**20%**
Saturated Fat 5 g	**25%**
Cholesterol 30 mg	**10%**
Sodium 660 mg	**28%**
Total Carbohydrate 31 g	**19%**
Dietary Fiber 0 g	**0%**
Sugars 5 g	
Protein 5 g	

Vitamin A 4%	•	Vitamin C 2%
Calcium 15%	•	Iron 4%

* Percent Daily Values are based on a 2,000 calorie diet. Your daily values may be higher or lower depending on your calorie needs:

	Calories:	2,000	2,500
Total Fat	Less than	65 g	80 g
Sat Fat	Less than	20 g	25 g
Cholesterol	Less than	300 mg	300 mg
Sodium	Less than	2400 mg	2400 mg
Total Carbohydrates		300 g	375 g
Dietary Fiber		25 g	30 g

Calories per gram:
Fat 9 • Carbohydrate 4 • Protein 4

% **Daily Value**
A percentage of day's intake in a serving, based on a 2,000-calorie diet.

Daily Value chart
Recommended daily intake of key nutrients, for both 2,000- and 2,500-calorie diets. Your calorie needs may be more or less than this amount.

Calories chart
Number of calories per gram of fat, carbohydrate, and protein.

Sample food label. Most foods are required by law to list nutrition facts. When selecting foods, pay attention to (1) serving size, (2) calories per serving, (3) total fat per serving, and (4) sodium. Source for label: U.S. Food and Drug Administration.

DASH Diet

In a landmark hypertension study called DASH (Dietary Approaches to Stop Hypertension), researchers at several medical centers studied the effects of eating more fruits, vegetables, whole-grain foods, and low-fat dairy products on hypertension. People in the study group who ate 4 to 5 fruit servings, 4 to 5 vegetable servings, and 2 to 3 low-fat dairy servings (nonfat milk, low-fat or nonfat yogurt) on a daily basis and limited their daily total fat intake to no more than 26 percent of calories lowered blood pressure dramatically.

For all participants, both those with and those without hypertension, the DASH diet lowered systolic pressure an average of 5.5 mm Hg and

> ## The DASH Way of Eating to Lower Blood Pressure
>
> Include these foods daily to help lower blood pressure:
>
> - 4 to 5 vegetable servings; 1 serving is 1 cup of a leafy vegetable, $\frac{1}{2}$ cup cooked vegetable, 6 ounces vegetable juice
>
> - 4 to 5 fruit servings; 1 serving is 6 ounces fruit juice, 1 medium fruit, $\frac{1}{4}$ cup dried fruit, $\frac{1}{2}$ cup fresh, frozen, or canned fruit
>
> - 7 to 8 whole-grain servings; 1 serving is 1 slice bread, $\frac{1}{2}$ bagel, $\frac{1}{2}$ cup dry cereal, $\frac{1}{2}$ cup cooked grain (such as rice) or pasta
>
> - 2 to 3 servings of low-fat or nonfat dairy foods; 1 serving is 8 ounces skim milk, 1 cup yogurt, $1\frac{1}{2}$ ounces low-fat cheese

diastolic pressure 3.0 mm Hg. In men and women with hypertension, the reductions were even more striking: 11.4 in systolic pressure and 5.5 mm Hg in diastolic pressure.

Overall, the DASH researchers estimated that Americans could reduce atherosclerosis by 15 percent and strokes by 27 percent by doubling their intake of fruits, vegetables, and low-fat dairy products and by cutting dietary fat.

Exercise

Lack of time is probably the most common excuse for not exercising. But exercise should not be put off. The heart depends on exercise for good health. In addition to increasing HDL cholesterol, the benefits of regular exercise include the following:

- Increasing functional capacity, the heart's ability to use oxygen more efficiently

- Decreasing blood pressure, by as much as 8 to 10 points in both systolic and diastolic pressure

- Helping prevent the onset and progression of type 2 diabetes

- Curbing the temptation to smoke

- Aiding in weight loss

To reap the most heart benefits, moderate-intensity exercise should be engaged in for at least 30 minutes each day. As an alternative, the same benefits can be gained by accumulating 30 minutes in 10-minute increments throughout the day.

Moderate-intensity exercise is also called aerobic exercise. Aerobic exercise increases the rate and depth of your breathing, raises your heart rate, and uses the large muscle groups. Examples include walking, swimming, jogging, dancing, and hiking. More strenuous exercise, such as stair-climbing and running, is not necessary to realize cardiac benefits.

Exercising at moderate intensity translates into working at 60 to 70 percent of age-predicted maximal heart rate. This target heart rate is 220 minus your age. If you have not been exercising, start slowly—aim for a heart rate lower than your target heart rate to avoid muscle injury and overtaxing the heart and lungs.

No matter how great the motivation to engage in aerobic exercise, the heart and lungs cannot meet the demand immediately. The cardiovascular system and muscles also perform better and are less likely to suffer negative effects when 5- to 15-minute warm-up and cool-down periods are included.

Begin with shorter bouts of exercise, say 15 to 20 minutes of exercise every other day. Progress by 3- to 5-minute increments per week until you reach the goal of 30 minutes of exercise each day.

The easiest exercise to start and stick with is a regular program of walking. Begin at a slow leisurely pace, where you notice no increase in heart rate and do not break a sweat, for 5 to 10 minutes. For the next 15 minutes, step up the pace just to where you notice the difference; then stroll leisurely again for 5 to 10 minutes.

Your exercise routine should be varied. Cross-training, or engaging in two or three different activities, is advantageous. A combination of walking, swimming, and cycling strengthens several muscle groups. Always consult a doctor before beginning any kind of strenuous exercise program.

Using Aspirin Preventively

Your doctor may prescribe a regular or baby aspirin daily to reduce myocardial infarction risk. For some people this is a very effective preventive therapy. Aspirin, a platelet-aggregation inhibitor, helps prevent blood from clotting. Overzealous blood clotting contributes to the blood clots that can cause myocardial infarction or occlusive stroke.

As helpful as aspirin is at the appropriate dose, it can be dangerous at higher doses; some people cannot tolerate aspirin at all. Aspirin can cause severe and potentially life-threatening bleeding problems and can increase the risk of a hemorrhagic stroke (a very rare event). Aspirin should only be taken under a doctor's supervision, with regular checkups to monitor the therapy. (See Aspirin Cautions, page 41.)

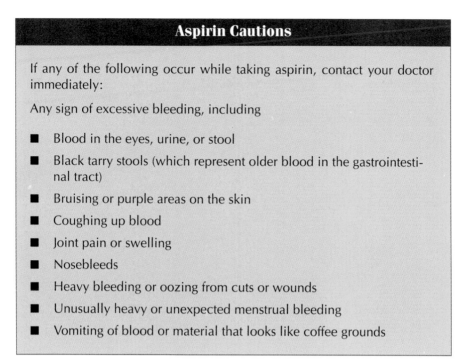

Aspirin Cautions

If any of the following occur while taking aspirin, contact your doctor immediately:

Any sign of excessive bleeding, including

- Blood in the eyes, urine, or stool
- Black tarry stools (which represent older blood in the gastrointestinal tract)
- Bruising or purple areas on the skin
- Coughing up blood
- Joint pain or swelling
- Nosebleeds
- Heavy bleeding or oozing from cuts or wounds
- Unusually heavy or unexpected menstrual bleeding
- Vomiting of blood or material that looks like coffee grounds

Aspirin is available in many forms, including tablets, suppositories, capsules, gum, and effervescent tablets. Your doctor or pharmacist can help find the form that best suits your needs.

Medication Compliance

Advancing drug research has yielded many effective medications that help control the conditions associated with CAD. Among them are antihypertensives, which bring blood pressure into the normal range; antiarrhythmics, which control an erratically or rapidly beating heart; and cholesterol-lowering medications, which help lower total and LDL cholesterol (see High Blood Cholesterol, page 21).

While the goal of any lifestyle-modification program is to reduce the need for medications, this is not always possible. It is important to take medications as they are prescribed, changing the dose only under a doctor's orders—do not take a little extra because the prescribed amount seems to offer such great benefits. Because some is good does not mean that a lot is better.

The same is true of vitamins and minerals. A doctor may prescribe vitamins such as folate and B_6. Again, the recommended doses should not be exceeded.

Stress Management

In this instant society, a few buttons on a machine are pushed and cash is retrieved from the bank at any hour of the day or night; an entire document is sent around the globe with a computer keystroke; fresh produce is delivered to Wisconsin from California overnight. This increased reliance on rapid technology has added to the level of stress in our society.

The heart is often the target of stress. During a stressful situation, heart rate increases and blood pressure rises. Blood vessels can narrow and cholesterol levels may rise. Some studies suggest that stress, and especially its hostility component, contributes to the initial development of atherosclerosis; other studies have found that stress can contribute to the acceleration and complication of CAD.

Stress often comes from overcommitment—at work, home, or in the volunteer sector. It may be difficult to say no to new projects or committees or to set limits on your social life, but you should be better able to enjoy the activities you do participate in if you can reduce your stress level.

Managing stress in the workplace is most difficult, because many situations are outside your direct control. A few simple actions may help eliminate stress from the work environment, including:

■ Switching from caffeinated to decaffeinated coffee or herbal tea

■ Leaving work at lunchtime; going for a short walk or relaxing somewhere outside your work environment

■ Practicing stress-reduction techniques (see below)

Stress-Reduction Techniques

■ Deep breathing: Stress causes muscles to tense up, including those that control breathing. Shallow breathing can result. Although the body begs for more oxygen to fuel the stress response, it cannot get it through shallow breathing. To compensate, breathing becomes very fast, which extends the stress reaction.

    The stress reaction can be reduced with deep breathing. Close your mouth and breathe in through the nose. Inhale deeply as you count to 10 and then exhale for 10 seconds. Repeat once or twice.

■ Focused imagery: Tune out stress by tuning into a relaxing image. Close your eyes and create a paradise in your imagination. Maybe

(box continues)

Stress-Reduction Techniques *(continued)*

you are on a beach in Hawaii, or skiing down fresh powder high in the Alps, or cruising on the French Riviera. Create the ultimate image, complete with the smell of sea air and the whooshing sound of skis plowing through fresh snow. When stress strikes, bring that image alive in three dimensions—sight, smell, and sound.

■ Biofeedback: With training, you can learn to slow heart rate and lower blood pressure. Generally, a psychologist specially trained in biofeedback techniques can train you to "talk" to your body. In most cases, the psychologist attaches you to machines that monitor pulse and blood pressure during training. Ask your doctor to recommend a qualified professional.

CHAPTER 3

What Is Heart Disease?

Introduction

When people think of heart disease, a heart attack may be the first disorder they envision. Clinically called a myocardial infarction, a heart attack tends to be severe, dramatic, and intense. A myocardial infarction occurs when a section of heart tissue dies due to severe disruption of blood flow to the area.

However, a myocardial infarction is only one type of heart disease. Under the umbrella term "heart disease" are a number of other conditions, including atherosclerosis (narrowing and hardening of the arteries), coronary artery disease (atherosclerosis of the arteries supplying the heart), angina pectoris (chest pain), congestive heart failure (a condition in which the heart loses its ability to pump effectively), aneurysm (blood clot that forms in a bulge in a vessel wall), stroke (brain attack), congenital heart disorders (heart disorders that are present at birth), valve disorders, and arrhythmias (disorders of the heart's rhythm).

In each disorder, the health and functioning of the entire cardiovascular system—heart, arteries, and veins—and such vital organs as the brain, lungs, and kidneys are at issue.

Who Has Heart Disease

According to 1999 estimates, approximately 58.8 million Americans have one or more types of heart disease.

- Hypertension (high blood pressure)   50 million
- Coronary artery disease   12 million
- Myocardial infarction   7 million
- Angina pectoris   6.2 million
- Congestive heart failure   4.6 million
- Stroke   4.4 million
- Rheumatic heart disease (see page 118)   1.8 million
- Congenital heart disorders   1 million

With so many Americans suffering from one or more types of heart disease, also called cardiovascular disease, a greater understanding of heart health and heart disease is necessary. Not only may "heart disease" be confused with "heart attack," but also heart disease tends to be associated with older men. The truth is that heart disease can and does affect women as often as it does men. Since 1984, more women have died each year of cardiovascular disease than have men (see Additional Risk Factors in Women, page 20, and Symptoms of CAD in Women, page 87). Children also suffer from several forms of heart disease (see Chapter 10, Pediatric and Congenital Heart Disease).

Cardiovascular disease is the leading cause of death for both men and women. Each year, these diseases claim the lives of more than 500,000 women and more than 450,000 men. More people die of heart disease than of the next sixteen causes of death combined.

The numbers speak for themselves:

- Before age 60, 1 man in 3 and 1 woman in 10 can expect to develop some major cardiovascular disease.

- Over time, the incidence of cardiovascular disease becomes equal in men and women; 20 percent of males and females have some form of cardiovascular disease.

Statistics concerning children and heart disease in the United States show:

- Cardiovascular disease is the third leading cause of death for children younger than 14 years and the fifth for children and young adults between the ages of 15 and 24 years.

- Approximately 36 percent of young athletes who die suddenly have an undiagnosed or undertreated heart problem.

- About 32,000 babies each year are born with congenital heart defects.

Each year, thousands of people die or suffer disability as a result of some form of cardiovascular disease. Finding out that you have or are at risk for developing some form of heart disease is a challenge. Techniques for diagnosis and treatment continue to grow more accurate and effective. With greater awareness, knowledge, and a commitment to a healthy lifestyle, you can become an effective advocate for your health and increase the chances that your heart will beat vigorously for a very long time.

Types of Heart Disease

The following pages provide a brief overview of the major types of heart disease. With each description, the page or chapter numbers for further information are indicated.

Atherosclerosis and Related Conditions

Whereas in children, most heart problems are due to congenital defects, in adults, many cardiovascular problems arise from atherosclerosis. Atherosclerosis occurs when the normally smooth inner lining of the arteries becomes thick and uneven, restricting blood flow. With age, the arteries naturally lose elasticity, thicken, and harden (a process called arteriosclerosis). As it roughens, the lining of an artery attracts white blood cells, which cluster and entrap oxidized low-density-lipoprotein (LDL) cholesterol (see Understanding Cholesterol, page 23). These fat-containing cells accumulate into fatty streaks and absorb calcium deposits, cellular waste, and fibrin (a protein formed during blood clotting) at the site, forming scablike deposits called plaque along the arterial lining.

As plaque accumulates, the innermost layer of the artery, called the endothelium, thickens. If the wall becomes sufficiently thick, the artery begins to close, reducing the amount of blood and, with it, the amount of oxygen that can be delivered to the body's tissues and organs. In addition, plaque deposits can rupture, causing hemorrhaging (bleeding) at the site.

When blood flow is obstructed or compromised and the body's tissues are deprived of the nutrients and oxygen they need to function, they are at risk for damage or death. Ischemia is a local and temporary blood deficiency. When blood flow is cut off for an extended period of time, areas of tissue die; this is called infarction. When atherosclerotic plaque sufficiently narrows the coronary arteries so oxygen to the heart muscle is obstructed, angina pectoris (chest pain) or myocardial infarction may occur. For more information on atherosclerosis, see Chapter 5, Coronary Artery Disease.

Coronary Artery Disease

Atherosclerosis occurs most frequently in the coronary arteries, which branch off the aorta and supply oxygen to the heart, and in the surrounding larger arteries. When plaque builds up within the coronary arteries and these arteries become blocked, the resulting condition is called coronary artery disease (CAD), the most common cause of death in the United States. The heart receives less oxygen, causing damage that then spreads through the myocardium, the heart muscle. For more information on CAD, see Chapter 5, Coronary Artery Disease.

Two conditions are directly related to CAD:

■ *Angina Pectoris.* When the myocardium receives an inadequate supply of oxygen, the result is angina pectoris, or chest pain (see also page 85). Angina is most commonly caused by a narrowing in the coronary arteries, or by coronary artery disease. It can also result from coronary spasm, in which the blood flow in the arteries is pinched off, heart valve malfunction, or a congenital heart defect.

■ *Myocardial Infarction.* A myocardial infarction occurs when the flow of oxygenated blood to the heart is cut off, causing injury to all or part of the myocardium (see also page 82). Most commonly caused by coronary artery disease, myocardial infarction can also be a result of a coronary spasm.

Congestive Heart Failure

Congestive heart failure is almost always a serious and frequently life-threatening condition. When the heart is unable to pump adequate amounts of blood—and with it, oxygen—to the tissues, fluid accumulates (congestion) in the veins as blood returning to the heart backs up. Often developing after the heart has been working at an accelerated pace for a long period of time, congestive heart failure can be a result of hypertension (high blood pressure) or blockage in the coronary arteries. For more information on congestive heart failure, see Chapter 8, Heart Failure.

Aneurysm

A blood vessel wall may balloon out at a certain point, and an aneurysm, a blood-filled sac that is formed by the stretched wall, may form. An aneurysm can occur in any blood vessel but is most commonly found in an artery. Usually a result of atherosclerosis coupled with hypertension, an aneurysm forms at weakened places along the artery wall.

An aneurysm may also be due to a congenital defect, infection, trauma, or an inherited disease such as Marfan syndrome (see page 130), in which a section of the aorta is dilated. Aneurysms occur most commonly in the aorta (aortic aneurysm), in the abdominal area below the kidneys (abdominal aneurysm), and in the chest cavity (thoracic aneurysm). The danger of an aneurysm lies in the possibility that it will burst, flooding the area with blood. If an aneurysm on a large blood vessel or the heart wall bursts, the resulting hemorrhage can be fatal. For more information on aneurysm, see page 198.

Stroke

The term stroke describes a cascade of events that occur when the blood supply to a part of the brain is obstructed. The three basic types of stroke are as follows:

■ *Cerebral thrombosis,* the most common form of stroke, in which a clot develops in a cerebral artery (an artery that supplies blood to the brain) narrowed by atherosclerosis

■ *Cerebral embolism,* which is caused when a piece of the plaque or a blood clot attached to the lining of a blood vessel breaks free, travels through the bloodstream, and lodges in a cerebral artery

■ *Cerebral hemorrhage,* which occurs when a cerebral artery bursts, flooding brain tissue with blood and causing blood loss and pressure on brain tissue; usually caused by a head injury or an aneurysm

For more information on stroke, see page 194.

Cardiovascular Conditions Unrelated to Atherosclerosis

Congenital Heart Disorders

Congenital heart disorders are present at birth and occur when the heart or surrounding blood vessels fail to develop normally during fetal maturation. Many congenital disorders interfere with the way blood flows through the heart chambers. Usually diagnosed before birth, immediately after birth, or during childhood, some congenital defects are not identified until adolescence or early adulthood. For more information on congenital defects, see Chapter 10, Pediatric and Congenital Heart Disease.

Valve Disorders

Valve disorders occur when the heart valves do not function correctly. The disorder may be congenital or develop later in life. Congenital valve defects include abnormal bicuspid aortic valve, in which the valve has two instead of three leaflets, and mitral valve prolapse, a generally benign condition in which the leaflets of the mitral valve flop back into the left atrium when the heart contracts.

Infection, myocardial infarction, and trauma may also damage the valves and cause valve disorders that may include the following:

■ *Valvular stenosis*—the opening of the valve is smaller than normal, limiting blood flow

■ *Valvular regurgitation*—the valve leaks, permitting blood to trickle backward across the valve, thus diminishing the supply of blood that flows forward

For more information on valvular defects, see Chapter 6, Diseases of the Heart Valves.

Arrhythmias

Arrhythmias are disruptions in the heart's normal rhythm. As many as 1 in 1,000 Americans have some type of arrhythmia, which varies in type and severity. Symptoms include fainting, palpitations (see page 152), shortness of breath, and chest pain; in rare instances arrhythmia can be fatal.

A number of factors can trigger arrhythmia, including stress, caffeine, tobacco, alcohol, diet pills, and cough or cold medicines. In some instances, other conditions, such as hypertension, disrupt the normal rhythm of the heart. Some arrhythmias are congenital.

For more information on arrhythmias, see Chapter 7, Rhythm Disorders.

Preventing and Living with Heart Disease

Heart disease, although the number one cause of death of both men and women in the United States, is an active area of research with new methods of detection and treatment developed and older methods improved each year. A diagnosis of heart disease, even congenital heart disease, has a better prognosis now than ever before, and rehabilitative techniques following heart surgery (see Chapter 11, Recuperation and Rehabilitation After Heart Surgery) have also become more advanced. With proper treatment and lifestyle adjustments, many people with heart disease lead productive and full lives.

CHAPTER 4

Diagnosing
Heart Disease

Introduction

Two key elements are involved in the diagnosis of heart disease: the doctor, who evaluates your symptoms, your medical history, your physical exam, and your test results; and the diagnostic tools themselves. Both of these elements are crucial to an accurate diagnosis. A doctor may be able to form a possible diagnosis or even several based on a description of your symptoms and a physical exam but will often rely on diagnostic tests for confirmation. These tests require an experienced doctor to order the correct procedure and interpret the results.

How to Select a Doctor and Hospital

Primary Care Doctors

Many times, diagnosis begins with the primary care doctor. The doctor's training, expertise, hospital affiliation, and access to resources will determine which diagnostic techniques will be employed and how extensive the diagnostic process will be. The primary care doctor will also decide when and if a specialist needs to be consulted. Having a skilled doctor and a good medical relationship is essential to good heart health.

In many instances the first indication of heart disease is an acute symptom—myocardial infarction (heart attack), stroke, or congestive heart failure. In a medical emergency, the choice of a doctor may not be possible. It may be the doctor at the nearest hospital emergency room or on call when symptoms appear who oversees diagnosis and treatment, at least in the early stages. Once the wheels are set in motion by an emergency, you may find yourself moved along, possibly with very little active participation.

Consequently, it is important to be thoughtful about all aspects of your health and medical care long before a crisis occurs. This means choosing a reliable, skilled doctor as your primary health care provider and building a solid medical relationship that allows for questions and provides comprehensive answers and that encourages you to be actively involved in your own health.

With a strong doctor-patient relationship, it is more likely that you and your doctor will be able to anticipate heart problems and work together to keep your heart healthy. And should a medical emergency occur or a complicated health problem arise, it is less likely that you will be swept along by the course of events.

Your choice of a doctor and hospital is influenced by a number of factors. You may choose a doctor who is a friend, who has treated your family for years, or who has been referred by friends. You may want to use a hospital that is close to your home or one that has a specific religious affiliation. However, medical choices are increasingly being shaped by the choice of health insurance.

If, for example, you have a traditional health insurance (indemnity) plan, you can see any doctor and use any hospital that you want. However, this type of plan tends to be expensive, and preventive care, such as immunizations and health screenings, is often not covered. Typically, there is a deductible that is paid out-of-pocket, after which the insurance company pays only a percentage of medical costs.

Today, though, most people are members of managed care plans, in which they are directed to specific networks of health care providers. These plans are likelier to cover some form of preventive care, and out-of-pocket costs are generally low. In many managed care plans, a primary care physician manages all of a patient's health care needs.

Different types of managed care plans allow various degrees of choice in selecting a primary care doctor. In some plans, you must select a primary care doctor from a specific organization. Other types of plans allow you to select a primary care doctor from different doctor groups. Still others allow you to select a doctor outside the network if you are willing to pay more out of your own pocket.

Many health plans use a process called utilization review to ensure that medical services are being used efficiently. Utilization review sometimes includes requiring a second opinion on some surgical procedures and always includes prior approval for elective hospital admissions.

The primary care doctor is usually either an internist who provides general medical care for adults, a family practitioner who provides general medical care for children and adults, or a pediatrician who provides general medical care for children. The primary care doctor decides when and what specialized medical, diagnostic, or treatment services are needed and either provides these services or makes a referral to the appropriate provider.

Specialized Medical Care

While it is always a good idea to approach issues of health and medical care with thought and prudence, it is especially important when you need specialized medical care for a complex health condition, such as heart disease. Then, finding the right match between you, your condition, the doctor, and the hospital becomes even more significant. The more complex your medical problem, the greater the differences in quality become, and the more they matter. Therefore, you will want access to specialists and perhaps to an academic medical center, or teaching hospital (see page 59), which can provide treatment based on the most up-to-date research and education.

Specialists involved in treating heart conditions include the following:

- *Cardiologists,* doctors who specialize in the diseases of the heart and blood vessels

- *Thoracic and cardiovasular surgeons,* doctors who specialize in treating the organs of the thoracic (chest) cavity—the heart and lungs—and the pleura (the membrane surrounding the lungs and thoracic cavity)

- *Pulmonologists,* doctors who specialize in the diseases of the lungs

In general, when the condition is serious, the diagnosis may be more extensive. Often, the treatment is more complicated as well. Therefore, when choosing a doctor or hospital, factors such as credentials, experience, outcome, and track record tend to matter more. For example, a surgeon who performs a complex procedure routinely is likely to have a higher rate of success than is a surgeon who performs it rarely. Furthermore, the complication rate for a particular procedure may be lower when the hospital is equipped to respond to all potential treatment needs and related complications.

Because a complex medical problem or multiple medical problems may require specialists or an appropriate academic or teaching hospital, you may want a health plan that allows easy access to high-quality specialized care. Each health plan differs in its requirements for seeing a specialist. Some doctors in a managed care plan refer to specialists only inside the plan but may allow referrals to specialists outside the plan for rare conditions. In other plans, you may have to pay all or a higher percentage of the doctor's fee if you see an outside specialist.

No matter how extensive or limited your options, choosing specialized medical care involves thought and a bit of research. Doctors vary in quality due to differences in training and experience; hospitals differ in the number of services they offer. There are a number of objective measures, or quality indicators, that can help you compare health care providers and services (see below and Factors to Consider, page 57).

Questions to Ask When Seeking Specialized Medical Care

When you have received a diagnosis of heart disease that requires specialized care, you should ask the following questions to assure yourself that the doctor and hospital you choose are of high quality and experienced in treating your condition.

- Is the doctor board certified in the specialty of internal medicine and the subspecialty of cardiology? If a surgeon is needed, is he or she board certified in surgery and the subspecialty of thoracic surgery? With which hospital is the doctor affiliated?

- If a specific procedure has been recommended, how many times has the doctor performed that procedure? How often has that procedure been performed in the hospital you are considering?

- Is the hospital accredited by the JCAHO (see page 58)?

- If anesthesia is necessary, how experienced is the anesthesia staff in the procedure you are considering?

- Is the hospital equipped with a full range of specialty departments in the event that complications arise from related conditions?

- Is an experienced heart surgery team available in the hospital in the event that emergency surgery becomes necessary?

- Does the hospital have a full range of diagnostic services (see Techniques for Diagnosing Heart Disease, page 63)?

- Does the hospital have a special unit for treating heart failure patients?

- Is the hospital associated with a teaching program (see page 59)?

- Does the hospital have fully accredited residency training programs in heart specialties?

- Does the hospital conduct research or clinical trials related to heart disease?

- What are the mortality and complication rates for the procedure you are considering?

You may also want to check and see if the hospital has performed patient satisfaction surveys, and evaluate the results.

In addition to evaluating a doctor based on objective criteria such as credentials and experience, you may also use subjective criteria—your feelings—to guide you as you choose a doctor. Trust your own judgment. The most productive doctor-patient relationships are founded on comfortable rapport and good communication. As you interview doctors or as you reconsider the match between you and your current doctor, ask yourself a number of questions:

- Are you comfortable with the doctor's manner and treatment style?

- Does the doctor seem genuinely interested in you and your health concerns?

- Do you feel comfortable talking about any concern you have—including sexual questions, bowel and urinary habits, and emotional problems?

- Can you ask questions and understand the answers, and when you do not understand, can you ask for clarification?

- Is the doctor aware of the latest developments in cardiac medicine?

How to Find a Pediatrician and Children's Hospital

When it comes to health care for a child, most parents rely on a pediatrician or family doctor to provide preventive, or well-child, care and to treat illnesses. The pediatrician or family doctor generally follows the child from infancy into adolescence.

Pediatrics is the medical specialty concerned with the care of children. In addition to having a thorough knowledge of general medicine, a pediatrician is trained to understand and address children's physical, emotional, and developmental issues. A family doctor, while not trained exclusively in pediatrics, is qualified to provide health care for children as well as for other family members.

A child's primary health care provider conducts routine examinations, offers information on nutrition and safety, monitors development and growth, gives immunizations against infectious diseases, and treats illnesses and injuries. However, if a child develops a more complicated or serious health problem, such as a heart condition that calls for more extensive diagnostic and treatment procedures, the doctor should refer the child and family to a specialist or team of specialists at a hospital or medical center.

If a child has a heart condition, the primary care doctor will likely manage the diagnostic process and treatment. The child and her family should also be referred to a pediatric cardiologist to confirm diagnosis and to review a treatment plan. In some cases, the child's particular problem is better managed by a specialist. The child's pediatrician will stay informed about the child's condition and continue to offer guidance. The specialist conducts an independent examination and evaluation and reports the findings to the primary care provider.

Sometimes parents also feel that they would benefit from a second opinion, especially when a recommendation for surgery has been made. An independent consultation may be helpful when parents are not comfortable with the pediatrician's treatment recommendation, when they have questions about the way in which the problem is being handled, when their questions are not being answered adequately, or when the child does not seem to be responding to treatment.

Whenever a major medical procedure is proposed, a second opinion should be sought. In most cases, the child's physician will suggest another doctor to provide consultation. Otherwise, parents can ask their own doctors for a referral. (See Seeking a Second Opinion, below.)

When a child needs to be hospitalized, in many cases treatment will be provided at the local hospital with which the doctor is affiliated. However, in some cases, the child will be referred to a children's hospital or a children's unit at a specialized heart clinic. There are a number of hospitals throughout the country that are dedicated to providing specialized health care to children.

Because children's hospitals specialize in pediatric health problems, they can be especially effective in diagnosing and treating more complicated medical problems such as childhood heart conditions. Moreover, many children's hospitals house and fund research and teaching that focus on diseases and issues that touch the lives of children.

Finally, a number of specialized treatment centers concentrate on specific health problems, such as heart disease, and many of them have special pediatric units. If your child has been diagnosed with a serious heart condition, talk to your child's doctor about choosing the most appropriate treatment center.

Seeking a Second Opinion

Most doctor-patient relationships work well. There may never be a need to seek another opinion—that is, until a more serious or complicated medical condition arises. Even then, in all likelihood, what your doctor tells you about your condition and your treatment options will make sense to you. However, in some cases, you may find that you are unclear about what is being recommended or whether those recommendations are the only or the best options for you.

Especially now, when it is so easy to access medical information in books and on the Internet, you may find yourself wondering and perhaps worried as you try to sort out the best options for you and your condition. While you do not want to hop from doctor to doctor, you do want to feel that the lines of communications are open and clear and that you can trust your doctor's treatment guidance.

If, for example, you develop a complex medical condition, or if your doctor recommends treatment or surgery that you have questions about, it is a good idea to get a second opinion. Many health plans actively encourage or even require second opinions in such cases and then often review the treatment recommendation themselves. If your doctor is unable to address your questions and your anxieties adequately or, having read and done research, you find yourself questioning your doctor's judgment or approach, then it may be a good idea to seek a second opinion.

There are other things to watch for: if your doctor does not seem to take your concerns seriously; if your doctor cannot arrive at a definitive diagnosis even after a battery of tests has been performed; if your symptoms are getting worse and not responding to treatment, despite consultation with your doctor; or if you are repeatedly hospitalized for the same or a related condition.

Most doctors are responsive when a patient expresses a wish to seek a secondary consultation. While you may worry about hurting your doctor's feelings, chances are that with a little diplomacy, you will not. In the event that your doctor cannot understand your wish to explore options more fully, you may in fact be better served by another doctor.

When it comes time to seek out an independent consultation, your doctor may be willing to recommend a consulting doctor. However, you may be referred to someone who holds very similar views. You can ask other doctors in your community—including your child's pediatrician—for a referral. In addition, you will likely find other doctors in your HMO listing or the Directory of Medical Specialists. Most health plans cover second opinions under certain circumstances. Be sure to check the health plan's policy on reimbursement for a second opinion.

Factors to Consider
Credentials

Consider the credentials of both your doctor and the hospital with which your doctor is affiliated. Nationally recognized medical professional organizations review and accredit doctors and hospitals alike. In order to receive credentials, doctors and hospitals must meet certain standards in health care delivery.

For doctors, board certification or the international equivalent indicates that they have achieved a certain level of training in their specialty areas. A national board establishes standards for each specialty. Doctors who are board certified in their specialties must have at least five years of training beyond medical school, practice for a specified number of years in that specialty, and pass a strenuous examination in their specialty area. Cardiologists should be board certified in the specialty of internal medicine and the subspecialty of cardiology. A thoracic and cardiovascular surgeon should be board certified in surgery and the subspecialty of thoracic surgery.

In order to retain board certification, doctors attend continuing medical education programs throughout their careers. While some excellent doctors are not board certified, board certification is generally a good indicator of a doctor's competence and experience.

The Joint Commission on Accreditation of Healthcare Organizations (JCAHO) is the nationwide accreditation body for hospitals. The JCAHO periodically conducts extensive inspections of hospitals to determine if they meet specific health and safety requirements. Only those that meet these requirements can receive and maintain accreditation. Although accreditation is voluntary, most hospitals go through the process. If the hospital you are considering is not accredited, it is important to know why. For information about a hospital's accreditation status, call the JCAHO at (630) 792-5000.

Experience

The number of years a doctor has been practicing medicine may or may not be a factor in the doctor's ability to provide effective diagnoses and treatment. Generally speaking, whenever there is a specialized medical problem or a need for surgical care, the more experience the doctor and hospital have with the necessary procedures, the better the results will be. An experienced surgeon who has handled many similar cases is likely to be better prepared for any complications that may arise during an operation. The American College of Cardiology (ACC), the American Heart Association (AHA), and the American College of Physicians (ACP) recommend that a cardiologist perform a minimum of 75 angioplasty procedures as the primary operator a year. According to the ACC, the AHA, and the ACP, a hospital should perform at least 200 balloon angioplasties a year. According to the Report of the Inter-Society Commission for Heart Disease Resources, a catheterization laboratory should perform a minimum of 300 procedures a year. The American College of Surgeons recommends that a hospital perform at least 150 open-heart surgeries a year; other organizations give guidelines of 200 to 300.

Range of Services

Whenever you consider using a doctor or purchasing a health plan, consider the affiliated hospitals and the range of services available, especially if you have a more complicated medical condition.

Hospitals with a broad range of services—specialty departments, for example, with many diagnostic and treatment options—are often preferable for complex medical conditions. The more services that are available within one facility, the more able the hospital is to respond promptly to any complications that may arise.

In addition, some hospitals are set up to handle related conditions. In these treatment centers, doctors and other health care professionals from different specialties collaborate to anticipate and manage related prob-

Teaching, Education, and Research Centers

Whenever health care professionals are engaged simultaneously in patient care, research, and teaching, they are able to share knowledge, research, and clinical findings. Moreover, they are able to apply that knowledge directly to patient care. In other words, there is an almost immediate transfer of basic scientific knowledge from the laboratory to care delivery at the patient's bedside.

Academic medical centers, or teaching hospitals, combine patient care with research and education. Very often, research or clinical trials related to a specific condition are conducted in teaching hospitals. These hospitals usually have a fully accredited residency training program in certain areas. In addition, professionals at teaching hospitals may also be exposed to the newest treatments and forms of technology.

This combination of treatment, research, and technology may also be responsible for lower mortality rates: According to a 1989 study, private, not-for-profit teaching hospitals had lower mortality rates than did other types of hospitals. Although the reasons for these lower rates are not altogether clear, the advantages of teaching hospitals, as noted above, are quite clear.

lems. Immediate access to a full range of specialty departments can prove critical, especially when the condition is serious, such as in the case of heart disease.

Finally, because there may be more than one way to treat your medical condition, choosing a hospital that can diagnose and treat your condition in a number of ways increases the chances that the treatment you receive will be the most effective.

Patient Satisfaction

While it is no doubt helpful to ask friends, family members, and colleagues what they think of a particular hospital, people's individual opinions are often shaped by a variety of personal factors unrelated to the quality of care. Patient satisfaction surveys allow you to judge quality based on many people's experiences and may provide a more objective measure.

Most hospitals routinely take surveys to assess patient satisfaction and then use the results to try to improve their services. Patient satisfaction generally reflects the personal side of care: How attentive are the doctors and nurses? Do they listen, answer questions and explain treatments? How much time does the doctor spend with the patient? Is the hospital clean? Is the food good? In many ways, patient satisfaction information may predict your experience in a particular hospital. However, be aware that patient satisfaction may not be related to the quality of medical care.

Outcomes

All people who undergo treatment for heart conditions assume, or at the very least hope, that afterward their symptoms will abate, and they will be able to resume a reasonably active life. While the chances for this kind of positive outcome are affected by the patient's age, general health at the time of treatment, and the medical condition being treated, a number of indicators can give a rough measure of a treatment's success in terms of the doctor and the facility.

It is always helpful and often reassuring to find out how well other patients respond to treatment or recover from the surgery that you are considering. The mortality rate, or the percentage of deaths associated with a certain procedure, can indicate risk. A joint ACP, ACC, and AHA Task Force on Clinical Privileges in Cardiology has developed an expected procedural mortality rate of 1 percent for angioplasty. According to several large studies, currently accepted guidelines in mortality rates for bypass surgery are at 2 percent. Another sensitive measure of quality is the morbidity rate, the rate of complications such as infection or rehospitalization, following treatment.

The hospital may be able to provide you with information concerning patients' health status and quality of life following treatment. Questions such as how soon, on average, patients are able to return to work, or perform the usual activities of daily living, or how many report being free from pain soon after an operation, are good indicators of the doctor's or hospital's effectiveness.

It is important, however, when you look at these data, to compare outcomes for patients most like yourself in order to get an idea of what your outcome is most likely to be. At the same time, rates may be reported differently from hospital to hospital, so the comparison may not be so straightforward.

Nevertheless, any procedure carries with it certain risks. The more serious the illness, the higher the risk. However, the chances that your condition will be accurately diagnosed and successfully treated can increase significantly if you choose a hospital with a good track record—especially for those procedures you are considering.

Empowering Yourself as a Patient

There is little question that if you have heart disease, being involved in your own care during and following treatment can be crucial to recovery and health. And, preventing heart disease is as important a part of health care as treating it. Whereas in the past the traditional doctor-patient relationship involved an all-knowing doctor and a passive, compliant patient, today all aspects of health care—from prevention to treatment to aftercare—necessitate that you, the patient, take an active part in your own health care.

Educating Yourself About Your Condition

As a consumer of health care services, you will be making decisions about your care and about what resources to use. In order to become a shrewd and effective partner in your own health, it is best to educate yourself. First, learn your own risk for heart disease through a comprehensive risk-factor analysis. Do you have a family history of heart disease? Who in your family has had a serious heart condition? Find out whether such risk factors as hyperlipidemia (high cholesterol levels), obesity, hypertension (high blood pressure), or diabetes run in your family.

Whether you have a family or personal history of heart disease, other risk factors, or simply want to take steps to minimize your risk, there are many ways of educating yourself. The American Heart Association and other medical organizations publish newsletters and provide informational services.

There are also numerous medical Web sites, making it increasingly possible for anyone, regardless of education or background, to gather substantial information, develop understanding and explore medical options. Web sites sponsored by the US government such as Healthfinder (www.healthfinder.gov), the National Institutes of Health (www.nih.gov/health), and the National Library of Medicine (www.nlm.nih.gov) are good sources. The American Heart Association (www.americanheart.org) and the Cleveland Clinic Web page (www.clevelandclinic.org/heartcenter) offer data about heart health and disease. Each site is linked to other relevant sites. Remember that anyone can post health care material, which may consist of personal opinions, incorrect information, or a biased sales pitch, on the Internet. Stick to sites sponsored by reputable organizations, universities, or the government.

Of course, your doctor is a valuable resource. Regular visits to your doctor provide regular opportunities to diagnose health problems and assess risk, as well as to gain useful information on good preventive care. By being informed, you can enter as a fully active participant in your own health when you walk into your doctor's office.

Taking Your Blood Pressure

The force or pressure with which the blood courses through the cardiovascular system both affects and indicates the health of the heart. Although it varies from person to person and within the same person according to time of day and in response to emotional and physical stress, healthy blood pressure averages around 120/80 mm Hg (the unit of measure mm Hg indicates how high in millimeters your blood pressure is able to raise a column of mercury). The first number corresponds to systolic pressure, the pressure created while the heart pumps blood into the arteries; the second number, diastolic pressure, indicates the pressure as the heart fills with blood for the next beat.

A diagnosis of high blood pressure is generally made when the reading is consistently higher than 140/90 mm Hg. Whenever blood pressure is elevated, the heart works harder than it should, straining the heart muscle and the arteries.

During most routine medical visits, your doctor measures and records your blood pressure using a sphygmomanometer (blood pressure cuff) and stethoscope. For a number of reasons, most often to monitor the effect and dosage of medications, your doctor may also recommend that you keep track of your own blood pressure.

In order to track your blood pressure, always measure around the same times each day. It is usually best to measure your blood pressure at times when you are relaxed, unless your doctor instructs you otherwise. Because blood pressure is not static—it rises in response to activity and stress and falls during periods of rest—variations in the readings occur. In addition, caffeine, smoking, and a full bladder can affect blood pressure.

Your doctor may advise you to make allowances for these variables and to avoid coffee or other stimulants around the time you are to use the monitor. Each reading should be recorded in a log, as should any activities that seem to trigger higher readings so that you can review your blood pressure pattern with your doctor at your next office visit.

A standard home blood pressure kit contains a sphygmomanometer with an attached rubber sack and stethoscope. Place your arm at heart level on the arm of a chair or on a table. If you are right-handed, take the pressure in your left arm; if you are left-handed, take the pressure in your right. Wrap the cuff tightly around your upper arm with the rubber bladder against one of the large arteries. The bottom of the cuff should be about an inch above your elbow. As you pump air into the bladder, the pressure in the cuff becomes higher than that in the artery. When the gauge reads

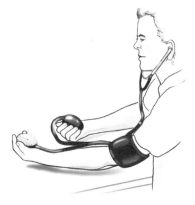

Proper position for taking blood pressure. Using a stethoscope and sphygmomanometer, you can monitor your blood pressure at home. Your arm should be level with your heart during the test.

approximately 30 mm Hg above the expected reading, stop pumping. Placing the stethoscope at the bend in your arm, you should hear no pulse in the artery. Deflate the bladder slowly, about 2 or 3 mm Hg per second. Record the reading at the first beat you hear, which occurs when the heart contracts and the blood rushes through the aorta and the pulmonary artery. This is the systolic pressure. Continue to deflate until there is no pulse sound, which occurs as the heart relaxes and the chambers fill with blood, and record the second number. This is the diastolic pressure.

Newer digital blood pressure monitors that do not use stethoscopes are available and generally easier to use. When a digital monitor is turned on, it automatically pumps up, then slowly releases. The systolic and diastolic pressures are displayed digitally; the heart rate is displayed in beats per minute.

Checking Cholesterol

Two tests are used to measure cholesterol levels. A finger-prick test can be done in the doctor's office or at places such as a health fair or shopping mall. A baseline lipoprotein profile, or lipid profile, is a more extensive blood test performed by a medical lab. Just who should be screened for cholesterol and how often is subject to controversy.

The American Heart Association (AHA) and the National Heart, Lung, and Blood Institute's National Cholesterol Education Program (NCEP) recommends that everyone have a baseline lipid profile at age 20 and then again every 5 years until age 60. The NCEP recommended screening includes total cholesterol levels and high-density lipoprotein (HDL) cholesterol profiles in all adults (see Chapter 2 for more information on cholesterol).

Whether someone should have subsequent periodic screenings is based on results. The AHA and NCEP recommend that even people at lowest risk for coronary artery disease (those with a total cholesterol lower than 200 mg/dL and HDL lower than 35 mg/dL) be screened again at least every 5 years. After 60, measuring cholesterol is optional, since at this age the effect of reducing cholesterol does little to correct coronary artery disease.

Techniques for Diagnosing Heart Disease

In the past decade, the diagnostic techniques used to determine whether a person has heart disease and if so, the type and extent of the disease have become increasingly sophisticated and effective. In most cases, more effective and precise diagnosis translates into more effective treatment—treatment that is more precisely tailored to an individual's particular condition.

Because diagnostic procedures can map problems so precisely, when treatment is needed—whether angioplasty (page 96) or valve replacement (page 122), or even open-heart surgery—doctors generally know what they will find before they begin. As a result of a range of diagnostic techniques, there is now little guesswork involved in treating heart disease.

Accurate diagnosis also helps to shape aftercare. And many of the same diagnostic tools are being used, even when there is no explicit heart disease, to detect conditions that could set the stage for future heart problems, thus increasing the likelihood that heart disease can be circumvented or, at the very least, its impact minimized.

Describing Your Symptoms

Most diagnostic examinations begin with your description of your symptoms. Symptoms, such as pain, pressure, discomfort, and any distinctive signs you may notice, are your body's way of calling attention to a problem. The specific symptoms or group of symptoms and their severity vary from person to person and from condition to condition.

Whereas for one person with a particular condition the discomfort may be unbearable, for another, it may be hardly noticeable. However, since pain is a subjective experience, and each person has a personal level of tolerance for pain and discomfort, the intensity of the sensation is not always a barometer of the severity of the condition. A person can have a heart condition that is well advanced, for example, and yet feel very little discomfort. On the other hand, someone can experience severe chest pain for no apparent reason.

Your doctor will ask you to describe any unusual discomfort you have. If your doctor does not ask, and you notice any disquieting or persistent sensations, bring it to your doctor's attention. Is your pain localized—that is, centered in one specific area of your body—or does it radiate out? Is it acute and sharp or dull and achy? Is the discomfort persistent, or does it diminish when you rest? Are there specific times during the day or night when the discomfort seems particularly keen?

As a rule, different heart conditions are signaled by slightly different symptoms. A myocardial infarction, or heart attack, occurs because part or all of the heart muscle sustains damage when the flow of oxygenated blood to the heart is cut off. Symptoms can include intense chest pain or prolonged, heavy pressure that radiates to the left shoulder and arm, the back, and even the teeth and jaw.

Men typically have a sensation of weight or pressure centered in the chest. Women often experience different types of symptoms, including burning sensations in the upper abdomen or midsternum. Difficulty breathing, sweating, nausea, vomiting, fainting, and lightheadedness may also occur along with the discomfort.

Angina pectoris, a symptom of coronary artery disease (CAD), occurs when the heart muscle is temporarily deprived of oxygen because the blood supply to the heart is insufficient for its current level of work. The

Cardiac Differences Between Men and Women

The 1949 Framingham Heart Study was the first research study to follow women over an extended period. Very quickly, it exposed the myth that heart disease is largely a male issue.

One of the more startling discoveries was that 45 percent of the women studied with symptomatic heart attacks died within one year as opposed to 10 percent of symptomatic men. This may be due, in part, to the fact that symptoms that are common to men are used as the standard. For men, heart disease most often announces itself in left-side chest pressure—"an elephant sitting on my chest."

On the other hand, women suffering from heart problems typically experience burning sensations in midsternum (under the breastbone) or upper abdomen. These sensations are often coupled with sweating, light-headedness and nausea. However, too often these symptoms are discounted or confused with indigestion or signs of menopause. As a result, studies show that as a group women delay in seeking treatment, usually much longer than men with similar heart-related symptoms. And women tend to be more tentative in reporting symptoms to their doctors. Doctors order ECGs or other cardiac diagnostic tests less often for women than for men.

Just as there are differences in the way men and women experience and report heart-related symptoms, there are differences in the effectiveness of some diagnostic tests according to gender. Some tests are not as accurate for women. The exercise stress test (see page 67), for example, is seldom accurate enough to be the sole diagnostic test for CAD in women.

In about one-third of all women, the exercise stress test indicates abnormalities when there are none. During exercise, a typical healthy woman can produce heart rhythms that resemble the rhythms characteristic of CAD. This may be due to fluctuations in estrogen levels. An exercise stress test may be sufficient to rule out heart disease, or it can be used to measure a woman's capacity for exercise and strenuous activity, but it cannot stand alone in diagnosing the presence of CAD.

In a slightly different way, doctors and technicians tend to be careful when using and interpreting echocardiography (see page 71) results in women. While this test is usually reliable for women, breast tissue can conceal or blur the heart, making it difficult to obtain clear, conclusive pictures.

primary sign of angina is chest pain during or after physical exertion or stress. In many instances, symptoms—including dull aching, tingling, burning sensation, tightness, squeezing, heaviness, constriction, pressure, anxiety, or shortness of breath—are relieved when the exertion or stress eases up.

Vasospastic angina, a type of chest pain that occurs when blood flow to the heart is blocked by a spasm in the coronary artery, causes a consistent racing sensation in the chest, especially at night, that can disrupt sleep.

Mitral valve prolapse, a common heart abnormality, can sometimes cause a sharp, achy, passing pain, usually occurring on the left, below the breastbone. In some instances the pain is dull and persistent, and in some instances, it can produce a pounding sensation, dizziness, and fatigue. Other valve diseases can prompt breathing difficulties with exertion or even during normal activities or when lying down. Relatively common signals of valve defects are palpitations (the feeling that the heart skips a beat or flip-flops in the chest), edema (swelling around the ankles, feet, or stomach), weakness, dizziness, faintness, and chest tightness and/or pain, pressure, or discomfort that lasts anywhere from a few seconds to a few hours.

The Physical Examination

After you describe your symptoms and the general state of your health, your doctor will examine you. The examination will include checking to see if there is a blue tinge to your skin especially around your fingernails and lips, which suggests a lack of oxygen; checking to see if your skin feels warm or cold to the touch; noting edema, or swelling, around the ankles, which could mean that not enough blood is reaching the area; and checking for an even or erratic pulse.

Cardiac auscultation—using a stethoscope to listen closely to the sounds the heart makes as it contracts and relaxes—is one of the simplest and oldest diagnostic techniques. By listening to your heartbeat, your doctor will be able to evaluate its rate and rhythm. Is it too fast or too slow? Is the pace even and appropriate? Are there skips, runs, or murmurs in the valves and occasionally in the heart muscle?

Normally, the blood flows silently and smoothly through the vessels. Does the blood flow sound turbulent, which could indicate a murmur? Is there a whooshing noise, perhaps an indication that blood is leaking backward because the mitral valve between left atrium and left ventricle does not close sufficiently when the ventricle contracts? Does it sound uneven and spasmodic, which could be a sign that hardened plaque along the vessel walls has caused partial occlusion of the arteries?

Noninvasive Tests

Depending on what your doctor hears, other tests may be recommended. The majority of tests are noninvasive; that is, they can be performed without penetrating the body. In general, noninvasive tests carry little risk and are pain-free. Invasive tests are those that penetrate the body. Because invasive tests carry slight risks and can be uncomfortable and more expensive, they are used less often and only when a more precise diagnostic picture is needed.

Stress Tests

A stress test, also called an exercise stress test, provides information about the way the heart responds to physical exertion. During a stress test, an ECG (see below), echocardiogram (see page 71), or nuclear scan (see page 74) is performed in combination with exercise, since an ECG or echocardiogram taken when the heart is at rest does not always accurately reflect the presence of heart disease.

By stimulating the heart through the use of a treadmill, stationary bicycle, or medication, a stress test may produce subtle changes, which give a more complete picture of the heart's fitness and health. Abnormalities may be revealed that show inadequate blood flow to the heart, which indicates a significant risk for myocardial infarction, especially during intense physical exertion.

An exercise stress test is most commonly evaluated with an ECG. During the test you are instructed to exercise on a treadmill or stationary bicycle while being closely monitored through an ECG. In addition to suggesting the presence of CAD, this test can also identify abnormal heart rhythms, evaluate the effectiveness of your current cardiac treatment plan, and help you develop an appropriate exercise program.

First, your heart's functioning is recorded through ECG while you are at rest. Next, you begin exercise on a treadmill or a stationary bicycle for about 7 to 12 minutes, gradually increasing your rate of exertion.

While it is normal for your heart rate, blood pressure, breathing rate, and perspiration to increase during the test, report any discomfort you feel in your chest, arm, or jaw; any breathing difficulties; dizziness; or lightheadedness. The lab personnel will watch for any symptoms or changes in the test results that suggest the test should be stopped.

A stress test can also be used with an echocardiogram or as part of a nuclear scanning test. In cases in which actual exercise is inadvisable or impossible, a stress test is performed with medications to stimulate the heart in ways that resemble the stimulation produced by exercise (see page 76).

Electrocardiogram

As a rule, an electrocardiogram (ECG or EKG) is the first test a doctor uses to determine whether a myocardial infarction (heart attack) has occurred. An ECG evaluates the electrical activity generated by the beating heart. Because it can measure changes in the heart's activities, it can detect signs of a previous myocardial infarction or of a developing one. It can also recognize the onset of another attack and therefore is often used to monitor high-risk patients.

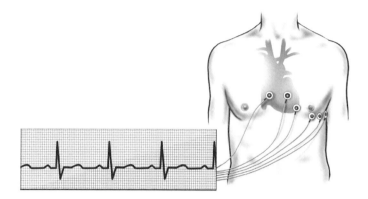

An electrocardiogram (ECG or EKG) monitors heart rhythm. Electrical sensor pads, or electrodes, are placed on the arms, legs, and across the chest. The ECG records the heart's electrical impulses as wave patterns on a strip of paper.

Simple and painless, an ECG uses twelve electrical sensor pads, or electrodes, that are placed on the arms, legs, and across the chest. Conductive jelly is dabbed at each point on the bare skin before the electrodes are attached.

As it detects the heart's electrical impulses, an ECG records the rhythms in wave patterns on paper. This graph indicates the size of the cardiac chambers, the contractions of the atria and the ventricles, and the period of rest and electrical restabilization between beats. Any abnormality in the heart's electrical conduction is revealed in characteristic changes in the ECG wave patterns. These changes can suggest that the heart has been damaged by infarction or ischemia (lack of oxygen).

While the ECG indicates abnormalities in the heart's pulsations, it does not pinpoint the exact nature or cause of the abnormality. Although changes in the heart's wave pattern are often indicative of heart disease, they can also be caused by changes in levels of blood hormones, salts, or other chemicals in the blood.

Holter Monitoring

A Holter monitor is a portable ECG monitor that records the heart's rhythm and can detect such abnormalities in rhythm as flutters and skipping. A Holter monitor helps doctors determine how serious an abnormal rhythm is and whether it requires treatment. Worn in a shoulder sling and attached to the chest by five leads for 12 to 48 hours, a Holter monitor measures the heart's electrical activities. When a flutter, flip, or skip

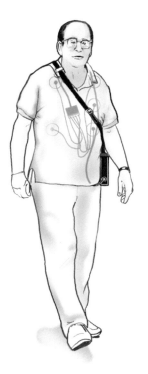

Holter monitor. This portable ECG is able to monitor heart rhythm for up to 48 hours. Electrodes are attached to the chest underneath clothing and the monitor is carried in a shoulder sling.

is felt, the wearer presses a button that relates sensation to actual activity. Many people also keep a diary to note when their symptoms occur and what they were doing at the time.

X-rays

Among the oldest diagnostic tests, x-rays show a visual profile of internal organs and can indicate conditions such as heart enlargement or fluid accumulating in the lungs as a result of heart failure. X-rays can pick up congenital conditions or defects. Sometimes, x-rays are used as an adjunct to other tests, such as catheterization (see page 76) (in which case, the procedure is considered invasive).

Magnetic Resonance Imaging

Magnetic resonance imaging (MRI) is a technique that combines computer technology, high-intensity magnetic fields, and radio waves to create sharp, clear images of the body's internal tissues. In particular, it can depict soft tissues that x-rays cannot.

When used to evaluate heart tissue, MRI can provide legible pictures of the heart muscle and the coronary vessels that supply the heart with

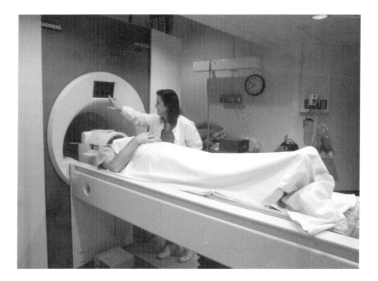

A magnetic resonance imaging (MRI) test is used to evaluate heart tissue. MRI can reveal the size and functioning of the heart's chambers, the thickness of the heart walls, and any congenital defects. An MRI scanner is a long tube that scans the body, producing cross-sectional images of the body's tissues.

blood. MRI can also detail the size and the functioning of the heart's chambers and the thickness of cardiac walls. It can also reveal the presence of any congenital defects.

An MRI scanner is a long tube that scans the body, as you lie on a platform, either in an open or enclosed unit. The procedure usually takes between 30 to 45 minutes. MRI can transmit cross-sectional images or "slices" of the cardiac muscle on film, thus providing three-dimensional or two-dimensional pictures from different angles.

Positron Emission Tomography

Positron emission tomography (PET) is a noninvasive technique for imaging internal body tissues and examining activities inside the body. PET differs from such imaging techniques as CT (see page 73) or MRI in that it can map the metabolic activities associated with the anatomic structures.

In PET, short-lived positron-emitting isotopes are injected into a vein. The interaction between the isotopes and body tissues allows images to be tracked and provides information on heart muscle metabolism. A device called a PET scanner then generates three-dimensional images.

PET scans are particularly useful for distinguishing between a healthy, well-nourished heart muscle and one that is oxygen deprived. It provides information that cannot be gained through MRI or CT about the viability and normality of cardiac tissues.

Specifically, this type of test helps doctors identify areas of CAD. During an emergency, PET can locate areas of heart tissue that may be suffering from ischemia because of a myocardial infarction but are not yet dead.

Echocardiography

An echocardiogram, also called a transthoracic echocardiogram or echo, is a graphic outline of the heart's movement created through ultrasound, or high-frequency sound waves. During an echocardiogram, ultrasound waves sent through the myocardium echo off the dense tissue, creating a shadow picture of the heart's valves and chambers (the same procedure is used to picture a fetus during pregnancy). This test works to evaluate the heart's pumping action; detect abnormalities in valve size, shape, and function; and show the direction of blood flow.

Echocardiography is used for a wide range of diagnostic purposes:

- To assess the overall function and efficiency of the heart and valves

- To determine the presence of valve disease, myocardial disease, pericardial disease, cardiac masses, and congenital heart disease

- To follow the progress of valve disease

- To evaluate the effectiveness of medical or surgical treatment in determining location and degree of blockage

One type of echocardiogram uses Doppler ultrasound. The test uses ultrasound waves and a sensitive microphone to detect sounds of turbulence or reduced blood flow in arteries, which may indicate blockages. The sounds are translated into images that appear on a monitor or can be printed on paper. In color Doppler, the sounds are translated into images that use color to indicate the direction and velocity of blood flow.

Another variation of the echocardiogram called a stress echocardiogram may be used to render a more detailed picture of the heart's health. Unlike an echocardiogram that is performed while the heart is at rest, exercise echo is performed while the heart is responding to exertion. This method is more proficient at evaluating the presence of CAD. The test, which takes about 40 minutes, begins with an echo image of the heart at rest. Then through exercise on a treadmill or stationary bicycle, you push the heart to its peak rate. When you are off the machine, a second echo image is taken. By comparing the two images, blockages in coronary arteries can be inferred. (See Stress Tests, page 67.)

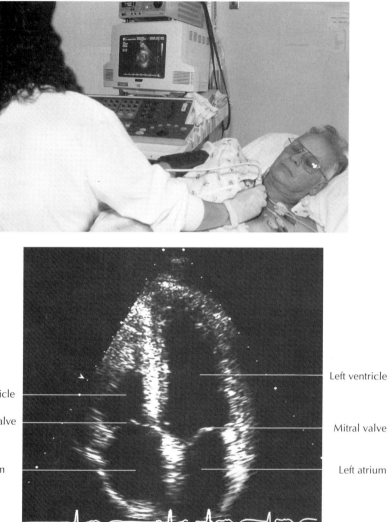

Transthoracic echocardiogram. This type of echocardiogram is taken using an ultrasound transducer (a device that produces high-frequency sound waves) placed on the outside of the chest. The sound waves are translated into an image of the heart's valves and chambers. The test is used to evaluate the heart's pumping action, detect valve abnormalities, and show the direction of blood flow. As in this scan, the position of the heart is often shown upside down (note that the ventricles appear on top of the atria). The orientation of the scan depends on the position of the transducer during the test.

Ultrafast Computed Tomography Scan

A standard computed tomography (CT) scan uses computerized x-rays to image thin cross sections or slices of the heart muscle and blood vessels that are displayed on monitors. An x-ray machine rotates as you lie face up on a table. As it scans, typically over a period of 10 to 15 minutes, the CT machine gathers information about the heart's anatomy and functioning, the efficiency of blood flow through the arteries, and the degree to which the arteries have narrowed.

However, because the heart and circulatory system are in constant motion, a CT scan is not always able to capture clear images. A technique called ultrafast CT is being used more widely to determine the presence of coronary calcification, calcium deposits that accumulate in and block arteries. Ultrafast CT is used for diagnosing CAD.

Sometimes, a dye or contrast medium is injected into the vein, which enhances the images. As the dye circulates, it may produce a warm sensation. Some people experience nausea, vomiting, or a metallic taste from the dye.

Invasive Tests

Blood Tests

Usually in a routine examination—and certainly to assess cardiovascular risk—the doctor takes a blood sample and sends it to a laboratory to be tested. Blood tests provide an easy, cost-effective way of diagnosing many cardiac conditions, including myocardial infarction and atherosclerosis. Blood tests can help the doctor make an early diagnosis, and therefore facilitate timely and aggressive treatment when appropriate. In addition, people with suspected atherosclerosis who are at risk for myocardial infarction are often monitored through the use of blood tests.

A number of blood tests can detect signs of heart problems, including injury to the myocardium indicating that a myocardial infarction has occurred. Blood tests confirm the presence of heart damage in the early stages, for example, in an emergency room, intensive care unit, or urgent care setting. These tests are also called heart-damage markers or cardiac enzyme tests.

When the heart has been damaged, enzymes that prompt healing are released into the bloodstream. A commonly used blood test measures levels of the enzyme creatine kinase, or CK. About six hours after a myocardial infarction begins, CK blood levels increase, peaking about 18 hours after the attack and returning to normal in 24 to 36 hours. Because blood tests can detect and assess the presence of CK, the extent and damage of the myocardial infarction can be identified, and aggressive treatment can be started early, possibly limiting the damage incurred by the infarction.

A blood test to detect elevated CK levels may be negative if it is performed prior to 6 hours after a myocardial infarction. Tests may be then performed serially to determine myocardial damage.

Another blood test measures the level of troponins, proteins that affect myocardial contractions. High blood levels of troponins, specifically troponin T (cTNT) and troponin I (cTNI), indicate muscle damage. A troponin test can be used to identify the risk for later heart problems as well as to evaluate existing damage. Other tests measure blood cholesterol levels; electrolytes, such minerals as sodium, potassium, calcium, and magnesium, that affect cardiovascular function; and thrombocytes (platelets), cells that aid the blood's ability to clot.

Invasive Stress Tests

Nuclear scanning is a diagnostic technique in which a small amount of a radioactive substance is injected into the body, and a scanner, or special camera, detects the radiation released by the substance and produces a computer image of the heart. Because blood does not show up on the scanner, the radioactive substance acts as a tracer for blood, providing information about heart function and blood flow.

Thallium Stress Test. A thallium stress test (also called a perfusion scan or test) is a type of nuclear scanning technique that uses the radioactive substance thallium. A thallium stress test combines nuclear scanning with exercise on a treadmill or stationary bicycle to assess heart function and determine if there is adequate blood flow to the myocardium.

At the start of the test, you are asked to exercise; when you have reached the maximum level of stress, a small amount of thallium is injected into a vein. The thallium travels through the bloodstream, reaching the coronary arteries and then the cells of the heart muscle. A camera detects the distribution of thallium in the myocardium. Because the thallium works as a tracer to indicate the areas of the myocardium that blood is reaching, regions that show less thallium have a loss of perfusion, or blood flow.

During the exercise portion of the test, alert the lab personnel if you experience angina, jaw or neck pain, lightheadedness, or breathing difficulties. You will also be tested a few hours after exercise to see how the blood flows when you are at rest.

Your test may indicate that your blood flow is normal during rest but that during exercise, your heart muscle is not receiving enough blood. Or your blood flow may be restricted at all times, due to blockages or narrowing of the arteries. If you have suffered a previous myocardial infarction, the test may show areas where there is no thallium, indicating damaged cells.

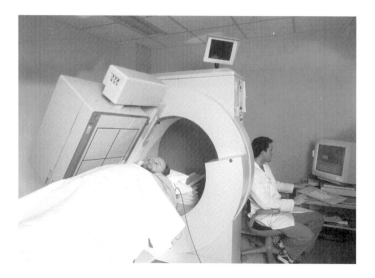

A nuclear scanning camera records images of the heart after a small amount of a radioactive substance is injected into the bloodstream. The camera traces the movement of the dye through the heart and reveals areas of reduced blood flow.

Radionuclide Ventriculogram. In this nuclear scanning test that evaluates ventricular function, a radioactive dye is injected into a vein, and a scanner records its movement through the heart's ventricles, or pumping chambers.

The test can be used alone or with a stress test (see page 67). There are two types of radionuclide ventriculograms: a MUGA (multigated acquisition) scan and a first-pass study. In a MUGA scan, blood is withdrawn and mixed with the radioactive substance technetium in a syringe, where the technetium binds to the red blood cells. Because of this binding, when the mixture is re-injected into the body, the technetium stays in the bloodstream for several hours, instead of being absorbed into the body's tissues, so that a series of images can be taken over time.

In a first-pass study, technetium is injected directly into a vein and circulates through the heart only once before it is eliminated. In the computer images produced by the scanner, the dye shows how much blood is pumped through the heart and how well the ventricles are pumping.

Three key measures of ventricular function are

■ *Ejection fraction,* the proportion of blood volume that the ventricles pump out of the chamber during systole (contraction). For example, if there are 100 milliliters of blood in the ventricle at the end of diastole (expansion) and 60 milliliters are pumped out during systole, the ejection fraction is 60 percent. A normal ejection fraction is 50 percent or higher.

■ *Stroke volume*, the amount of blood a ventricle pumps out during a single contraction. Normal stroke volume for an adult is about 90 milliliters.

■ *Cardiac output (CO)*, the amount of blood a ventricle pumps out of the heart in one minute. This is equivalent to the heart rate—the number of times the heart beats in a minute—times the stroke volume. A normal cardiac output is about 5 liters.

The ejection fraction gives an indication of the strength of the ventricle. If the ventricle is weakened, its ability to squeeze out enough blood for circulation through the body may be adversely affected. The ejection fraction must be evaluated in terms of the volume of blood going through the heart. If the stroke volume or cardiac output is inadequate, heart failure is possible even if the ejection fraction is normal.

Dipyridamole and Dobutamine Stress Tests. If it is inadvisable or impossible for you to exercise on a treadmill or stationary bicycle for a stress test, a medication, usually dipyridamole (Persantine) or dobutamine (Dobutrex), is used to prompt changes similar to those induced by exercise in the heart's blood flow. These medications can be used together with an ECG, echocardiogram, or thallium stress test.

Although these procedures are generally painless, occasionally both dipyridamole and dobutamine cause a warm, flushing feeling, and in some cases, a mild headache. These symptoms or any chest discomfort, excessive shortness of breath, or irregular heartbeats should be reported to the stress lab personnel immediately.

Catheterization

Catheterization is a procedure in which a catheter—a long, slender, flexible, hollow tube—is inserted inside the arteries or chambers of the heart. This test is used primarily to check internal pressures in the heart, to measure blood flow, to assess valve leakage, and to examine the arteries for blockage. More than two million cardiac catheterizations are performed in the United States each year, the majority in an outpatient setting.

The procedure is generally painless, although you may feel a slight pressure or some discomfort. You are given a mild sedative to help relax, but you remain awake throughout the procedure. The catheter is threaded through an artery in the arm or groin with a thin, flexible wire. The doctor then uses x-ray equipment to guide the catheter toward the heart. When the catheter reaches the heart, the wire is removed, leaving the catheter in place. The catheter then sends information back to a machine that measures blood and oxygen in the heart chambers.

A catheter is used in a procedure called angiography to create x-rays, still photos, or moving images of the heart's chambers. A special fluid called contrast medium or dye is injected into the artery through the

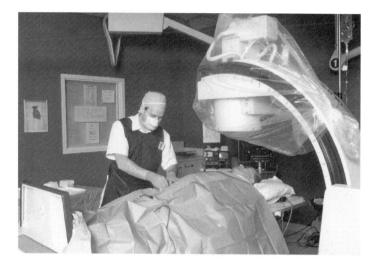

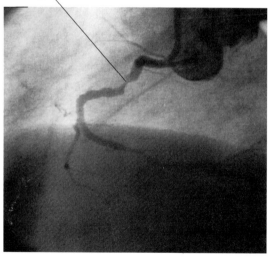

Blockage

Cardiac catheterization, also called coronary arteriography or coronary angiography, is used to evaluate the coronary arteries. A contrast dye is injected into an artery through a catheter (a long, hollow tube inserted into a vein and advanced to the heart). The dye then creates a silhouette on an x-ray that reveals blockages or narrowed areas in the coronary arteries. Doctors can also use this test to evaluate the pumping strength of the heart and to detect valve abnormalities.

catheter. The use of these dyes allows for detailed evaluation of parts of the heart, including the vessels. Angiography can delineate size and shape as well as detect blockages or other abnormalities in arteries anywhere in the body.

When catheterization is used to assess the coronary arteries, it is called coronary arteriography or cardiac catheterization. The catheter is usually inserted into the femoral artery in the groin and advanced until it reaches the coronary arteries. Contrast dye is then injected through the catheter, and a silhouette becomes visible on an x-ray.

The contrast material is photographed as it moves through the heart's chambers, valves, and major vessels. From these photographs, doctors can tell whether the coronary arteries are narrowed, whether the heart valves are working correctly, and whether the strength of the heart muscle is adequate.

Catheters are generally left in the body for a short time. In rare cases, they can cause infection, or blood clots form around them. Occasionally, these blood clots obstruct local circulation, causing damage to the arterial tissue. Rarely, a catheter breaks or punctures an artery.

Electrophysiology Studies

Electrophysiology studies (EPS) are used to map the origin of arrhythmias (see Chapter 7, Rhythm Disorders). This test is performed in a manner similar to cardiac catheterization. You are conscious but sedated; a catheter is wired through a vein in the arm, leg, or upper body and placed in the heart. The heart's pattern of electrical activity is recorded and evaluated. The heart can also be stimulated electronically during the test to elicit the arrhythmia, which aids the doctor in determining the origin of the arrhythmia.

EPS are performed when an arrhythmia has not been responsive to treatment, when it is severely disabling, or when there appears to be a risk of sudden cardiac death.

Transesophageal Echocardiogram

A transesophageal echocardiogram (TEE) is a type of echocardiogram that provides clearer images of the heart's movement because the sound waves are transmitted from inside the body. During TEE, an ultrasound transducer, which produces high-frequency sound waves, is positioned on an endoscope, a long, thin, flexible tube about $1/2$ inch in diameter. The probe is placed down the throat. From the esophagus, the transducer provides pictures of the heart's valves and chambers. TEE allows a close evaluation of the heart's pumping action without interference from the ribs or lungs. This is especially helpful in viewing otherwise obscured parts of the valves.

TEE is often used when the results from standard echocardiogram studies are not sufficient. Sometimes, TEE is combined with Doppler ultrasound or color Doppler (see page 71) to evaluate blood flow across the heart's valves. This test is used to assess the overall function of the heart's valves and chambers; to determine the presence of valvular heart disease, myocardial disease, pericardial disease, cardiac masses, and congenital heart disease; to evaluate the effectiveness of valve surgery; and to evaluate abnormalities of the left atrium.

There is some discomfort involved in TEE. Usually, the throat is anesthetized and a doctor gives a mild sedative intravenously, which occasionally causes drowsiness. You lie on your left side on an examina-

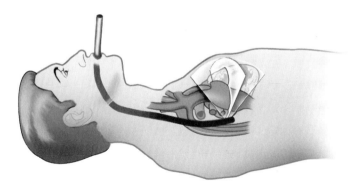

Transesophageal echocardiography (TEE). Like transthoracic echocardiography, a TEE uses sensitive microphones to pick up ultrasound waves and create an image. In this test, the transducer is attached to the end of an endoscope, a long flexible tube, and placed down the throat. A TEE provides clearer images of the heart than does a transthoracic echocardiogram.

tion table, a dental suction tip removes secretions, and the endoscope is inserted into your mouth and swallowed. Once it is in the esophagus, the endoscope does not interfere with breathing. Heart rate, blood pressure, and oxygen levels are closely monitored during and immediately after the exam.

The test typically lasts 90 minutes. Afterward, there may be temporary soreness or numbness in the throat. Once sedation has worn off, normal activities can be resumed, although driving is not advised.

CHAPTER 5

Coronary Artery Disease

Introduction

Like all the body's organs, the myocardium (heart muscle) requires a constant supply of oxygen and nutrients to remain vigorous and functioning. The heart receives oxygen and nutrients in the blood through a specialized network of arteries called the coronary arteries.

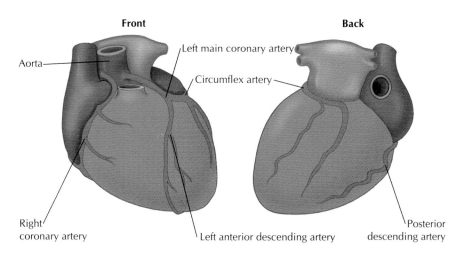

Locations of the coronary arteries. The coronary arteries deliver blood carrying oxygen and nutrients to the heart muscle.

This network includes two major coronary arteries called the left main coronary artery and the right coronary artery that fork from the point at which the aorta meets the left ventricle. Blood vessels called the circumflex artery, the left anterior descending artery, and the posterior descending artery branch off from the left and right coronary arteries and wrap around the myocardium. When the arteries of the heart are healthy, they have a smooth lining that ensures unrestricted blood flow.

Often as a result of long-standing lifestyle practices, the coronary arteries become clogged with plaque—clusters of cells, fats, and cholesterol that accumulate along the arterial walls. The blood supply to the heart is impeded, or it can become blocked temporarily or reduced over an extended period of time. This disease process, called atherosclerosis, causes the arteries to narrow and harden. The resulting condition, known as coronary artery disease (CAD), also called ischemic heart disease, is chronic and advances over time.

When blood flow is consistently insufficient or temporarily cut off, the heart muscle becomes starved for oxygen. This condition is called ischemia. Ischemia—a local or temporary deficiency in the blood supply—can produce angina (chest pain).

However, if the blood supply to the heart is completely obstructed or cut off abruptly, the muscle cells are at risk of irreversible injury, and the tissue can die. Consequently, a myocardial infarction (heart attack) can occur. In a myocardial infarction, an area of the myocardium has been permanently damaged. The extent of the damage determines whether the myocardial infarction will be fatal.

In most people, CAD begins in young adulthood, gradually developing throughout life. The effects of CAD—angina or myocardial infarction—occur between the ages of 50 and 70 (and generally 10 years later in

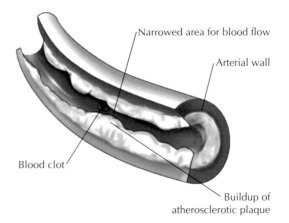

Atherosclerosis is the buildup of fatty material called plaque on the walls of the arteries. Atherosclerosis of the coronary arteries is called coronary artery disease (CAD).

Narrowed area for blood flow

Arterial wall

Blood clot

Buildup of atherosclerotic plaque

A

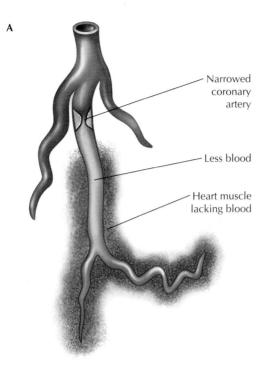

Narrowed coronary artery

Less blood

Heart muscle lacking blood

B

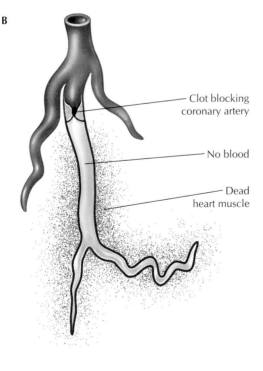

Clot blocking coronary artery

No blood

Dead heart muscle

(A) Ischemia—reduced blood flow through the coronary arteries—causes a lack of oxygen in the myocardium (heart muscle) and angina (chest pain) results. (B) Myocardial infarction—death of the heart tissue cells—occurs when blood flow to an area of the myocardium is cut off or severely reduced.

Scope of Coronary Artery Disease in the United States

Although CAD is the single largest cause of death in both men and women in the United States—accounting for nearly one-half of all fatalities—medical advances and public health awareness have resulted in a dramatic 60 percent decline in the CAD fatality rate since 1950. Better control of risk factors, improved medical and surgical treatment for myocardial infarctions and strokes, and a dramatic drop in cigarette smoking are the major reasons for this significant decrease.

Despite these changes, the incidence of CAD continues to increase. Some facts about CAD include the following:

- About every 30 seconds someone in the United States suffers a coronary event.

- In 1996, more than 240,000 men and 230,000 women died of CAD.

- Risk factors between individuals can vary dramatically. For example: Between the ages 35 and 74, a black woman is 72 percent more likely to die of CAD than is a white woman.

- As many as 12 million people—5.8 million men and 6.1 million women—who are alive today have a history of myocardial infarction, or angina, or both.

women). In the United States, approximately 1 million people develop significant CAD each year. Ischemic heart disease—disease that results from inadequate coronary artery blood flow—is the most common cause of death in industrialized nations.

As plaque accumulates along the artery wall, a rupture or tear of the diseased wall can occur. This causes blood clots to form and further impede or abruptly interrupt blood flow. These clots can lead to a myocardial infarction. A stationary clot that obstructs blood flow in a coronary artery is called a coronary thrombus or coronary occlusion. Pieces of atherosclerotic plaque that break off and travel, wedging somewhere else in the heart's circulation, are called emboli.

Sometimes, a coronary artery can contract temporarily or go into spasm, disrupting blood flow to part of the heart muscle. Coronary artery spasm can occur in blood vessels that appear normal. However, it usually occurs when the artery is partially blocked by atherosclerosis. In approximately two-thirds of all cases, there is severe coronary blockage in at least one major vessel, and the spasm occurs at the site of the obstruction. A severe spasm can lead to myocardial infarction.

Angina Pectoris

Coronary artery disease can eventually lead to a condition known as angina pectoris. Angina pectoris is the medical term for chest pain or discomfort that occurs when the heart muscle receives insufficient blood flow. Angina generally occurs after a period of physical exertion or emotional stress. (A variation of angina—variant, or Prinzmetal's, angina—is a form that generally occurs while a person is at rest; see below.) As strain increases, the heart muscle is unable to obtain the amount of blood and consequently oxygen it needs to meet the increased demand. Angina affects men most frequently after the age of 30 and women after menopause (see Symptoms of CAD in Women, page 87).

Angina is marked by:

■ Tightness, fullness, or pressure just beneath the sternum (breast-bone)

■ A sensation of constriction, heaviness, and burning that may radiate to the neck, throat, left shoulder, or left arm, typically lasting a minute or two, although it may last as long as 15 minutes

■ Occurrence with physical or emotional stress and relieved with rest

Variant Angina

Variant angina (also called vasospastic or Prinzmetal's angina) is usually caused when a muscle spasm in one or more coronary arteries blocks blood flow to the heart by narrowing the vessel. However, about two-thirds of people with variant angina have severe coronary atherosclerosis in at least one vessel. Although generally associated with severe spasm, variant angina may also occur without symptoms.

This is a rare type of angina and almost always occurs when the body is not placing demands for oxygen on the heart—during sleep, for example. Variant angina may awaken a person with a sense of anxiety; a dull pain that radiates to the back and arm may also be experienced.

During the acute phase of the disease, up to 20 percent of people with variant angina experience a myocardial infarction. Treating the atherosclerosis relieves the angina.

Often, variant angina is smoking-related. Emotional factors and exposure to the cold may also be involved. A doctor may perform an ergonovine test to confirm coronary spasm (see page 89).

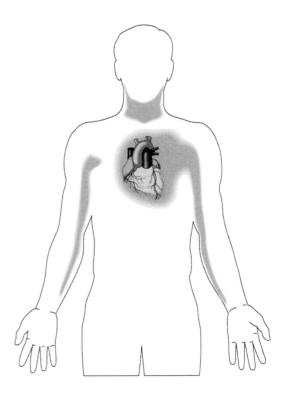

Angina (chest pain or discomfort) may radiate to the neck, throat, left shoulder, or left arm. (Adapted with permission from *Cleveland Clinic Heart Advisor*, Vol. 1, No. 6, June 1998, Torstar Publications, Inc. All rights reserved.)

If serious arrhythmias (heart rhythm disturbances) develop during angina, the risk of sudden death increases significantly. Whenever a person with stable angina (pain that follows a predictable pattern in terms of frequency and the factors that precipitate it) begins to experience chest pain or discomfort more frequently, pain or discomfort that seems to be prompted by even mild exertion or stress, or pain that disturbs sleep, the condition has progressed to *unstable angina*, which could signal an important change in status, requiring immediate medical attention.

Angina pectoris usually occurs when blood flow to the heart, while adequate for normal activity, is not sufficient when greater demand is placed on the heart such as during unusual physical activity or emotional stress. Angina can be prompted by such activities as heavy lifting, strenuous exercise, or rigorous sports; by indigestion after a large meal; by extreme temperatures; by sexual activity; or by emotional upset.

During these times, the heart muscle naturally hastens its pace to accommodate a greater need for oxygen. If the coronary arteries have become narrowed and rigid and are therefore unable to accommodate the increase in blood flow, chest pain can result. In this way, angina can be a clue that CAD is present.

87

Symptoms of CAD in Women

Each year, more than 250,000 women in the United States die as a result of heart disease. Many of these deaths would be prevented if CAD was not considered a "man's disease."

Studies show that doctors have been more likely to dismiss a woman's symptoms as indigestion or perimenopausal symptoms and not to look for CAD as aggressively in women as they do in men. A woman's symptoms tend to be less likely to be identified as heart-related. Women are also less likely to recognize symptoms in themselves and seek treatment.

The symptoms of CAD, and especially of myocardial infarction, can be significantly different in women than they are in men. Recognizing these symptoms can make women more effective partners in fighting CAD.

On average, the symptoms of CAD appear 10 years later in women than in men. Women tend to have myocardial infarctions 10 years later than men do.

The most common symptoms of heart disease in women are:

- Pain or pressure over the chest that travels into the arm or jaw

- A burning sensation in the chest or upper abdomen

- Shortness of breath, irregular heartbeat, dizziness, sweating, fatigue, and nausea

When angina occurs regularly and is not directly linked to physical activity, it may signal an impending myocardial infarction. A person experiencing angina attacks in any form should consult a doctor.

Medications are available to dissolve clots that block the coronary arteries or to thin the blood. Procedures such as coronary balloon angioplasty (page 96) can unblock areas in the arteries and coronary artery bypass surgery (page 100) can reroute blood supplies around blockages. These treatments are used only after the problem has become acute. But without significant lifestyle changes, the disease process usually continues unchecked.

Risk Factors for Coronary Artery Disease

To some extent, whether a person develops CAD is determined by a number of lifestyle factors. Many heart problems can be addressed effectively through preventive measures. In order to minimize the likelihood of developing CAD or to limit its severity, it is crucial to become aware of the risk factors for CAD.

While there are many specific causes of CAD, several factors greatly increase the risk of developing the disease. The more risk factors a person has, the greater the likelihood of developing CAD. They include:

- Smoking (affects 25 percent of the US population)

- High blood pressure (affects 20 percent)

- Elevated blood cholesterol (affects 50 percent)

- Sedentary lifestyle (affects 60 to 80 percent)

- Obesity (affects 30 to 40 percent)

For more information regarding risk factors, see Chapter 2, Keeping the Heart Healthy.

Detection and Diagnosis

If severe chest pain occurs, the activity that may have triggered the pain should be stopped at once. Stopping physical activity should relieve the discomfort because the strain on the heart will be eased and its need for oxygen reduced. Next, the doctor should be contacted. If the discomfort does not diminish quickly with rest, or if the frequency or severity of the attacks increases, *immediate* medical attention should be sought.

If the doctor suspects that there is a risk of CAD or if symptoms of angina or myocardial infarction have been experienced (see The First Signs of Myocardial Infarction, page 89), a battery of diagnostic tests will be conducted. Most of these tests can be done either before or after a myocardial infarction. The doctor will probably order an electrocardiogram (ECG or EKG; see page 67) or blood tests to rule out possible myocardial damage (see page 73). Other tests that may be ordered include the following:

- *Echocardiography,* which examines heart's structure and function through the use of ultrasound (see page 71)

- *Stress tests,* which can detect, through graded exercise, any limitation in the heart's function and capacity (see page 67)

- *Holter monitor examination,* a 24-hour ECG that provides a long-term picture of heart activity (see page 68) to detect heart rhythm disturbances

The First Signs of Myocardial Infarction (Heart Attack)

The following signs—when not provoked by physical activity or emotional stress—are fairly clear warnings of a myocardial infarction:

- Intense or persistent pressure, pain, or tight, full, squeezing sensations centered in the chest that last more than a few minutes

- Pain that radiates out from the chest to the shoulders, neck, arms, teeth, or jaw

- Chest discomfort or a burning sensation in the upper abdomen or midsternum (breastbone) coupled with lightheadedness, fainting, sweating, nausea, vomiting, or shortness of breath

Without exception, a myocardial infarction is a medical emergency. If you have severe chest pain that lasts for more than 30 minutes, or if you have CAD and your pain is not relieved by nitroglycerine, you could be having a myocardial infarction. If you experience any of these symptoms, stay calm but seek help immediately. Call 911 and calmly and clearly describe the nature of the problem to the dispatcher and give your name, address, and telephone number. Early treatment is essential. Every minute counts. (See Thirty Minutes to Treatment, page 279.)

The sooner you can receive lifesaving treatment with clot-dissolving medications or by catheter opening of the blocked artery, the greater your chances that the myocardium can be saved.

- *Coronary angiogram,* specialized x-rays of the heart that use dye injected through a catheter to develop a roadmap of the heart's arteries (see page 95)

- *Nuclear scanning tests,* which create a computer image of the heart muscle using a short-lived radioactive substance injected into a vein (see page 74)

In cases of coronary artery spasm, an ergonovine test, in which the drug ergonovine is administered to induce coronary spasm, is both sensitive and useful. Occasionally, voluntary hyperventilation or coronary injections of acetylcholine are used to provoke variant angina, in order to measure the severity of the reaction.

What About Sex?

One of the most tenacious myths about heart disease is that having a heart condition means curtailing or abandoning an active sex life. Another myth is that resuming sexual relations after angina or myocardial infarction creates a risk of another myocardial infarction, stroke, or sudden death. But there is no reason to forgo sexual activity after recovery from myocardial infarction or heart surgery. For the most part, after a reasonable time elapses (about a month), and with awareness of individual responses to physical exertion, most heart patients should be able to return to a satisfying and active sex life.

Factors that are not purely physical can affect sexual arousal and enjoyment during recovery from a serious heart condition. For example, any sexual problems that were present before may well resurface afterward. They may even become amplified. Some people worry about their ability to perform sexually after recovering from myocardial infarction or angina. This preoccupation can hinder their performance or enjoyment.

Moreover, any major health problem can bring on depression, which in turn can interfere with sexual interest and ability. Symptoms of depression develop in approximately 20 percent of people immediately after a myocardial infarction. Talking to a doctor can help mitigate these factors and soften their impact on sexual activity. If they persist, and cause problems in a relationship, the professional assistance of a counselor or therapist may be helpful.

People can enjoy sexual activities and simultaneously address any fears. First, regular and appropriate exercise and physical activity will help maintain and improve overall stamina and strength. Sexual activity will be less taxing if it occurs at times of rest and relaxation. The doctor may recommend taking certain medications before sexual relations. Any concerns about sexual activity should be discussed with a doctor. (For information about sexual relations during postoperative recovery, see page 240).

Medications

CAD is a progressive process. Although medications and sophisticated direct procedures may be necessary to address acute problems, without significant change in unhealthy habits, the underlying disease process will most likely continue. Therefore, even when more direct treatment methods are used, effective and long-term treatment will always include lifestyle modifications.

Treatment aims at both controlling symptoms and slowing or arresting the atherosclerotic process. The method of treatment chosen for active and acute symptoms of CAD depends on many factors—primarily the degree to which the heart muscle has been damaged. If blood flow has been temporarily blocked, as in angina, and if the blockage is less than 70 percent, medications are usually the first line of treatment.

Vasodilators

Vasodilators cause blood vessels to relax, which in turn opens and enlarges the lumen (the inside of the vessels). Blood flow is improved, allowing more oxygen and nutrients to reach the heart muscle.

Nitroglycerin, a coronary vasodilator, is the most common pharmacologic treatment for acute attacks of angina—it is used in 90 percent of all cases. Nitroglycerin works both to dilate, or widen, the arteries, increasing blood flow to the heart muscle itself and also to relax the veins, curtailing the amount of blood that returns to the heart from the body. This combined action alleviates the stress on the heart's pumping action.

Usually administered in pill form, dissolved under the tongue, or as a spray atomized under the tongue, nitroglycerin works quickly—usually in less than a minute—to ease discomfort. Long-acting nitrate preparations are often used to maintain vasodilation throughout the day (doses as high as 90 to 120 milligrams may be used). Nitroglycerin can cause headaches in some people, although this side effect is usually mild. The combination of nitrates and sildenafil (Viagra, the popular impotence treatment) is potentially lethal (see Viagra, below).

Viagra

A treatment for male impotence (erectile dysfunction), sildenafil (Viagra) has achieved wide popularity. However, when a person is taking medications containing nitrates, including nitroglycerin, Viagra can cause a potentially lethal drug interaction; for some, the combination can produce life-threatening hypotension (low blood pressure). As a result, Viagra should not be considered by anyone who is undergoing chronic nitrate drug therapy or who is taking short-acting nitrate-containing medications.

In addition, people considering Viagra should consult the doctor if they

- Have active coronary ischemia, even if they are not taking nitrates

- Have congestive heart failure or even mild hypotension

- Are taking erythromycin, cimetidine, or protease inhibitors, which can prolong Viagra's half-life (the rate at which Viagra is broken down by the body)

To date, there is no evidence that using Viagra in combination with heparin, beta blockers, calcium-channel blockers, narcotics, or aspirin causes significant interactions. For people who experience recurring mild angina while using Viagra, non-nitrate anti-anginal agents, such as beta blockers, should be considered.

Calcium-Channel Blockers

Calcium-channel blockers are often prescribed for angina, sometimes in combination with nitrates. Calcium-channel blockers curb calcium absorption in cells; calcium contributes to contraction of the vessels. As the normal flow of calcium through heart channels is interrupted, the arteries dilate and blood flow increases. This group of medications, including nifedipine (Adalat, Procardia) and verapamil (Calan, Isoptin, Verelan), is especially effective in treating hypertension and some arrhythmias (abnormal heart rhythms), as well as angina.

Calcium-channel blockers can also help prevent the coronary spasms that prompt variant or Prinzmetal's angina (see page 85). These drugs are usually used along with nitrates. Because Prinzmetal's angina tends to be episodic, use of calcium-channel blockers is typically tapered off after 6 to 12 months of treatment.

Beta Blockers

Beta blockers reduce the heart's demand for blood by inhibiting the stimulating effects of the hormone epinephrine (adrenaline) on the heart. This medication lowers heart rate and blood pressure, easing the propulsion of blood through the myocardium. Some beta blockers not only slow blood flow but also dilate the blood vessels. Therefore, they can significantly slow the progression of heart failure and improve the chances of surviving myocardial infarction. In addition, by blocking excessive release of epinephrine, beta blockers can improve the pumping action of the left ventricle.

Beta blockers are seldom prescribed for people with severe, unstable heart failure, asthma, diabetes, or severe bradycardia. In some cases, they cause fatigue and depression, and they can lessen sexual desire.

Thrombolytics

Thrombolytics work to dissolve thrombi, or blood clots, that form in the blood vessels, which are responsible for most myocardial infarctions. By doing so, thrombolytics restore blood flow. Studies show that prompt administration of thrombolytics—within a few hours after myocardial infarction—reduces damage to the myocardium and decreases fatalities. Once the clot is dissolved, healthy circulation is restored. Thrombolytic agents are administered intravenously (through a vein).

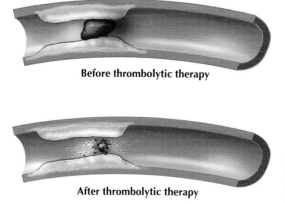

Before thrombolytic therapy

After thrombolytic therapy

Thrombolytic medications work to dissolve blood clots in the blood vessels.

ACE Inhibitors

Traditionally used to lower high blood pressure and to treat a number of heart-related problems, these medications block the activation of angiotensin, the enzyme that causes blood vessels to constrict. Studies show that ACE inhibitors block inflammation of the blood vessels.

Chelation Therapy

Chelation with ethylenediamine tetracetic acid (EDTA) is an accepted treatment for heavy metal poisoning, such as lead poisoning. Injected into the blood, this agent binds to the metals. In this way, the heavy metals can be removed from the body in the urine.

Recently, chelation therapy has been touted as a treatment for CAD. However, there is no scientific evidence to indicate any benefit from this form of therapy. The Food and Drug Administration (FDA), the National Institutes of Health (NIH), the American Heart Association (AHA), and the American College of Cardiology (ACC) agree that no adequate, controlled, published studies using currently approved scientific methodology support the use of chelation therapy. A recent scientific study of chelation therapy determined that it was no more effective than a placebo in treating men and women with certain forms of cardiovascular disease.

The real danger in using chelation therapy, or any form of unproven treatment, is that it may prevent people from seeking and receiving well-established and effective treatment.

Anticoagulants

Platelet Blockers

Platelet blockers are used to avert myocardial infarctions and strokes in people at risk of these events. These agents act as platelet aggregation inhibitors—they help reduce the tendency of the blood to form clots. In this way, their use can reduce the risk of myocardial infarction. Aspirin is the most widely used platelet blocker. Clopidogrel (Plavix) and ticlopidine (Ticlid) are two other platelet blockers that may be prescribed as an alternative to aspirin. Even stronger platelet blockers such as glycoprotein IIb–IIIa inhibitors (ReoPro) are used temporarily during angioplasty and stenting.

Minor side effects of platelet blockers can be minimized. Stomach upset can be mitigated by taking medication with food or just after a meal. Alcoholic beverages should be avoided, as alcohol can worsen stomach upset. Judgment should be exercised whenever activities that require alertness are performed, such as driving a car, until the effects of the drug are clear.

Blood Thinners

Blood thinners also work to keep the blood from clotting, although they work by a different mechanism than platelet blockers. A common blood-thinning medication is heparin. Heparin, used intravenously, provides strong blood thinning during a cardiac event such as myocardial infarction or the need for angioplasty. Another commonly used agent is warfarin (Coumadin). However, because warfarin is a powerful medication, which requires frequent blood testing and adjustments, it is used most commonly for heart valve disorders and for fibrillation (heartbeat irregularity).

Cautions

Because these medicines can increase the risk of bleeding, the doctor may stop treatment before any dental or surgical procedures and advise against activities that may result in injury.

It is also important to consult the doctor about taking any of these medications (including aspirin) during pregnancy or when breastfeeding. If you are taking a blood-thinning drug (such as warfarin), or medication for gout or diabetes, or if you have any bleeding problems, consult your doctor before using a platelet blocker.

Catheter and Surgical Interventions

One of the most remarkable aspects of modern medicine is the progress in techniques for treating CAD. These advances have saved hundreds of thousands of lives and have allowed these people to live longer and healthier lives.

Limited forms of CAD are sometimes treated with angioplasty, a procedure that clears plaque from the coronary arteries. More severe forms may require coronary artery bypass graft (CABG) surgery (see page 100), in which a surgically implanted shunt diverts blood flow from the aorta past an obstruction.

Before performing either of these procedures, doctors locate the blockage's exact location within the coronary artery. A diagnostic x-ray procedure, called coronary angiography, is performed. A long, thin plastic tube called a catheter is threaded through an artery in the arm or leg and forwarded into the coronary arteries. A liquid contrast dye is then injected through the catheter, and high-speed x-ray films track the course of the liquid. This technique locates and measures precisely the blockage in the artery.

Another procedure, intravascular ultrasound (IVUS), offers a more comprehensive view of the artery. A miniature sound probe on the tip of a coronary catheter is threaded through the coronary arteries and produces extremely detailed images of the interior walls of the blood vessels.

Choosing Between Angioplasty and Bypass Surgery

Most blockages are treated with medication and lifestyle modifications. However, if coronary angiography reveals a more severe blockage in one of the coronary arteries, more direct intervention may be necessary to open the artery. In cases where plaque has narrowed the diameter of a coronary artery by more than 50 percent, angioplasty (see page 96) or bypass surgery (see page 100) will likely be considered.

Deciding between angioplasty, a nonsurgical interventional procedure, and coronary artery bypass graft (CABG) surgery, an open-heart operation that creates a detour around the narrowed or blocked part of the artery, can be difficult. This decision is directed by a cardiologist, who considers the patient's age and overall health, as well as the number and severity of the blockages. In general, angioplasty and CABG surgery appear to yield comparable results over time. However, several factors determine why angioplasty may be chosen.

Why Angioplasty May Be Chosen

In many cases, angioplasty is the first step taken when it appears that medications are not relieving angina. Angioplasty is relatively quick, safe, and effective. Patients tend to recover from it quickly.

Angioplasty can often be performed at the same time as a diagnostic procedure, cardiac catheterization (see page 76). When this happens, the procedure is extended only by an hour or two, and the patient generally goes home the next day. The discomfort is minimal and risk of a serious complication following the procedure is usually less than 1 to 2 percent. Most patients who have angioplasty experience long-term success, although restenosis (see page 98) occurs in 25 to 33 percent of patients.

Angioplasty is most commonly performed when the blockage is in a single vessel and can be easily reached. However, more and more often it is also being performed when there are multiple blockages in two vessels. Sometimes, it is performed in emergency situations to open a clogged artery after a myocardial infarction has occurred.

Why CABG Surgery May Be Chosen

When three or more coronary arteries have become seriously narrowed, CABG surgery is more likely to be performed (see also When Is CABG Surgery Necessary?, page 101). This is because the more arteries that are involved, the greater the chance are that one will reclose (see Restenosis, page 98), which necessitates repeat angioplasty. Also, if an artery is fully blocked, it may not be reopened by balloon angioplasty or stenting, and this may necessitate surgical bypass.

Angioplasty

The term angioplasty comes from the Latin "angio," meaning blood vessel, and "plasty," meaning "to mold or shape." Medically referred to as percutaneous transluminal coronary angioplasty (PTCA), angioplasty is a group of invasive techniques used to reshape the inside of the coronary arteries.

In balloon dilation or balloon angioplasty, a catheter with a small balloon (approximately 3 millimeters in diameter) at its tip is inserted into

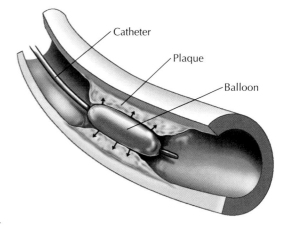

Balloon angioplasty is a procedure to open clogged arteries. A catheter fitted with a balloon at its tip is inserted into an artery (usually in the groin) and advanced to the heart. Upon reaching the area of blockage, the balloon is inflated, which breaks up the plaque and opens the artery.

Catheter

Plaque

Balloon

Mason Sones, MD: The First Cardiac Catheterization

Cardiac catheterization for either diagnosis or treatment would not be possible without the contributions of Dr. Mason Sones, a cardiologist at the Cleveland Clinic. In 1958, Dr. Sones was inadvertently responsible for the first selective coronary angiogram. While performing an aortogram (a procedure in which x-ray pictures are taken of the aorta following an injection) on a 26-year-old patient suffering from rheumatic heart disease, he accidentally injected contrast dye into the right coronary artery.

The patient suffered no ill effects, and Dr. Sones recognized the benefits of creating clear, detailed pictures of the coronary circulation. Based on his discovery, he designed catheters and developed techniques to x-ray the various coronary arteries. Out of this accident arose the knowledge that would change cardiology and that paved the way for further advances in documenting coronary artery blockages.

an artery in the leg or arm and moved to the precise location of the blockage within a coronary artery. The balloon is inflated for 1 to 2 minutes; as it expands, it compresses and redistributes the atherosclerotic plaque, opening the artery. The balloon is usually inflated and deflated several times.

About half a million people in the United States undergo coronary angioplasty each year. In general, angioplasty is safe, with a mortality rate of less than 1 percent. As with any invasive procedure, there are some risks, although complications are rare. Even though anticoagulant agents are used, a thrombus can form near the blockage being treated, potentially leading to a myocardial infarction. More rarely, a patient develops irregular heartbeats or arterial spasms. Because the patient is closely monitored during the procedure, these problems are usually quickly detected and corrected.

Stents

Since their introduction in the early 1990s, stents have revolutionized interventional cardiology. These metallic wire mesh tubes are inserted after balloon angioplasty to form a scaffold in severely blocked arteries. The use of stents can also limit the incidence of restenosis (reclosing of the artery) that occurs after balloon angioplasty or other catheter procedures. However, restenosis may occur with the stent procedure, and 10 to 20 percent of people experience significant renarrowing within 6 months after angioplasty with conventional stents (see Restenosis, page 98).

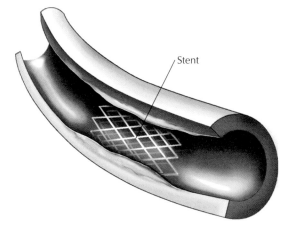

Stent

After the clearing of a blocked artery, a stent, a wire mesh tube, may be inserted to keep the artery from reclosing.

Restenosis

Stenosis is the medical term that refers to a condition, usually the result of disease, that causes a vessel to become abnormally narrow. Whenever a coronary artery becomes clogged, usually by the atherosclerotic buildup of fat, cholesterol, and other substances, to the point at which blood flow is constricted, it is said to be stenosed.

The most common procedure for reopening a stenosed coronary artery is balloon angioplasty (see page 96). However, in about 10 to 20 percent of all instances, the artery renarrows within six months of angioplasty. This reclosure is called restenosis.

In most cases, restenosis occurs without a clear cause. Sometimes, though, restenosis develops because the artery was slightly damaged during the angioplasty. Once the arterial wall is damaged, plaque is more likely to build up around the site.

Restenosis is more likely to occur in people with type 1 (insulin-dependent) diabetes and in those who do not make appropriate lifestyle modifications to reduce the risk of atherosclerosis. If a person smokes and eats a diet rich in fats, atherosclerosis may well reclose a newly cleared artery. When an artery becomes restenosed, a second angioplasty may be necessary.

Less commonly, restenosis can occur after CABG surgery (see page 100). And, stenosis may occur in the grafted blood vessel. As with other stenosed arteries, angioplasty or bypass surgery may be needed to reopen the grafted segments.

In order to decrease the chances of restenosis, doctors have developed improved forms of angioplasty. For example, stents—collapsible supports used to prop up an artery—are used when arteries restenose repeatedly (see Stents, page 97).

Because these stainless-steel cylinders prop the artery open as it heals and combat restenosis, they appear to reduce the need for subsequent bypass surgery.

A collapsed metal stent is positioned over a balloon catheter and transported to the blockage. As the balloon inflates, the coil expands. It is then locked in place to create a rigid support within the artery. It remains as a permanent scaffold, facilitating blood flow to the heart muscle.

Typically, platelet blockers or blood-thinning agents are prescribed after a stent procedure. Although a magnetic resonance imaging (MRI) scan should not be done without a cardiologist's approval for 6 to 8 weeks after a stent procedure, airport or store detectors do not pose any problems in relation to the stent.

Treated Stents

Because restenosis occurs within 6 months in approximately 15 to 25 percent of conventional stent procedures, doctors have begun to use specially treated stents to reduce restenosis rates. Stents covered with heparin, a natural blood clot-resistant substance, appear to be effective in preventing clot-related complications within 30 days after being placed.

Irradiated Stents

A small wire treated with a radioactive substance traditionally used to curb the growth of cancer cells is effective in curbing the growth of cells within blood vessels that can follow stenting or balloon angioplasty. Radioactive seeds of iridium-192 are temporarily implanted inside stents, exposing the cells in the artery wall to ionizing radiation. After 20 to 30 minutes, the seeds are removed, leaving no radioactivity in the body. The amount of radiation is equivalent to that received during routine angioplasty when the catheter and blood vessels are viewed through x-rays. This appears to reduce restenosis significantly.

Coronary Atherectomy

In the late 1980s and early 1990s, several newer catheter technologies, called atherectomy or atheroma removal procedures, have been developed to remove the blockage. Unlike angioplasty, which uses a balloon to compress the plaque against the artery wall, atherectomy is ablation, or cutting away, of the blockage. Atherectomy appears both to clear the coronary artery and may reduce the rate of restenosis under certain circumstances. Directional and rotational atherectomy are two types of this technique.

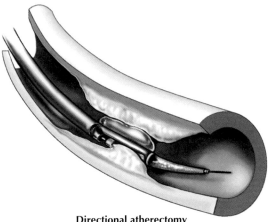

Directional atherectomy

Atherectomy is a procedure to cut away plaque from blocked arteries. There are two types of atherectomy, directional and rotational. Directional atherectomy uses a razorlike device attached to the side of a balloon to shave plaque away. Rotational atherectomy uses a high-speed diamond-shaped drill to break up plaque.

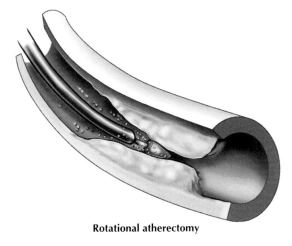

Rotational atherectomy

- *Directional atherectomy* uses a razorlike device attached on the side of a balloon to shave the deposits away.

- *Rotational atherectomy* employs a high-speed diamond-tipped drill to pierce fatty deposits. This technique is especially effective in treating plaque that has become calcified.

Coronary Artery Bypass Graft Surgery

Coronary artery bypass graft (CABG) surgery is what is commonly known as open-heart surgery. Bypass surgery does not eliminate the blockage or address the underlying disease process. It creates a detour to reroute the blood around the blockage, using blood vessels from other parts of the body. The benefits and risks of open-heart surgery versus minimally invasive techniques need to be weighed carefully; a decision as to which one is the best treatment must be made with the consultation of a cardiologist or heart surgeon on a case-by-case basis (see Minimally Invasive Techniques, page 104).

Because most occlusions occur in the first centimeter or two of the major arteries feeding the heart and only rarely affect smaller branches, the surgeon is able to directly maneuver around the area of the blockage. Generally, a blood vessel is taken from the chest or leg. It is attached at one end to the aorta and grafted at the other end onto the coronary artery below the blockage. The new segment allows sufficient blood to flow to nourish the heart muscle once again. Blood volume and pressure are restored to the myocardium, and usually chest discomfort is relieved.

CABG surgery is an effective treatment. Each year, almost half a million coronary bypass operations are performed in the United States. Bypass surgery significantly relieves chest pain and other related symptoms that do not otherwise respond to medication.

When Is CABG Surgery Necessary?

If CABG surgery is a viable option, the cardiologist will discuss the reasons it is needed. In general, the following occurrences indicate that bypass surgery may be the best treatment:

- A critical narrowing of the left main artery, the vessel that supplies the most blood to the main section of the myocardium, or heart muscle

- Severe angina that does not respond to medication

- Blockages in three or more coronary vessels

Rene Favaloro, MD: The First Coronary Artery Bypass Graft

During the 1960s, Dr. Rene Favaloro pioneered CABG surgery as a treatment for angina pectoris. A surgeon at the Cleveland Clinic, Dr. Favaloro was the first to describe CABG surgery as a treatment for CAD. By the mid-1970s, bypass surgery had become a readily accepted form of therapy throughout the United States. Today CABG surgery is performed routinely and safely at cardiac centers and at many community hospitals around the world.

- Repeated angioplasty and repeated restenosis after angioplasty
- Blockage in a graft created in previous bypass surgery

The Procedure

Typically, open-heart CABG surgery takes anywhere from 3 to 6 hours, during which time the patient is fully anesthetized. The operation begins by opening the front of the chest. The sternum (breastbone) is split vertically with a specialized saw called a reciprocating saw, and a winchlike device spreads open the split sternum. The soft tissues covering the heart, as well as the pericardium, the membrane around the heart, are cut away.

Next, the surgeons "harvest" the conduits, the blood vessels to be used to create the bypass. The internal mammary artery from the chest wall has the highest patency rate (likelihood of remaining open) and is the most frequently used vessel; it is used in 90 percent of bypass procedures in the United States. The great saphenous vein from the inside of the calf or thigh is the next most often used (see Selection of Conduits, page 103).

In coronary artery bypass surgery, the blood flow through the coronary arteries is diverted so that arterial blockages are bypassed. The internal mammary artery from the chest wall is the most frequently used blood vessel for bypass. The lower end of the internal mammary, or thoracic, artery is detached and reattached to the coronary artery below the area of blockage. Blockages may also be bypassed by taking a blood vessel from the chest or leg and attaching it to the aorta at one end and below the area of blockage in the coronary artery at the other end.

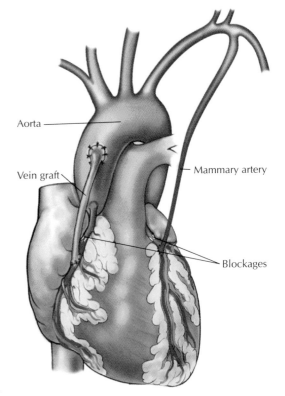

Aorta

Vein graft

Mammary artery

Blockages

Selection of Conduits

In the past, veins taken from the groin or leg were favored for CABG surgery. The greater saphenous vein, a long straight vein running from inside the ankle bone up to the groin, was used almost exclusively to bypass the blockage. This vein is the right size, shape, and length for use as a bypass conduit.

Today, surgeons use arteries more frequently because they do not seem to close as quickly after surgery as do veins. The internal thoracic (internal mammary) artery, which winds inside the chest wall beneath the sternum, seems to be the best artery for CABG surgery. Studies show that the internal thoracic artery is more resistant to atherosclerotic buildup than the native coronary arteries. By detaching the lower end of the internal thoracic vessel, the surgeon transplants the thoracic artery to the surface of the heart.

The radial artery in the arm, the gastroepiploic artery to the stomach, and the inferior epigastric artery to the abdominal wall are also used to create detours around blocked coronary arteries. If a patient needs more than one bypass graft, the surgeon will most likely use the thoracic artery and the leg vein.

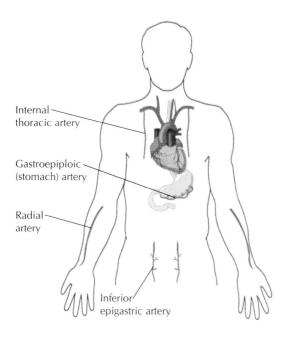

Internal thoracic artery

Gastroepiploic (stomach) artery

Radial artery

Inferior epigastric artery

The most commonly used blood vessels for coronary artery bypass surgery are the internal mammary artery, the radial artery in the arm, the gastroepiploic artery to the stomach, the inferior epigastric artery to the abdominal wall, and the saphenous vein from the leg. (Adapted with permission from *Cleveland Clinic Heart Advisor*, Vol. 2, No. 1, January 1999, Torstar Publications, Inc. All rights reserved.)

During CABG surgery, the patient's vital functions are fully supported by artificial circulation while the heart is at rest, in a procedure called cardiopulmonary bypass. A mechanical device pumps the blood and maintains the appropriate oxygen level. As the blood circulates through the machine, it can sometimes be refrigerated, lowering the body temperature.

A vascular clamp is applied to the aorta, separating the blood flow to the heart from that to the rest of the body. A cold potassium solution is then injected into the coronary arteries, which immediately renders the heart motionless, cold, and relaxed.

The surgeon begins to work on the surface of the heart, making a small incision in the front wall of the coronary artery. For each intended bypass, the opening is expanded with specialized scissors and the donor vessel sewn on.

After all the grafts are in place, an electric shock is delivered to restart the heart's pulsations. The vascular clamp is released, once again allowing blood to flow into the coronary arteries. The heartbeat is then restored and the circulation transferred back to the heart and lungs. The pumping equipment is removed and the anticoagulant is chemically reversed with the drug protamine. The chest cavity is closed, and the operation is completed.

Postsurgery Hospital Stay

Recovering from open-heart surgery usually takes several days; you will probably spend about 24 hours within an intensive care unit (ICU). If you undergo surgery, you may wake up in the ICU. You will likely be attached to a tube to help you breathe for the first 24 hours after the operation. Typically, you are given drugs to control pain and an anticoagulant agent—generally aspirin—to prevent blood clotting. For the first day, you are fed through an intravenous tube. By the second or third day, you are encouraged to sit up, walk a bit, and eat regular food. Throughout, your heartbeat is monitored continuously.

With rising costs and vigilant insurance providers, most people are home within a week of their surgery—assuming, of course, that there are no complications or apparent risks involved. Two or three weeks after surgery, you will return to the hospital to be examined.

Minimally Invasive Techniques

In the past, the only technique for CABG surgery was to operate through an open chest using cardiopulmonary bypass with the appropriate replacement vein or artery. Today new, less invasive options are being developed and are proving successful for a number of patients. In most instances, these techniques reduce discomfort, the likelihood of complications, length of hospital stay, cost, and stress on the patient.

Although the vast majority of CABG operations are still open-heart procedures, minimally invasive techniques are now commonly utilized and

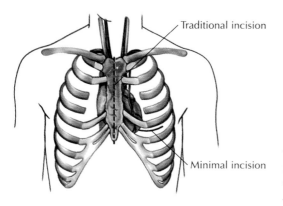
Traditional incision

Minimal incision

Minimally invasive surgery involves a smaller incision, fewer risks, and a shorter recovery time than the traditional open-heart surgery.

will likely continue to increase in the future. Three forms of less invasive coronary bypass surgery are used: PortCAB, MIDCAB, and OPCAB.

The PortCAB Procedure

The PortCAB procedure (also called port-access CAB) is performed through a small incision on the front of the chest. The PortCAB technique is useful for single- or multi-vessel grafting. It allows access to the front and back of the heart, while with the MIDCAB procedure only the front is accessible. During the procedure, the heart is stopped and a cardiopulmonary bypass machine (heart-lung machine) is used to circulate the blood. But unlike traditional open-heart procedures, in which the aorta is clamped off and circulation maintained through large bypass tubes, in PortCAB, a cardiopulmonary bypass machine is attached through the groin. A specially designed catheter is threaded through blood vessels in the groin and advanced to the heart. A balloon on the tip of the catheter is inflated, effectively blocking the aorta from the inside. The heart is then stopped, and multi-vessel bypass is performed on the totally motionless heart.

The MIDCAB Procedure

The MIDCAB, or minimally invasive direct CAB, can be performed with the heart beating using a stabilizing device. The procedure involves a 5- to 8-inch incision in the chest wall. Using special retractors, the internal thoracic artery is mobilized from the chest wall and then bypassed to the front artery of the heart. Special stabilizers have been developed to allow accurate sewing while the heart is beating. A forklike device applies pressure on either side of the artery to be bypassed, immobilizing the area. As it braces the heart, this stabilizing platform allows for more precise, controlled grafting of the internal thoracic artery directly onto the heart's left anterior descending artery. Another stabilizer, the Octopus system, uses small vacuum suction cups to grip and immobilize the area around the vessel being bypassed.

The advantages of the MIDCAB are the smaller incision and avoiding cardiopulmonary bypass; however, the disadvantage is that only the front of the heart is accessible to the surgeon. The best candidates for the MIDCAB procedure are people with a blockage in the left anterior descending coronary artery on the front of the heart.

The OPCAB Procedure

The OPCAB, or off-pump, procedure evolved from the MIDCAB. The procedure is performed through an incision that allows for complete access to the heart, but the bypasses are done without the use of cardiopulmonary bypass. The same stabilizers used in the MIDCAB can be used to bypass any vessel of the heart. The OPCAB is useful for people with multiple blockages.

The MIDCAB and OPCAB are known as beating heart procedures because the heart is not stopped to do the bypasses. Because these two

---

Transmyocardial Revascularization

Transmyocardial revascularization (TMR) or laser revascularization is a procedure that uses lasers to carve a series of channels in the heart muscle to increase blood flow. TMR can either be performed in the catherization laboratory by a trained interventional cardiologist or by a cardiac surgeon in the operating room. In the operating room, a laser is inserted into the chest cavity through a surgical incision on the left side of the chest.

Between heartbeats, the surgeon uses a laser to bore from 20 to 40 holes, each 1 millimeter in diameter, through the heart's left ventricle. After the chamber is filled with blood, so that the inside of the heart is cushioned and protected, the surgeon seals the outer openings by using a laser to flatten the holes on the outside. Oxygen-rich blood then flows through the myocardium.

Preliminary studies show that 80 to 90 percent of patients who have undergone TMR experience such a reduction in severe chest pain that they are able to live relatively normal lives. While it will not replace coronary artery bypass or angioplasty as the most common method of treating CAD, there are instances when TMR is a safe, effective way to restore blood flow to the myocardium.

TMR may be used

■ For a person at very high risk of a second bypass or angioplasty

■ When blockages are too difficult to treat with bypass

techniques do not require cardiopulmonary bypass, they may hasten recovery and reduce the risk of stroke and blood transfusions.

Success Rates of CABG Surgery

As a rule, patients who are in good overall health do very well after CABG surgery. For younger people otherwise in good health, the mortality rate for open-heart CABG surgery is about 2 percent. People older than 70 may be at slightly increased risk of complications, as are those with impaired ventricular functioning (poor pumping), diabetes, or kidney disease. In general, women are at a slightly higher risk than are men of serious complications after open-heart surgery. Recovery for people who undergo repeat procedures or who have other procedures performed simultaneously tends to be a bit slower.

Although bypass surgery is largely effective in relieving symptoms of coronary artery disease, 10 to 15 percent of bypass grafts become blocked within a month of surgery. Mammary artery grafts have a slightly lower rate of stenosis. Platelet antagonists help keep grafted vessels open longer.

People who smoke, who eat diets rich in fat, who do not manage their hypertension and blood cholesterol levels, and who lead a sedentary lifestyle are at higher risk of complications and for graft reclosure. Because surgery does not correct the underlying atherosclerotic process, people who adopt a healthier lifestyle tend to experience fewer complications.

A person at higher risk of serious complications, whose problem is especially complicated, or who is undergoing a repeat procedure may want to consider undergoing surgery at a specialized heart center or cardiology department in a large medical center instead of going to a community hospital.

Reoperations

Although most CABG surgery is successful and the grafts hold out over time, in the first year after surgery as many as 24 percent of patients report a recurrence of angina. Within 5 years, almost one-half of all bypass patients report significant chest pain. Within 10 years, 12 to 15 percent have symptoms severe enough to warrant a second operation. Fifteen years after bypass surgery, 30 percent require a second operation.

A number of factors can make repeat surgery necessary. The single most important factor is the type of blood vessel used in the first operation. Patients with vein grafts have a higher and earlier chance of needing a second operation than do those with arterial grafts. Also, the younger the patient, the more likely that he or she will eventually need a new graft.

Complications

An increased risk of stroke is the most serious complication associated with this type of treatment. The older the patient, the higher the risk of any complication.

Autologous Blood Transfusions in Surgery

Although in many instances open-heart surgery does not require blood transfusions, complications can arise in which a patient needs extra blood. To reduce the risk of blood transfusion reactions and to eliminate the already minimal risk of contracting viral diseases like acquired immunodeficiency syndrome (AIDS) or hepatitis through blood transfusions, autologous blood transfusions—banking one's own blood for use in later transfusions—may well be a suitable option to consider before open-heart surgery.

If the patient and doctor agree that this type of transfusion is appropriate, blood collection can begin up to 6 weeks before surgery. Donating blood is a painless process, taking up to 20 minutes at each session. Blood can be stored in liquid form for 42 days. If the blood is not used during the operation, it is discarded.

Other possible complications are rare and include myocardial infarction, lung problems, and bleeding disorders. In addition, whenever a cardiopulmonary bypass machine is used, neurologic changes can occur. These are usually experienced as mental difficulties, such as memory loss, personality shifts, inability to focus, or unclear thinking. In most cases, these neurologic problems are temporary.

The Future

As the population ages, coronary artery disease will affect more people. At the same time, more and better diagnostic and treatment methods are being developed. Many techniques of the future are being used today in limited circumstances. New medications—new thrombolytic drugs, for example—work more effectively to dissolve thrombi. Investigations into the role of genetic growth factors in promoting angiogenesis mean that eventually it will be possible to generate a new collateral circulation network to counteract the ravages of atherosclerosis.

As the effectiveness and applications of less invasive techniques in both diagnosis and treatment widen, more patients suffering from CAD will benefit from them. The therapeutic use of catheters to treat blockages will increase, and new catheter design will allow for more efficient coronary angiography and angioplasty. Lasers and ultrasound will be used more extensively—ultrasound will be used to deliver medications directly to the blocked areas. In addition, gene therapy and other techniques will be used more extensively to prevent and treat restenosis.

CHAPTER 6

Diseases of the Heart Valves

Introduction

The heart's system of four one-way valves ensures that blood moving from one part of the heart to the next and out of the heart to the body travels in the correct direction—and only in that direction.

The heart has four main valves:

- *Mitral valve*: The valve controlling blood flow from the left atrium to the left ventricle

- *Tricuspid valve*: The valve controlling blood flow from the right atrium to the right ventricle

- *Aortic valve*: A very strong valve regulating blood flow from the left ventricle into the aorta, the large artery that distributes blood flow throughout the body

- *Pulmonic valve* (also called the pulmonary valve): The valve controlling blood flow from the right ventricle to the lungs

Each valve is composed of leaflets and an annulus. The leaflets are strong, thin pieces of tissue that swirl shut with remarkable efficiency. The annulus, a ring of fibrous tissue attached to the leaflets, helps maintain the valve's shape. The mitral and tricuspid valves are supported by tough, fibrous strings called chordae tendineae, which are attached to papillary muscles, part of the inside wall of the ventricles. The chordae tendineae and papillary muscles keep the leaflets stable against any backflow of blood.

Each valve snaps shut after allowing just the right amount of blood to flow from one location to the next. The orchestration of valve openings

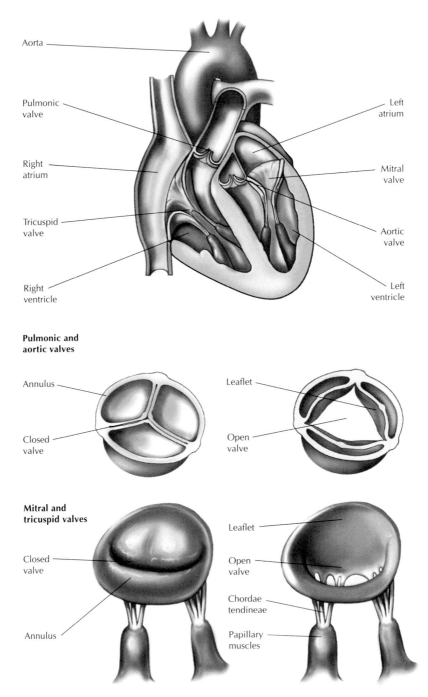

The location and structure of the heart's valves. The valves consist of leaflets and an annulus. The leaflets are strong, thin pieces of tissue that form the opening and closing of the valve. The annulus is a ring of fibrous tissue attached to the leaflets that helps maintain the valve's shape. The mitral and tricuspid valves are supported by tough, fibrous strings called chordae tendineae, which are attached to papillary muscles, part of the inside wall of the ventricles.

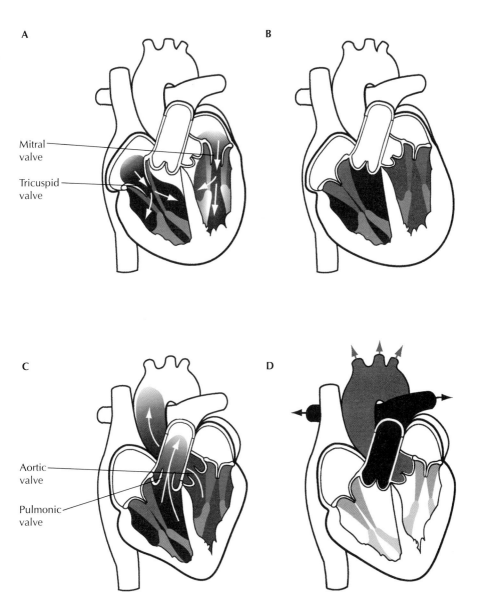

(A) Blood flows from the right atrium to the right ventricle and from the left atrium to the left ventricle through the open tricuspid and mitral valves respectively. (B) When the ventricles are full, the tricuspid and mitral valves close to prevent blood from flowing backward during ventricular contraction. (C) When the right ventricle contracts, the pulmonic valve opens to allow blood to be pumped out into the pulmonary artery and to the lungs. Similarly, the contraction of the left ventricle causes the aortic valve to open allowing blood to be pumped through the aorta and out to the body. (D) After ventricular contraction, the pulmonic and aortic valves snap closed to prevent blood flowing backward into the ventricles.

and closings prevents blood from flowing back. By listening through a stethoscope, a doctor can hear the clamping shut of each valve, which makes the heartbeat's well-known "lub dub" sound.

Serious disorders of the valves are rare. An estimated 2 percent of the American population has some problem with the aortic valve, approximately 5 percent with the mitral valve, and fewer than 1 percent with the tricuspid or pulmonic valve. Not all these people require surgical treatment and some may not even require medical treatment. Often, people with minor valve problems are simply observed over time by their doctor. People who have damaged, weakened, or replaced

Mitral Valve Prolapse

Mitral valve prolapse is the most common heart valve abnormality, affecting 3 to 5 percent of the adult American population; it is also the leading cause of mitral valve surgery in the United States. In many cases, though, people with mitral valve prolapse lead completely normal lives and do not need surgery.

In mitral valve prolapse, the valve has more leaflet tissue than is needed to function normally. When it opens, the mitral valve billows up like a parachute. Instead of lying flat when the valve closes, the extra tissue flops up through the valve, leaving tissue where it does not belong and preventing the valve from closing perfectly.

Heart specialists used to agree that people with mitral valve prolapse—even those without symptoms—should take antibiotics prophylactically before undergoing dental or surgical procedures. Valves with any amount of damage tend to attract bacteria that are in the bloodstream, and dental and surgical procedures often "loosen" bacteria at the site of the procedure, sending them into the bloodstream. (See Infective Endocarditis, page 113).

Today, heart specialists are not all in agreement about the need for prophylactic antibiotic therapy, but most still recommend it. People with mitral valve prolapse need to make sure that their dentist is aware of their condition and to discuss with their dentist the most appropriate prophylactic therapy before undergoing each dental procedure. The same is true for any surgical procedure, however minor.

Medical or drug treatment for mitral valve prolapse is usually not necessary unless a person develops secondary abnormalities, the most common of which is mitral valve regurgitation (leaking of the valve). Mitral valve prolapse with progressive mitral valve regurgitation may necessitate corrective surgery. People with mitral valve prolapse and mitral regurgitation may develop abnormal heart rhythms.

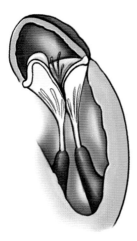

Mitral valve prolapse. The mitral valve's two leaflets are larger than necessary and billow (prolapse) into the left atrium with each heartbeat. Because of the prolapse, the leaflets may be unable to close properly, causing regurgitation (leaking).

valves are at risk, however, of developing endocarditis, an infection of the heart's lining, which can lead to further valve damage (see Infective Endocarditis, below).

The frequency with which valves are damaged is related to their anatomy and amount of work they do—which is why the mitral valve has a higher prevalence of problems than do other heart valves. This valve literally has a high-pressure job: Blood flows through it with greater force than it does through other valves (heart valves are exposed to pressure in the following decreasing order: mitral, aortic, tricuspid, and pulmonic). The mitral valve is thus under more pressure to clamp shut completely in order to prevent backflow.

Valves can exhibit many types of damage. With the mitral and aortic valves, this damage usually results in one of two relatively rare conditions: stenosis, or valve narrowing, and insufficiency, or "leaky" valves.

Mitral valves also suffer a slightly more common but generally not serious congenital abnormality called mitral valve prolapse. In the approximately 3 to 5 percent of the population who have this condition, the leaflets of the mitral valve prolapse, or sink into the upper chamber of the heart during the valve closing, allowing some blood to regurgitate, or flow backward into the left atrium (see Mitral Valve Prolapse, page 112).

Infective Endocarditis

Tissues made of endothelial cells line the inner surface of every body organ, including the heart. The exquisitely sensitive and complex endothelium in the heart, called the endocardium, smoothes out over large surfaces and pinches up to form and line the heart valves.

Normally, the endocardium is resistant to infection. However, if a valve has been injured or damaged, the body sends out platelets and fibrin to heal and scar over the area. Platelets are blood cells that form clots, a normal part of healing; fibrin is a body protein that helps in the clotting process. In people with valve damage, this attempt at self-healing may lead to infective endocarditis, because the thrombocyte-fibrin conglomerate is a magnet for any microorganisms circulating in the bloodstream.

Infective endocarditis is a different disease than it was in the past. Even the name for the disease has changed. Previously, infective endocarditis was called subacute or acute bacterial endocarditis because the most common—and almost exclusive—cause of an infected endocardium was bacterial, usually group A strep. Today, the endocardium can become infected by many types of bacteria as well as by other types of microorganisms, including viruses and fungi.

Endocarditis often causes no symptoms. At every moment, the body is host to bacteria and other microorganisms, and the immune system nearly always prevents them from multiplying sufficiently to cause infection. But as microorganisms gather on the scarred area of a valve, they can increase in number and cause an infection that damages the valve.

The microorganisms that cause endocarditis can originate from normal body flora—microorganisms that are always present in the body. Bacteria that caused no infection and no symptoms on the tooth or skin can be loosened during a minor procedure and travel silently to the small injury on the surface of the valve, where they can cause an infection. These infections occur rarely and randomly.

It is important that all infections in the body be treated early and completely, even in people who appear healthy. Often, a person who develops infective endocarditis does not recall having had a tooth abscess or skin infection. However, he or she could have had a minor (and unnoticed) injury to the mucous membranes lining the mouth, the gastrointestinal system, or the genitourinary system, which allowed bacteria to enter the body and attack the endocardium. The infection in the heart progresses silently and may not be recognized until symptoms arise.

Groups at Risk for Infective Endocarditis

At particular risk for developing endocarditis are people who have heart or valve structural abnormalities or prosthetic valves or are intravenous drug users:

■ *Pre-existing structural abnormalities in the heart or valves.* About three-fourths of people with endocarditis have a preexisting structural abnormality in the heart or valve. About 4.8 percent of people with aortic stenosis (narrowing of the aortic valve) will develop endocarditis. People with mitral valve prolapse are also at increased risk of endocarditis; studies reveal that a person with mitral valve prolapse has a five- to eightfold higher risk of having an endocardial infection than a person with a structurally normal mitral valve has.

■ *Prosthetic valves.* A growing cause of infective endocarditis is the increasing number of prosthetic valves implanted. People with these valves are more susceptible to heart infections because prosthetic valves attract bacteria that the body usually destroys before they can multiply sufficiently to cause an infection. About 1 to 4 percent of people with prosthetic valves develop infective endocarditis within one year of having their valve inserted; another 1 percent become infected during each year thereafter. Keys to prevention in people with prosthetic valves or valvular disease of any type are to maintain meticulous dental hygiene (see Importance of Dental Care, below) and to take antibiotics before or after certain medical procedures.

■ *Intravenous drug use.* Another cause of infective endocarditis is intravenous drug use. People who inject illicit drugs expose themselves to the types of microorganisms that travel to the heart and cause infective endocarditis. In these cases, the most common disease-causing organism is Staphylococcus aureus, which can infect normal heart valves.

Importance of Dental Care

People at risk for infective endocardititis are advised to maintain good care of their teeth and gums including regular dental checkups. Some research shows, however, that people with valve abnormalities avoid regular dental checkups and cleaning for fear that it will place them at risk of infection. In so doing, they are increasing the chance they will develop dangerously high levels of bacteria in their mouths. Careful, gentle, and meticulous daily oral hygiene and frequent visits to the dentist are necessary to prevent endocarditis in people who are at risk of this infection, but brushing too vigorously or using a toothpick or high-pressure water-cleaning device can drive these bacteria into the bloodstream and lead to endocarditis. Antibiotics are often prescribed before and after dental procedures to prevent the spread of bacteria to the damaged valve.

Diagnosing and Treating Infective Endocarditis

A person with infective endocarditis may show a variety of symptoms, depending on what parts of the heart are infected. The most common symptoms are fever, weight loss, red marks on the skin and fingernails, heart murmurs, and liver enlargement. Chills and night sweats are common.

Doppler echocardiography (see page 120) is the most important diagnostic test to confirm infective endocarditis. If Doppler echocardiography does not clearly show the damage, other tests may be ordered, including cardiac nuclear scanning (see page 74) and magnetic resonance imaging (MRI; see page 69). Blood cultures are important in diagnosing infective endocarditis. Blood is drawn, using a sterile technique, from three sites on the body. The blood sample is transferred to a culture medium, which facilitates the growth of bacteria; the bacteria can then be analyzed.

Because the microorganisms that cause infective endocarditis are potent and adhere stubbornly to the valve, endocarditis is treated aggressively. Intravenous antibiotic therapy, which is stronger than antibiotics taken by mouth, is often necessary. Many people can complete at least part of this intravenous therapy at home, with the help of a home-care nurse. Several weeks or even months of therapy may be necessary to eliminate the infection.

In some cases, surgery is necessary to either excise the infection or to repair or replace a valve damaged by infection. The cardiologist and surgeon work together to plan the surgery at a time when the infection is sufficiently controlled and before the damaged valve compromises heart function.

Aortic and Mitral Valve Stenosis

"Stenosis" is the Greek word for narrowing; simply put, a stenosed valve is one in which the opening of the valve has become narrowed. When this happens, the pressure with which blood flows through the valve is

Aortic valve stenosis

Mitral valve stenosis

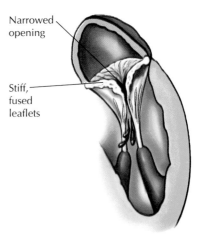

Narrowed opening

Thickened, hardened leaflet

Narrowed opening

Stiff, fused leaflets

Valve stenosis refers to the narrowing of the valve that can occur as a result of calcification (calcium deposits thickening and hardening the valve) or previous infection (which can cause the leaflets to become scarred). The normal valve opening in an average adult is about the size of a 50-cent piece. Valve stenosis can reduce the opening of the valve to the size of a dime or smaller.

decreased, limiting the heart's ability to pump blood to where it is needed. The degree to which blood flow is limited depends on how much the valvular opening has narrowed. Valvular stenosis may be caused by congenital defects, rheumatic fever, or calcium deposits on the valves that accumulate with age (calcification).

Signs and Symptoms

Because each valve controls blood flow through distinct parts of the heart, the symptoms a stenosed valve causes depend on which valve is affected.

Aortic Valve Stenosis

Aortic valve disease often develops silently, usually over the course of a number of years. For most people, aortic valve surgery does not become necessary unless symptoms occur. Once symptoms develop, a person is generally ill enough to require surgery fairly soon.

Shortness of breath and fatigue—signs of congestive heart failure—are generally the first symptoms in a person with aortic valve stenosis. Congestive heart failure occurs because not enough blood is able to exit the heart through the stenosed aortic valve to be pumped throughout the body. As a result, the body's cells do not receive enough oxygen. Congestive heart failure can rapidly become more severe; when it does, excessive amounts of fluid are retained and high blood pressure (hypertension) develops. For more information on congestive heart failure, see page 158.

The next most common symptom of aortic valve stenosis is angina, or chest pain, which generally occurs with exercise or exertion in about 35 percent of people with a stenosed aortic valve. Angina occurs as stenosis advances because the blood supply to the myocardium decreases. For more information on angina, see page 85.

Fifteen percent of people with aortic valve stenosis seek medical care because they experience syncope, a condition causing lightheadedness and faintness, usually during exercise or exertion. Syncope is a fairly common condition in the general population, and although it is one of the three common symptoms of a diseased aortic valve, most people with syncope do not have a diseased aortic valve.

Mitral Valve Stenosis

Whether a person with mitral valve stenosis experiences symptoms depends greatly on age. About one-half of younger people (average age 28) have no symptoms at the time they are diagnosed, often during a routine checkup or a visit to the doctor for another reason. Another 47 percent of this young population who have a stenosed mitral valve have only mild or moderate symptoms at the time they are diagnosed.

Studying a slightly older group of people with mitral valve stenosis reveals a different picture. The majority—approximately 86 percent of people with an average age of 42—experience symptoms such as shortness of breath with any type of exertion, spitting up blood, fatigue, foot and ankle swelling, and abnormalities of heart rate and rhythm.

A common abnormality in the heart rhythm of older people with mitral valve stenosis is atrial fibrillation, which is fairly serious and sometimes life-threatening. Because the heart beats erratically, blood does not flow smoothly and regularly. The time between some beats is long enough to allow blood to pool, which increases the risk of thrombogenesis, or blood-clot formation. The increased risk of blood clots is one reason why people with atrial fibrillation face a higher risk of stroke (see page 152).

Causes and Prevention

Rheumatic Fever

The most common cause of mitral valve stenosis is untreated rheumatic fever. By contrast, untreated rheumatic fever causes less than 20 percent of aortic valve stenosis. Sometimes, rheumatic fever strikes both the aortic valve and mitral valve, causing stenosis in both. Rheumatic fever is the result of a serious or untreated group A streptococcal infection, the type that causes "strep throat" and fever. Rheumatic fever is not an infection itself, but rather the aftermath of an immune reaction elicited by the presence of strep bacteria in the body.

Rheumatic fever causes inflammation of the body's connective tissues. Inflammation of the heart valves leads to scarring of the leaflets, which can narrow the valve and also make it difficult for the valve to close properly, causing leakage. When rheumatic fever causes permanent damage to the heart, the condition is called rheumatic heart disease.

Damaged heart valves due to rheumatic fever may show no symptoms for years, but eventually serious complications resulting from valvular inefficiency may arise. The most serious of these is congestive heart failure (see page 158).

Rheumatic fever is most common among children aged 5 to 15 years. The use of antibiotics to treat strep infection has reduced the incidence of rheumatic fever in the United States dramatically. The death rate of rheumatic fever and rheumatic heart disease has decreased by two-thirds (from around 15,000 to around 5,000) since 1950.

Rheumatic fever must be treated promptly and effectively. The general rule is to seek medical care and a throat culture for a sore throat that lasts more than 3 days, or sooner if the sore throat is accompanied by fever and headache. Even without a sore throat, a person with fever and a skin rash should seek medical care to determine whether there is a streptococcal infection.

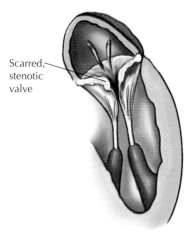

Scarred, stenotic valve

Untreated rheumatic fever can cause mitral valve stenosis. The leaflets become inflamed and then scarred, narrowing the opening of the valve.

If a strep infection is diagnosed, it is important to finish the entire course of prescribed antibiotic therapy. Because the sore throat clears up and many people feel better after a couple of days of starting antibiotic therapy, they may discontinue taking the antibiotics. Although the throat symptoms may not recur, the streptococcal bacteria multiply again once the antibiotic is no longer in the bloodstream and can continue to affect the heart or other organs.

Congenital Defects

The most common cause of aortic stenosis is a congenital defect in which the valve has two rather than three cusps (bicuspid aortic valve; see page 225), which occurs in approximately 1 percent of the population. While the condition is generally mild in children, it can lead to more serious problems in later years.

Idiopathic Aortic Valve Stenosis

Men are more commonly affected by idiopathic aortic stenosis (a stenosis of unknown cause) than are women; symptoms usually occur when men are in their 50s and 60s. In contrast, when aortic stenosis is caused by rheumatic fever, symptoms occur earlier, generally during the fourth decade of life.

Less Common Causes of Valvular Stenosis

Among other, less common causes of valvular stenosis are

■ Inborn errors of metabolism, such as Fabry's disease and Hurler-Scheie syndrome (both of which more commonly cause mitral rather than aortic valve stenosis)

- Autoimmune diseases, such as systemic lupus erythematosus and rheumatoid arthritis

Diagnosis

In diagnosing valve stenosis a doctor will perform a physical examination and record medical history. The doctor will ask about symptoms and listen to the heart by placing a stethoscope on several places on the chest and neck.

The heart sounds heard at different parts of the upper torso are distinct from sounds at other locations because of the way internal organs muffle or accentuate sound traveling through the chest. By listening at each place, the doctor can pick up the distinctive sounds of aortic or mitral valve stenosis.

A number of tests may be necessary to confirm the diagnosis and pinpoint the exact area and type of valvular damage; this is essential in assigning the optimal therapy. The tests include the following:

- *Electrocardiogram (ECG or EKG)*: When heart valves do not function properly, they may change the rhythm with which the heart beats as well as its speed. The ECG reveals these rhythm abnormalities by recording the electrical signals the heart produces and displaying them on a graph.

- *Chest x-ray*: A chest x-ray gives a clear picture of the size of the heart and some of the main blood vessels, such as the aorta. Aortic and mitral valve stenosis can cause enlargement of certain parts of the heart, which will show up on an x-ray, as will dilation, or enlargement, of the aorta, which can occur when the aortic valve becomes diseased.

- *Echocardiography*: This is a form of ultrasound that shows the structure and position of the heart in great detail. Often performed in conjunction with a Doppler study (see below), echocardiography can reveal the exact nature of the valve problem and show how the heart is pumping. An echocardiogram is often repeated at regular intervals after an initial diagnosis to assist doctors in deciding when to perform corrective surgery. Echocardiography is performed either transthoracically (across the chest wall) or transesophageally (the probe is placed down the person's throat). Transesophageal echocardiography is used when the infection cannot be viewed well from outside the chest.

- *Doppler echocardiography*: The Doppler portion of this test measures the pressure at which blood flows through the valves, which is important in judging how a diseased valve affects overall heart function.

- *Stress testing*: Because it may be necessary to determine exercise tolerance, doctors may perform a stress test (see page 67). Stress testing may be dangerous in people with significant symptoms associated with aortic valve stenosis, so a test using medications that prompt similar changes in the heart but does not require vigorous exercise, may be given instead (see Dipyridamole and Dobutamine Stress Testing, page 76.)

■ *Cardiac catheterization*: This test gives a direct view inside the heart through a tiny catheter, or tube, inserted into a vein (usually one in the groin) and advanced to the heart. Cardiac catheterization is often not necessary to determine the extent and severity of most valve disease. But because some valve disease, especially aortic stenosis, occurs at a time of life when coronary artery disease (CAD; atherosclerosis, or narrowing, of the coronary arteries) also occurs frequently, cardiac catheterization is often performed. Knowing whether or not CAD is present enables doctors to design the most appropriate surgery. When a person has CAD, heart surgeons may correct both problems at the same time, which is generally found to improve the success rate of valve surgery.

Treatment and Results

There are many effective treatment options for the small number of people with aortic or mitral valve stenosis. Many people never require surgical valve repair. Should reparative surgery become necessary, valves can be repaired or replaced, depending on the kind of valve involved, the type of damage, and whether the person has undergone previous valve surgery. If possible, repair is preferred because it has less of an impact on the patient.

While people with mitral valve stenosis are awaiting reparative surgery, medications can help relieve some symptoms and complications. Antiarrhythmic medications normalize the heart rhythm, and other heart medications can improve the heart's hemodynamic, or pumping, function. Anticoagulants (anti-clotting medications) help prevent thrombogenesis, or blood-clot formation.

Traditionally, valve surgery has been performed through a large incision down the center of the chest. Not only is the resulting scar cosmetically unattractive, but the size of the incision greatly increases the chances of operative complications, including bleeding and infection; it also delays healing and recovery and can result in pain. Recovery from open-chest surgery takes at least 6 weeks.

Advances in minimally invasive surgical techniques expand the options, reduce potential complications, and decrease recovery time significantly. People who have undergone minimally invasive surgery generally go home from the hospital sooner, and the procedure is less expensive.

The heart remained the last frontier in minimally invasive surgery for a few critically important reasons. No matter how small the incision, the heart must be paused or at least slowed for surgeons to operate on it successfully. Until recently, this remained an impossible task through the small incisions used in minimally invasive surgery.

Now, surgeons performing minimally invasive valve surgery have two choices: They can stop the heart and use a cardiopulmonary (heart-lung) bypass machine, which circulates the blood while the heart is being operated on, or they can insert the necessary equipment through tiny incisions, called ports. Alternatively, surgeons can quiet the vigor of a beating heart with suction devices, which slow movement just enough to perform the delicate surgery.

Establishing an adequate indirect view inside the heart was not possible until recent advances were made in the designs of endoscopes— tubes with a miniature camera and light source that are inserted inside the heart. The images picked up by the camera are displayed on screens in the operating room directly in front of the surgeon. These projected images allow the surgeon to operate without seeing directly inside the chest. Miniaturized surgical equipment is also inserted into the tiny ports. The surgeon operates by looking at the images and maneuvering the surgical equipment as needed.

In addition to images created by endoscopy, transesophageal Doppler echocardiography (page 120) performed during surgery offers an aid to surgeons not only in guiding surgical technique, but also in judging the condition of the valve after the procedure and before closing the incision.

With these advantages, minimally invasive surgery is the method of choice for people undergoing the first surgical procedure (called primary surgery) for the repair or replacement of diseased aortic and mitral valves. The mortality rate of minimally invasive valve procedures continues to fall as experience mounts and is now below one-half of 1 percent. People undergoing secondary, or repeat, valve surgery generally are not candidates for the minimally invasive approach because they have too much scar tissue inside the chest.

Surgery for Aortic Valve Stenosis. More than three-quarters of stenosed aortic valves are replaced rather than repaired, because very few people with a stenosed aortic valve have the type of damage that is amenable to repair. People who need a new aortic valve have a wide range of valve types available to match their needs.

The cardiologist analyzes each person's type of valvular damage, physical condition, age, total heart function, lifestyle, likelihood of reoperation, and whether lifelong anticoagulant therapy (necessary when some types of valves are implanted) is safe. Then, the cardiologist and cardiac surgeon choose the most suitable valve.

Replacement valves fall into two broad categories: mechanical valves (artificial valves) and biological valves (valves that are made of human or animal tissue). The type of valves available, and their advantages and disadvantages, include the following:

Mechanical valves

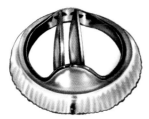

Bileaflet valve

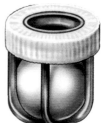

Ball and cage

Bioprosthetic valve

Homograft

Ross procedure

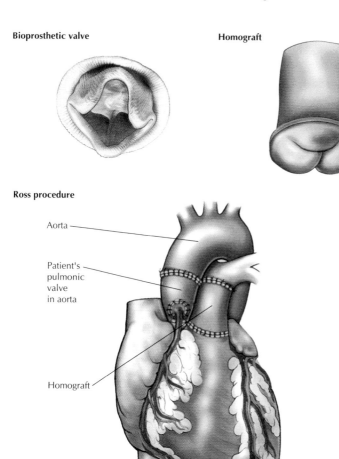

Aorta

Patient's pulmonic valve in aorta

Homograft

When valve replacement is necessary, the old valve is surgically removed and a new valve is sewn to the annulus. The new valve can be mechanical (either bileaflet or ball-and-cage types), bioprosthetic, or a homograft. In the Ross procedure, the patient's own pulmonic valve is removed and used to replace a diseased aortic valve. A homograph is then inserted to replace the removed pulmonic valve.

- *Mechanical valves.* Mechanical valves are available in a range of sizes, allowing the surgeon to match the patient's anatomy. Mechanical valves are easily implanted and they yield excellent hemodynamic function (ability of the heart to pump effectively). They are very durable and long-lasting, and rarely develop problems with structure or function. The most common problem with mechanical valves is thrombogenesis, or blood-clot formation, which tends to occur on the valve's surface. The body (rightly) perceives the valve as a foreign material and protects itself by clotting it over. This is why people with mechanical valves need life-long anticoagulant therapy, which greatly reduces the likelihood of thrombogenesis, but also increases the risk of bleeding.

    Two common types of mechanical valves are bileaflet and ball and cage. Bileaflet valves have two semicircular leaflets attached to a hinge. The leaflets swing open to allow blood to flow through the valve. The ball-and-cage valve is an older version of prosthetic valve. The ball moves up or down in the cage alternatively blocking blood flow or allowing blood to flow through.

- *Porcine bioprostheses.* Removed from a pig and preserved by freezing, porcine valves offer two choices in aortic valve replacement. Like mechanical valves, porcine valves are available in a range of sizes and are easily implanted. The risk of thrombogenesis in people with porcine valves is extremely low, which is why people who receive them do not generally need long-term anticoagulant therapy. The disadvantage is that porcine valves have a limited life span, approximately 8 to 10 years, after which they begin to deteriorate. A replacement implant is generally needed.

- *Pericardial bioprostheses.* Formed from bovine pericardial tissue (the tissue lining the heart of a cow), these valves offer several advantages. Hemodynamic function of pericardial bioprosthetic valves is generally excellent, and they rarely cause thrombogenesis, so anticoagulant therapy is generally unnecessary. Pericardial bioprostheses are generally more durable than porcine bioprostheses, although they may begin to deteriorate and need replacing after a decade.

- *Homograft valves.* A homograph valve is a human valve transplanted from a donor. The advantages are many, including excellent hemodynamic function, extremely low risk of thrombogenesis, and very low risk of infective endocarditis. Supply of aortic valve homografts is limited, and appropriate sizes are not always available. Homografts do deteriorate over time but are thought to be more durable than porcine bioprostheses. Implanting a homograph requires a technically advanced operation.

- *Pulmonary autografts.* An autograph is a valve transplanted from one position to another within the same person. In a technically challenging surgery, called the Ross procedure, surgeons move the valve from the pulmonary artery to the aorta and implant a pulmonary homograft to replace the pulmonic valve. The pulmonic valve is nearly identical to the aortic valve, thus preserving the circulation of the blood and nearly eliminating the risk of thrombogenesis. The disadvantage is that one abnormal valve is exchanged for two abnormal valves, with an uncertain long-term risk of valvular dysfunction. Occasional complications of the Ross procedure include aortic valve regurgitation (leaking) and pulmonic valve stenosis (narrowing).

Aortic stenosis often occurs at a time in life when people are more likely to have CAD. If bypass surgery becomes necessary before the aortic valve needs replacing, surgeons may replace the valve at the time of the bypass surgery, which helps avoid another operation in the near future. Because there is always a question of whether a new valve will ever be needed, doctors carefully weigh the pros and cons of prophylactic valve surgery.

Surgery for Mitral Valve Stenosis. Approximately two-thirds to three-quarters of people who need surgery for mitral valve stenosis undergo repair rather than replacement. Reparative surgery eliminates the need for an artificial valve, which is associated with its own set of problems, and also reduces surgical risk. Some people with mitral valve stenosis may be candidates for a less invasive procedure—percutaneous balloon valvuloplasty—which can open the obstructed mitral valve and prevent complications associated with a stenosed mitral valve (see Percutaneous Balloon Valvuloplasty, below).

Percutaneous Balloon Valvuloplasty

Percutaneous balloon valvuloplasty is a technique used to open obstructed valves (primarily mitral valves, and rarely aortic valves) that is far less invasive then reparative surgery. A catheter whose tip is fitted with an unopened balloon is inserted through a blood vessel in the groin, advanced to the heart, and then to the mitral valve.

At its target, the balloon is inflated with force, with the goal of forcing open the narrowed or stenosed mitral valve, thereby improving blood flow and heart function. The mitral valve opening usually increases significantly, abnormal pressure that often builds up in the heart when the mitral valve is stenosed decreases, and the heart is better able to pump blood.

Not everyone is a candidate for balloon valvuloplasty. Although the mitral valves of people chosen for this procedure are stenosed, the valves must not leak too much, must still be relatively thin (not thickened by disease) and minimally calcified, and must retain some degree of mobility. Two-dimensional echocardiography is a useful diagnostic tool in choosing those who will benefit from percutaneous balloon valvuloplasty.

How well a person does immediately after mitral valve replacement depends on the seriousness of valve disease and the degree of heart failure at the time of surgery. Doctors classify people with heart failure into one of four functional classes: Those in functional class I have the least serious form of heart failure, and those in class IV have the most severe form.

People who are in functional class I, II, or III heart failure have a more than 98 percent chance of surviving during surgery and the immediate postoperative period. If a person's heart failure has progressed to functional class IV, the survival rate drops to 75 percent.

This is one reason that reparative surgery for a stenosed mitral should be performed earlier rather than later. Some evidence suggests that early surgery not only improves long-term survival but also increases the success of valve repair (see Early Valve Repair Surgery, page 127).

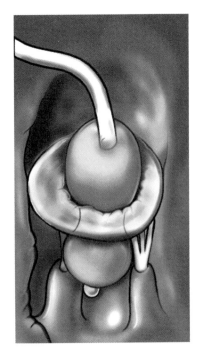

Balloon valvuloplasty is a treatment option in some cases of mitral or aortic valve stenosis. A catheter with a balloon at its tip is passed through the valve and inflated to widen the valve opening.

Early Valve Repair Surgery

One study designed to evaluate the success of earlier, rather than later, surgery in mitral valve repair showed that people whose surgery was performed sooner (they had less severe mitral valve disease and functional class I or II heart failure) had 100 percent survival at 11 years after surgery, and 97 percent were free from all complications.

In contrast, people who underwent mitral valve repair when they had serious valve disease and were in functional class III or IV heart failure had a 70 percent chance of successful repair. At 11 years, 13.9 percent of these people needed reoperation and 26.6 percent had suffered at least one complication.

Repairing a stenosed mitral valve depends on the specific type of damage to it. Surgery may be performed on several parts of the valve, including the leaflets and the tendons that hold them in place. The surgeon must have extensive experience in the multiple types of mitral repair technically possible, and the experience of the surgeon is one of the most important predictors of success.

Mitral and Aortic Valve Regurgitation

Valve regurgitation describes a valve that does not sufficiently close and, therefore, leaks. This can occur over time (chronic) or in a short period of time (acute). Acute valve regurgitation is generally more serious than chronic, necessitating emergency treatment.

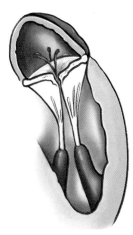

In valvular regurgitation (also called valvular incompetence or "leaky valve"), some blood leaks backward across the valve, so less blood flows forward. The heart muscle must work harder to circulate enough blood to the body.

Signs and Symptoms

Mitral Valve Regurgitation

Chronic Regurgitation. People with mild to moderate chronic mitral valve regurgitation may never have symptoms, and even those with moderate to severe disease can be symptom-free for decades. Yet their hearts gradually undergo changes caused by a leaky valve. The left side of the heart, both the atrium and ventricle, slowly stretches out.

Although the heart can compensate for these changes, after many years ventricular failure may occur, which leads to heart failure. A leaky mitral valve may also lead to atrial fibrillation (a rhythm abnormality), an increased risk of embolism (blot clot traveling in the bloodstream), and infective endocarditis (see page 113).

The first symptom that people with chronic mitral regurgitation experience is shortness of breath on exertion. With time, the shortness of breath becomes more severe, often occurring when the person is lying down; fatigue and weakness may accompany it. Swelling caused by accumulated fluid may develop in the legs and feet and sometimes in the abdomen.

Acute Regurgitation. Acute mitral regurgitation occurs if one of the chordae tendineae holding the valve in place suddenly ruptures. Unlike a slowly leaking valve, this rare sudden rupture causes an overload of blood into the left ventricle and left atrium, which have not stretched over time to accommodate extra blood, as they have in chronic mitral regurgitation.

As a result, people with acute mitral regurgitation suffer sudden and severe left ventricular failure. They may develop pulmonary edema (fluid buildup in the lungs; see page 158) and cardiogenic shock, in which the heart becomes unable to pump enough blood to the body, causing dangerously low blood pressure. Unlike people with chronic mitral regurgitation, those with the acute form are suddenly and severely disabled and must be hospitalized.

Aortic Valve Regurgitation

Like people with chronic mitral regurgitation, those with chronic aortic regurgitation can remain symptom-free for years. However, as the left ventricle becomes weakened by aortic regurgitation, shortness of breath and swelling of the legs and feet occur, increasing in severity as the ventricle becomes weaker.

People with aortic regurgitation may also suffer from angina, or chest pain. Another symptom is the unpleasant awareness of the beating of the heart and carotid artery pain (pain in the neck where the large blood vessel beats).

Causes and Prevention

Mitral Valve Regurgitation

The main causes of chronic mitral valve regurgitation are as follows:

- Mitral valve prolapse, the most common cause (see page 112)
- Inflammatory conditions, such as rheumatic heart disease (see page 118) and systemic lupus erythematosus
- Degenerative conditions, such as calcification of the mitral valve opening and Marfan syndrome (see page 130)
- Infections, such as infective endocarditis (see page 113)
- Structural valve problems, such as cardiomyopathy (see page 164), heart muscle dysfunction, or shortage of blood to the heart (ischemia)
- Congenital problems, including atrial septal defect (see page 223) and transposition of the great arteries (see page 214).

People whose mitral regurgitation is caused by ischemic heart disease generally have more serious and symptomatic disease. They are at greater risk of suffering a myocardial infarction (heart attack), which increases the regurgitation and decreases the functioning of the left ventricle.

Aortic Valve Regurgitation

Causes of aortic valve regurgitation include

- Bicuspid aortic valve (see page 225)
- Rheumatic heart disease (see page 118)
- Infective endocarditis (see page 113)
- Calcium deposits on the leaflets
- Marfan syndrome (see page 130)

Detection and Diagnosis

Physical Exam

A physical exam is crucial in diagnosing valve regurgitation. People with minor mitral regurgitation may have only a heart murmur, while those with more severe disease show the signs of left ventricular failure, including abnormal sounds and presence of fluid in the lungs, distended neck veins, liver enlargement, and swelling of the legs, feet, and abdomen.

Symptoms in people with acute mitral regurgitation are more dramatic and include a fast heart rate, a quickened rate of breathing, and a number of abnormal heart sounds heard through a stethoscope.

Marfan Syndrome

Marfan syndrome, which affects about 1 of every 20,000 people, is caused by a genetic mutation in cells that form connective tissue, which is found throughout the body. The resulting abnormalities most often strike the tissues that form the eyes, skeletal system, and heart.

A close look inside the heart by echocardiography reveals that between 80 to 95 percent of people who have Marfan syndrome show changes in heart tissues characteristic of the condition. Only about 40 to 60 percent have symptoms, the most common of which are mitral valve prolapse and problems with the aorta.

Typically in Marfan syndrome, the aorta dilates, or stretches in diameter. This problem can cause aortic valve regurgitation; it can also cause the aorta to rupture, a life-threatening condition.

A woman with Marfan syndrome who becomes pregnant is at increased risk of aortic dissection, in which the pressure of the flowing blood causes the arterial wall to split. This risk is especially heightened during the third trimester, delivery, and the first month after delivery. Doctors monitor these women throughout their pregnancies, especially during periods of high risk.

The characteristic murmur of aortic regurgitation is relatively loud and long, especially as the disease progresses. Blood pressure is abnormal and produces characteristic sounds that the doctor hears while measuring blood pressure.

Diagnostic Tests

People with suspected valve regurgitation undergo Doppler echocardiography (page 120), which can reveal abnormalities in valve formation, the size of the left atrium, the functional ability of the left ventricle, and how much blood is leaking backward. It also measures the pressure within various sections of the heart.

Cardiac catheterization (page 76) is generally not necessary to diagnose valvular regurgitation but is useful to identify the presence of CAD and to give the doctor more information about how the left ventricle is functioning.

Treatment and Results

Mitral Regurgitation

Antibiotic therapy to prevent infective endocarditis is often prescribed for people with chronic mitral regurgitation. Many people also need medications to correct the abnormal heart rhythm that results from the atrial fibrillation and anticoagulants to prevent the formation of blood clots, for which they are at risk. Other medications such as vasodilators, digoxin, and diuretics may be necessary to compensate for the failing left ventricle while surgery is awaited.

In people with acute mitral regurgitation, drug therapy is often administered intravenously. Emergency surgery to correct the underlying problem is almost always required in cases of acute mitral regurgitation.

Aortic Regurgitation

People with mild aortic regurgitation may not need treatment if they have no symptoms, but they should be monitored regularly by their doctor. If aortic regurgitation progresses to a more serious condition, medications to control resulting heart rhythm abnormalities or medications to assist the left ventricle may become necessary. In severe cases, surgery to replace the aortic valve may be needed.

Tricuspid and Pulmonic Valve Problems

Abnormalities of the tricuspid and pulmonic valves are much less common than those of the aortic and mitral valves.

Tricuspid Stenosis

The tricuspid valve can become stenosed from rheumatic heart disease; more than 90 percent of stenosed tricuspid valves are due to rheumatic fever (see page 118). The only other common cause of tricuspid stenosis is carcinoid heart disease, which is relatively rare. Carcinoid heart disease is not cancer, but a thickening of the heart muscle.

When just the tricuspid valve is stenosed, without mitral valve stenosis, a person feels tired and retains fluid; fluid retention may be the most bothersome problem.

Chest x-rays generally show an enlarged heart. In tricuspid valve stenosis, this enlargement is due to a stretched-out right atrium. ECGs (see page 120) show abnormalities specific to tricuspid valve disease. As with other valve disease, Doppler echocardiography is important to diagnosis and to revealing other causes that can mimic tricuspid valve disease, such as a tumor in the right atrium.

Diuretic medications can provide temporary relief for people with tricuspid stenosis. Eventually, the valve must be replaced or repaired; in some cases, stenosis can be corrected sufficiently by balloon valvuloplasty (see page 125). Surgeons can repair some tricuspid valves, opening them sufficiently with surgical techniques to avoid valve replacement. When the tricuspid valve must be replaced, surgeons can use a mechanical or a bioprosthetic valve (see page 122).

Tricuspid Regurgitation

A leaky tricuspid valve can occur for many reasons, including as a result of other heart conditions. CAD, high blood pressure, mitral regurgitation, mitral stenosis, and cardiomyopathy (see page 164) can eventually wear out the tricuspid valve, causing it to leak. Congenital heart problems, connective tissue diseases such as rheumatic fever or lupus, traumatic injury, radiation therapy, and infections can also stress the tricuspid valve to the point of leaking.

People with tricuspid regurgitation may notice a pulsation in their jugular vein or a pulsating right eyeball. Some people have no symptoms until the right ventricle starts to fail, and then they notice increasing fatigue and swelling in the legs, feet, and abdomen.

Doppler echocardiography is the most important test for diagnosing tricuspid regurgitation; chest x-rays and ECGs are also used. A pulse-wave or color Doppler reveals the misdirected blood flow and helps the doctor estimate the severity of the problem.

Treatment often entails valve repair or replacement, and the timing is dictated by the degree of heart failure that is experienced.

Pulmonic Valve Stenosis and Regurgitation

Congenital anomalies are the most common cause of pulmonic valve stenosis. Rarely, pulmonic stenosis occurs from rheumatic or carcinoid heart disease. Most people do not experience symptoms until the valve narrows severely; those who do notice symptoms may feel palpitations (the heart racing or jumping around irregularly) or chest discomfort.

Regurgitation in the pulmonic valve occurs for a variety of reasons, including infection, pulmonary hypertension (high pressure inside the lungs), rheumatic fever, rheumatoid arthritis, and Marfan syndrome (see page 130). Symptoms vary and generally relate to the cause of the leaky valve.

The three main diagnostic tests used are the ECG, chest x-ray, and Doppler echocardiogram.

The treatment of choice for pulmonic valve stenosis is balloon valvuloplasty (see page 125). Rarely, surgical repair becomes necessary; treating the underlying cause of pulmonic regurgitation usually solves the leaky valve problem without the need for repair or replacement of the pulmonic valve.

CHAPTER 7

Rhythm Disorders

Introduction

The heart's steady pumping is controlled by electrical impulses that signal the heart muscle to contract and expand in a cycle commonly called the cardiac, or heart, cycle. This cycle begins precisely at the end of one heart contraction and lasts to the end of the next contraction. The electrical impulses that initiate each contraction emanate from a part of the right atrium called the sinus node, or sinoatrial (SA) node. This cluster of cells functions as the body's natural pacemaker, which keeps the heart pacing at a particular rate.

After being spontaneously generated in the sinus node, these electrical impulses spread through the atrium to reach the atrioventricular (AV) node, an electrical relay station in the center of the heart where the two atria and two ventricles come together. There is a slight delay of the impulses at the AV node that allows the atria to contract slightly before the ventricles contract.

The impulses then move to a group of adjacent fibers called the bundle of His, which branch out into both ventricles. The muscle cells of the ventricles receive the electrical impulses that trigger the "pump." The average time it normally takes for these impulses to travel through the heart is one-fourth of a second.

The heart's electrical impulses can be recorded by a test called an electrocardiogram (ECG or EKG; see page 137). The impulses follow a prearranged pattern through the heart, which can be traced by specific wave patterns on the ECG. Cardiologists refer to three main components of the wave pattern:

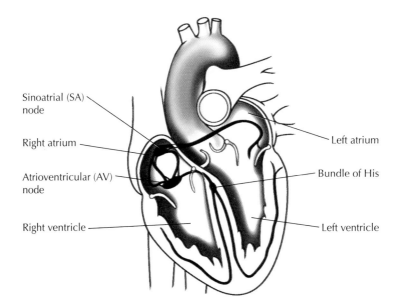

Sinoatrial (SA) node

Right atrium

Atrioventricular (AV) node

Right ventricle

Left atrium

Bundle of His

Left ventricle

Electrical impulses that control the heartbeat begin in the sinoatrial (SA) node in the right atrium. An impulse spreads from the SA node through the atrium to the atrioventricular (AV) node, an electrical relay station in the center of the heart. There the impulse is briefly delayed, allowing the atria to contract. From the AV node the impulse spreads to the bundle of His, a group of fibers which branch out to both ventricles. The muscle cells of the ventricles receive the impulse, stimulating the ventricles to contract.

- The P wave, which shows the impulse as it activates atrial contraction

- The QRS complex, which describes the impulse as it activates ventricular contraction

- The T wave, which represents the tail end of the impulse after which the ventricles relax

The heart's electrical system ensures that the heart beats rhythmically and evenly. For the most part, the heart beats in a fairly steady rhythm, generally between 60 to 100 beats per minute when a person is at rest. The number of times the heart beats per minute is called the heart rate, which varies by age, size, gender, and degree of athletic training. In general, women have slightly higher heart rates than men do.

Children, who have higher metabolic needs, tend to have the highest heart rate of all healthy people, approximately 90 to 120 beats per minute at rest. On the other end of the spectrum, well-trained athletes, whose

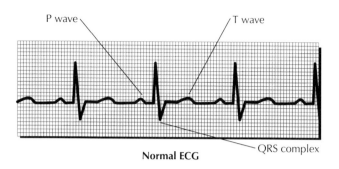

P wave

T wave

QRS complex

Normal ECG

The heart's electrical activity can be measured by a test called an electrocardiogram (ECG or EKG). The electrical impulses can be traced as specific wave patterns on the ECG. The P wave represents atrial activation. The QRS complex describes the electrical wave that activates ventricular contraction. The T wave represents the end of the impulse and ventricular relaxation.

---

hearts have become very efficient because of regular physical training, may have heart rates as low as 40 beats per minute at rest.

What Are Arrhythmias?

Normally, the heart beats in a steady, even rhythm with a predictable and repetitive amount of time between each beat. An arrhythmia is a disruption in either one or both aspects of normal heart rate:

- The rhythm, producing an uneven heartbeat
- The rate, causing very slow or very rapid heartbeat

Most people's hearts have "skipped a beat" on occasion—which may be perceived as a fluttering in the chest, or a pause followed by a sudden start, which some people describe as a leap in the chest. In some cases, these instances can occur 10 to 100 times per day but are harmless and do not need treatment. Sometimes, certain substances or medications can instigate arrhythmias, including caffeine, tobacco, alcohol, diet pills, and cough and cold remedies.

Some people, however, have an arrhythmia caused by coronary artery disease, hypertension (high blood pressure), or a previous myocardial infarction (heart attack). In general, arrhythmia that is associated with heart disease is more serious than arrhythmia that occurs in an otherwise healthy heart.

Overall, approximately 4.3 million Americans have some form of arrhythmia caused by a heart condition. Other medical conditions, such as thyroid abnormalities, anemia, bleeding, and fevers, can cause arrhythmia; stress can also instigate arrhythmia. Treating the underlying condition or alleviating the stress generally halts the arrhythmia.

After noting that the normal heart rate varies depending on levels of activity and general state of health, the three main types of arrhythmia include the following:

- Tachycardia: a rapid heartbeat, usually defined as a rate over 100 beats per minute

- Bradycardia: a slow heartbeat, usually defined as a rate under 60 beats per minute

- Fibrillation: a chaotic, random, very rapid heartbeat, which can reach as high as 300 beats per minute or more

Another means of categorizing arrhythmias is by where they originate in the heart. Those that begin in the atria, or the heart's upper chambers, are called supraventricular (above the ventricle; thus, in the atrium)

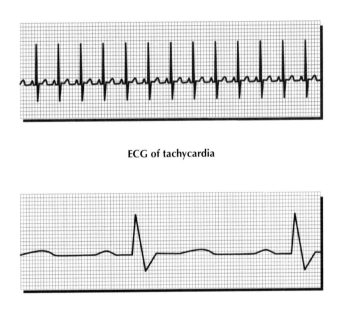

ECG of tachycardia

ECG of bradycardia

Tachycardia is a condition characterized by rapid heartbeat (over 100 beats per minute). Bradycardia is a condition characterized by slow heartbeat (under 60 beats per minute).

or atrial arrhythmias, while those starting in the lower chambers are ventricular arrhythmias. In general, the atrial arrhythmias are not life-threatening and are less serious than the ventricular arrhythmias. However, an atrial arrhythmia can become serious if it initiates a ventricular arrhythmia. Electrical impulses follow a set pattern through the heart, beginning in the atria; a rhythm disruption in the atria can affect the contractions of the ventricles. The most serious type of arrhythmia can cause cardiac arrest, a life-threatening situation in which the heart suspends its pumping action, or stops.

Symptoms of arrhythmia depend on the type of arrhythmia, its severity, how long it lasts, and how frequently it occurs. An arrhythmia may go unnoticed until a doctor discovers it during a routine physical exam. In other people, arrhythmia may be associated with symptoms of weakness, fatigue, chest discomfort, shortness of breath, or fainting and may be diagnosed before it causes any serious consequences. But sometimes arrhythmia is not diagnosed until cardiac arrest has occurred followed by resuscitation.

Diagnosing Arrhythmias

Electrocardiogram

An electrocardiogram (ECG or EKG) is a snapshot of the heart's electrical pattern at one point in time. Because ECG captures only a segment of electrical activity, it is not the most helpful test in diagnosing an arrhythmia. Arrhythmias occur sporadically, or usually at times other than when a person is lying in a doctor's office undergoing ECG recording. Arrhythmias, in fact, are more likely to occur when a person is active than at rest. Because of these factors, other diagnostic tests are often necessary. For more information on ECG, see page 67.

Stress Tests

An ECG may be performed in combination with a stress, or exercise, test. During a stress test, a person exercises on a treadmill while ECG is performed to evaluate the heart's rhythm under duress. For more information on stress tests, see page 67.

Holter Monitor and ECG Event Recorders

A useful test in diagnosing arrhythmias is the 24-hour ECG, or Holter monitor. For this test, a person is attached to a small portable ECG machine, which records the heart rhythm continuously for a longer period of time, usually 24 hours. For arrhythmic episodes that happen less frequently, such as once every few days or weeks, an event monitor can record the ECG when the patient pushes a button during the occurrence of a symptom.

Electrophysiological Studies

In many cases, the arrhythmia does not occur frequently enough to be documented with the Holter monitor or event recorder. In these cases, electrophysiological testing can provide valuable information. This form of testing, performed in a cardiac catheterization laboratory under careful monitoring, provides detailed information about the heart's electrical activity and allows the doctor to determine precisely where in the heart the arrhythmia originates and how serious it is.

Electrophysiological testing is performed under mild sedation by a cardiac subspecialist, the electrophysiologist. First, the doctor makes a small puncture of a vein in the groin area, into which catheters (long, thin tubes) with a tiny electrode on their tips are threaded through the vein and guided into the heart. These catheters are usually positioned at various places in the heart's right side.

Once in place, the electrodes transmit information to a computer about the heart's electrical activity and how that activity travels through the heart during each contraction. The pattern of electrical activity is visualized on a rhythm strip similar in appearance to an ECG strip. This rhythm strip may describe the arrhythmia sufficiently to provide a definite diagnosis and help the doctor prescribe treatment.

Electrophysiologists can deliberately elicit an arrhythmia using a programmed electrical stimulation. To do this, the electrophysiologist moves the catheter to various locations in the heart and delivers tiny pulses of electric current to the site, purposely eliciting the arrhythmia that the patient is experiencing.

Because this procedure is performed in a very controlled environment under continuous monitoring, the risk of complications is minimal, estimated at less than 1 percent in the hands of an experienced electrophysiologist. Even the initiation of arrhythmias that could cause cardiac arrest is quite safe in the laboratory as these are terminated quickly by the electrophysiologist.

Once an arrhythmia is elicited, the patterns of electrical activation recorded by the catheters can help the physician identify the source and mechanism of the arrhythmia. The studies also help the doctor plan potential treatment to cure or control the arrhythmia.

Major (Serious) Arrhythmias

Ventricular Tachycardias and Ventricular Fibrillation

The most serious arrhythmias are tachycardias or fibrillation that originate in the ventricles. Ventricular tachycardia can become ventricular fibrillation, in which the ventricles twitch rapidly but cannot pump blood. Ventricular fibrillation is fatal unless cardiopulmonary resuscita-

Cardiac Arrest

In cardiac arrest (also called sudden cardiac death), the heart's electrical system—its rhythm regulator—gives out and the heart mechanically stops, or arrests, its pumping action. Cardiac arrest is not the same as a heart attack, in which due to coronary artery blockage the heart muscle itself does not get enough blood and the heart tissue is damaged. During a cardiac arrest, the heart cannot pump, no oxygenated blood is distributed to the body (which means no oxygen reaches the brain), and a person loses consciousness. Cardiac arrest is nearly always fatal if the heart does not start again on its own or if successful resuscitation efforts are not begun.

An efficient emergency medical system (EMS) team can often reach a person in cardiac arrest within 5 to 10 minutes of its onset. Studies show that by this time, about 70 percent of people are in ventricular fibrillation (see page 138), and the remaining 30 percent have no heart rhythm at all. EMS teams use defibrillation, a means of shocking the heart out of the chaotic fibrillating pattern that occurs during cardiac arrest, to restore a normal rhythm.

Men between the ages of 50 and 70 with some underlying heart disease are most at risk for cardiac arrest. These heart diseases include the following:

- Atherosclerosis (narrowing of the arteries due to plaque buildup)

- Hypertension (high blood pressure)

- Cardiomyopathy (disease of the myocardium, or heart muscle)

- Congestive heart failure (a condition in which the heart muscle does not pump well enough to maintain normal body function; see page 158)

Although the majority of people who experience cardiac arrest do not have any distinctive symptoms just prior to their heart's stopping, a careful analysis of the days or hours immediately preceding the event may reveal that they did experience a set of nonspecific symptoms. These symptoms could have included chest pain, shortness of breath, or something as vague as fatigue.

Cardiac arrest has a definite circadian rhythm: It is more likely to occur at certain times of the day than at others. The incidence is lowest during sleep and rises rapidly soon after awakening.

Careful attention to any signs indicating a cardiac problem and assessing a person's risk for ventricular tachycardia are essential to help prevent cardiac arrest.

tion (CPR; see page 281) is administered. Ventricular tachycardias/fibrillation cause about 50 percent of all cardiac-related deaths. The most common cause of ventricular tachycardias/fibrillation is ischemic coronary artery disease, or coronary artery disease that significantly reduces blood flow to the heart muscle.

Risk Factors for Ventricular Tachycardia

People who have had a myocardial infarction, or heart attack, and are left with myocardial scars—scarred muscle tissue with poor blood flow—are at high risk for ventricular tachycardia. Often, there are small areas of healthy muscle tissue within these scars where electrical impulses generate normal activity. However, the scar tissue is interwoven with the normal tissue, and so the electrical impulses may take a winding or indirect route.

In addition, the normal cell-to-cell movement of electrical impulses may be slowed. Overall, electrical conduction tests of these scarred areas show low-energy and delayed signals that start and stop. This combination of abnormalities is thought to cause the ventricular tachycardia associated with scarred heart muscle after a myocardial infarction.

Factors that predict which people who have had a myocardial infarction will be affected by ventricular tachycardia include the following:

■ Severe myocardial infarction (and therefore larger areas of scarred heart tissue)

■ Ventricular dysfunction following myocardial infarction

Tests that measure ventricular function include the following:

■ Left ventricular ejection fraction—the amount of blood the left ventricle is able to pump out during a contraction, measured as a percentage of the total amount of blood in the left ventricle before contraction (see page 75)

■ New York Heart Association Functional Class—the degree of heart failure is judged by this standard scale, where functional class I indicates a minor degree of failure and functional class IV indicates the worst degree of failure

Other signs and symptoms that predict a person's risk for sudden ventricular tachycardia include syncope (fainting), indicating possible serious arrhythmias, and specific characteristics on special ECG recordings such as signal-averaged ECG (see page 141).

Treatment

Treatment for ventricular tachycardias include the following:

Signal-Averaged Electrocardiography

Signal-averaged electrocardiography uses a computer program to detect low-energy electrical impulses traveling through scarred areas of the myocardium. Signal-averaged ECG can detect impulses that are too weak to be detected by regular ECG. This test works by amplifying the sound of the impulses and reducing background electrical "noise." Like regular ECG, signal-averaged ECG is a non-invasive procedure and is particularly helpful in diagnosing ventricular tachycardias.

■ Implantable defibrillators

■ Radiofrequency ablation

■ Medications

Implantable Defibrillators. Implantable defibrillators are used to correct severe, potentially fatal ventricular arrhythmias. Implantable defibrillators have two main components. The first part is a pulse generator, which contains the electronic power sources and the memory, which is

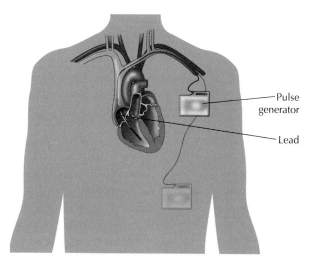

Implantable defibrillators may be used to correct severe ventricular arrhythmias. The defibrillator consists of two parts: a pulse generator, which contains the electronic power sources and the memory, and the lead wires, which connect to the heart. The pulse generator may be implanted in the chest wall or the abdomen.

When an implanted defibrillator detects a serious arrythmia, such as ventricular fibrillation, the device stops the arrythmia with an electrical shock that restores normal rhythm.

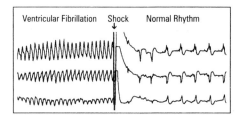

programmed to identify normal and abnormal heart rhythms. The second part holds the electrode system, leads or wires that connect to the heart. The current implantable defibrillators are powered by batteries that last between 5 to 7 years, depending on how they are programmed and activated in response to abnormal rhythms.

The defibrillator has three important tasks: First, it monitors the heart's rhythm and identifies arrhythmias as they occur. Second, it distinguishes between serious and nonserious arrhythmias. Third, when it detects a serious arrhythmia (such as one that can cause syncope or cardiac arrest), the defibrillator activates itself and stops the arrhythmia with an electrical shock that restores the heart to a normal rhythm. Modern defibrillators can also act as pacemakers (see page 145) to prevent bradycardia.

An implantable defibrillator is recommended for people who have had a myocardial infarction and are at high risk of cardiac arrest. Implantable defibrillators are also recommended in high-risk people who have heart disease of a genetic basis, such as hypertrophic cardiomyopathy (see page 165). Defibrillators are also recommended for those who have experienced at least one episode of ventricular tachycardia.

A recent, large multicenter study evaluated the effectiveness of the implantable automatic defibrillator in the prevention of sudden cardiac death caused by ventricular tachycardia in people who had had a heart attack, comparing it to standard drug therapy. This study found that people treated with the implantable defibrillator had approximately one-half the mortality of the drug-treated group.

Radiofrequency Catheter Ablation. In radiofrequency catheter ablation, the muscle fibers in which the abnormal rhythm starts are cauterized (using an electric current to destroy tissue) nonsurgically. Radiofrequency ablation is used alone in people without heart damage or in conjunction with other treatments in those with scarring due to previous myocardial infarction or in those with heart failure.

In the cardiac catheterization laboratory, the electrophysiologist identifies the area of abnormal conduction within the myocardium using a catheter with an electrode at its tip (see Electrophysiology Studies, page

138). Then, still using the catheter, the electrophysiologist delivers radiofrequency energy to the area destroying the abnormal tissue. The radiofrequency energy source heats only a very small portion of the myocardium under the catheter tip—generally, an area about 5 to 7 millimeters in diameter and 3 to 4 millimeters deep. The success of this technique in treating ventricular tachycardia depends on accurately identifying the area of abnormal tissue and is estimated at approximately 70 percent.

Medications. Medications are an important adjunctive therapy (a treatment used to support other treatments) for people with ventricular tachycardia who have underlying congestive heart failure and ischemia (lack of oxygen to the heart muscle). The medications often used in treatment include the following:

- Beta blockers, which block the effects of the hormone epinephrine (adrenaline). Beta blockers reduce the amount of oxygen the heart requires and cause the heart to beat slower and less forcefully, lowering blood pressure and heart rate.

- Amiodarone and sotalol, antiarrhythmics that help correct irregular heartbeat by decreasing the heart tissue's propensity for arrhythmia.

When cardiac arrest is due to ischemia (lack of oxygen) of the heart muscle, a person may have to undergo a surgical or nonsurgical procedure to revascularize, or restore blood flow to the heart. Such procedures include coronary artery bypass graft (CABG) surgery (see page 100) and angioplasty (see page 96).

Bradycardias

Sinus Node Dysfunction

Although sinus node dysfunction is the most common cause of bradycardia (slow heartbeat), it does not necessarily produce symptoms. The term refers to any abnormality in sinus node function that causes the heart to slow; it also refers to a condition in which the heart alternates between tachycardia and bradycardia (tachycardia-bradycardia syndrome, also called "sick sinus" syndrome; see page 144).

Heartbeat originates in the sinus node. This node is made up of nests of principal pacemaker cells, which spontaneously "fire" impulses that spread throughout the heart's electrical pathway. These pacemaker cells are cocooned within fibrous tissue. Previously, sinus node dysfunction was thought to occur almost exclusively because the fibrous tissue became fibrotic, or hardened. Today, cardiologists know that fibrosis is not the only cause of sinus node dysfunction.

Other causes of sinus node dysfunction include factors that cause an imbalance in the sympathetic and parasympathetic nervous systems; both influence heart rate, as well as other bodily functions. The parasympathetic nervous system exerts a slowing effect on the heart rate, while the sympathetic system tends to quicken it.

These systems exert their effect through the release of neurotransmitters and hormones. The parasympathetic system releases the neurotransmitter acetylcholine, and the sympathetic system produces epinephrine and norepinephrine, hormones that induce the "fight or flight" response. Balanced appropriately, these substances (along with others) produce a heart rate that is neither too fast nor too slow. But when one system produces too much or too little of its chemical, heart rate can become too rapid or too slow.

In addition to tachycardia-bradycardia syndrome, sinus node dysfunction can cause other types of bradycardia, including inappropriate sinus bradycardia, sinus arrest, and sinoatrial exit block.

Inappropriate Sinus Bradycardia. This type of bradycardia is diagnosed in people whose heart rate falls below 60 beats per minute persistently and does not increase with exercise. Doctors carefully distinguish this bradycardia from the normally slow, resting heart rates of athletes, as well as from the heart rates of people who experience low rates normally during sleep. Doctors implant a pacemaker when heart rate falls persistently during the day in nonathletes, especially when it causes fatigue or syncope.

Sinus Arrest. The terms sinus arrest and sinus pause are used interchangeably to refer to this condition that occurs because the principle pacemaker cells of the sinus node fail to activate. Sinus pauses of greater than 2 seconds but less than 3 seconds may occur incidentally, or by chance, in people with otherwise normal heart rhythms, and these pauses do not cause symptoms; this is especially true in well-trained athletes. When sinus arrest lasts for at least three seconds it may cause symptoms, such as dizziness or lightheadedness. Treatment, when necessary, most commonly consists of implanting a pacemaker.

Sinoatrial Block. This bradycardia occurs because the sinus impulse does not leave the sinus node region. When the condition is severe and causes symptoms, treatment consists of inserting a pacemaker (see page 145).

Tachycardia-Bradycardia Syndrome

In tachycardia-bradycardia syndrome, sometimes called "sick sinus" syndrome, the heart alternates between beating fast (tachycardia) and slow (bradycardia). The syndrome causes a specific set of symptoms

Pacemakers are small devices implanted into the chest wall that contain an electrical system capable of pacing the heart when the heart's own electrical system has problems. Some pacemakers pace only the ventricles and some only the atria; others are dual-chamber pacemakers, which can pace both chambers. Pacemakers are implanted under the skin near the collarbone, and leads, or wires, are connected to the heart's electrical conducting system usually through the veins (see illustration on page 146).

A person who has a pacemaker implanted generally stays in the hospital for a night after implantation, attached to a heart monitor so doctors can check the heart rhythm the pacemaker produces. Sometimes, they must also adjust the pacemaker settings.

Reasons for implanting pacemakers include the following:

■ Treatment of atrioventricular block (see page 148)

■ Treatment of sinus node dysfunction (see page 143)

If it has been recommended that you receive a pacemaker, you should choose a specialist with extensive experience in pacemaker implantation. The Pacemaker Training Policy Conference Group, a national advisory group on pacemaker implantation and use, recommends choosing a doctor who meets the following criteria:

■ Participation in at least 50 initial pacemaker implantations as the primary operator (it is further recommended that at least half of these involve dual-chamber pacemakers)

■ Participation in at least 100 pacemaker follow-up visits

■ Participation in at least 20 revisions of pacing systems

■ Thorough knowledge of treatment of pacemaker, as well as surgical complications and emergencies

Interference from outside electrical sources concerns many people with pacemakers. For the most part, electrical sources encountered in everyday life do not interfere with pacemaker function. The most common sources of electromagnetic interference for pacemakers are found within a hospital environment, including electrocautery (an electrical source used during surgery to stop bleeding), cardioversion (an electrical means of shocking the heart into a normal rhythm), and magnetic resonance imaging (MRI, an imaging test that uses magnetic forces). Because these instruments are regulated by trained hospital staff, they pose little threat to a person with a pacemaker, as long as hospital staff are aware of the pacemaker. People with pacemakers should also avoid very close contact with anti-theft devices, digital cell phones (although this issue is still under investigation; for safety, the cell phone should not be placed directly against the chest), high-output ham radios, and high-intensity radio waves, such as are found near large electrical generators or radiofrequency transmission towers.

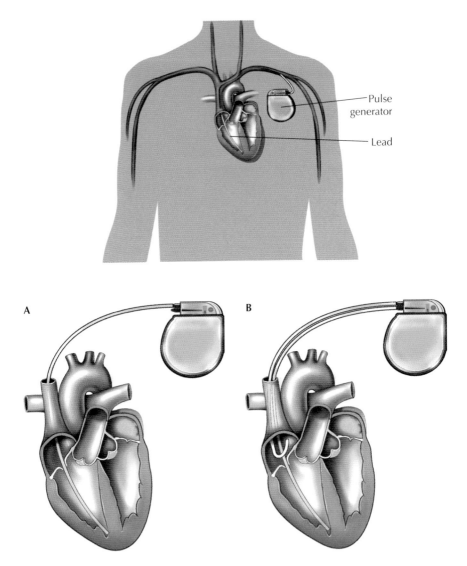

A pacemaker is a device implanted into the chest to control and prevent arrhythmias. Like an implantable defibrillator, a pacemaker consists of a pulse generator, containing power sources and a programmable memory, and a lead(s) that connect to the heart. A pacemaker can be (A) single-chamber or (B) dual-chamber, which can pace both chambers.

that can be due either to the tachycardia or the bradycardia and sometimes to both. The tachycardia portion of this syndrome usually originates in the atria and is usually paroxysmal (sudden or spasmodic) atrial fibrillation. While the overall incidence of tachycardia-bradycardia syndrome in the general population is not known, a Belgian study found that approximately 3 of every 5,000 people over the age of 50 were affected.

Symptoms include dizziness, confusion, fatigue, syncope, and congestive heart failure. Syncope is usually caused by atrial fibrillation that spontaneously stops and is then followed by a long pause or a significant period of bradycardia.

Doctors can sometimes diagnose the condition with 24-hour ECG monitoring or exercise testing and occasionally by testing the autonomic nervous system. In autonomic nervous system testing, doctors administer drugs that affect heart rate; the heart rate of people who have tachycardia-bradycardia syndrome responds characteristically. When people experience symptoms infrequently, electrophysiological testing may be necessary (see page 138).

Tachycardia-bradycardia syndrome can be due to intrinsic causes (conditions and diseases of the heart) or to extrinsic causes (some drugs and noncardiac conditions and diseases). The intrinsic causes include the following:

- Coronary artery disease (atherosclerosis, or narrowing, of the arteries supplying the heart)

- Cardiomyopathy (disease of the myocardium)

- Collagen vascular diseases (such as scleroderma or systemic lupus erythematosus)

- Inflammations of the heart, such as myocarditis (inflammation of the myocardium) or pericarditis (inflammation of the pericardium)

- Surgical trauma to the heart (especially after heart transplantation; occurs in approximately 45 percent of heart transplant patients)

- Congenital heart diseases (conditions present at birth); in some conditions tachycardia-bradycardia syndrome occurs as a result of corrective surgery

The most common extrinsic causes include the following:

- Cardiac drugs, including beta blockers, calcium-channel blockers, digoxin, some antihypertensive agents, and some antiarrhythmic drugs

- Noncardiac drugs, including lithium, cimetidine, amitriptyline, and phenytoin

- Hypothermia (excessive exposure to cold)

- Sepsis (a serious infection in the bloodstream)

- Abnormal levels (either high or low) of electrolytes—minerals normally present in the bloodstream—especially potassium

- Increased vagal tone, or too-strong impulses from the vagus nerve, one of the nerves that influences heart rate; well-trained athletes may have vagal tone that is too strong, causing bradycardias

Treatment depends on which portion of the condition causes symptoms. In some cases, treating the underlying problem or removing a causative medication may correct the problem. When the bradycardia produces symptoms not controlled by treating the underlying condition or eliminating the offending medication, a pacemaker may be needed. The bradycardia of tachycardia-bradycardia syndrome is the most common reason for implanting a pacemaker.

The tachycardia is often treated with antiarrhythmic medications, and careful selection is important to prevent other arrhythmias from developing. Many people need both pacing and medications to control the condition. Approximately 75 to 80 percent of people with tachycardia-bradycardia syndrome benefit from pacemaker implantation.

Atrioventricular Block

Another leading cause of bradycardia is atrioventricular block, or heart block. In this condition, an electrical impulse activated normally by the sinus node in the right atrium does not reach the ventricles, or pumping chambers. The signal is blocked in the atrioventricular node or in the bundle of His. Atrioventricular block can occur as first-, second-, or third-degree, in order of severity:

- In first-degree heart block, the impulse slows somewhat in the AV node but is not interrupted. A person rarely experiences symptoms because the heart rate does not drop.

- Second-degree heart block indicates interruption of some impulses as they conduct through the AV node. Second-degree heart block may produce symptoms of dizziness and even syncope because the heart rate tends to drop lower than in first-degree heart block. However, some forms of second-degree heart block cause no symptoms.

- In third-degree heart block, also called complete heart block, a person may still not have symptoms, although symptoms are more common. A person may be aware of a slow heart rate and a "heavy heart" feeling, and also may fatigue easily, have syncope, and develop heart failure.

Sometimes, but not always, first- or second-degree heart block may progress; when it does, people may experience a Stokes-Adams attack. This occurs as a result of a very slow or absent pulse and causes dizziness, syncope, and convulsions. Other symptoms that occur as the condition progresses include fatigue, difficulty in thinking clearly, dyspnea (shortness of breath) on exertion, angina (chest pain), and congestive heart failure. These latter symptoms generally occur because cardiac out-

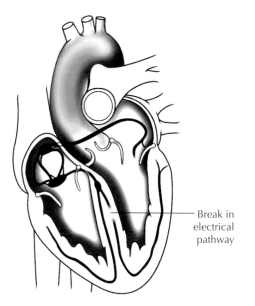

Break in
electrical
pathway

Atrioventricular block, or heart block, occurs when an electrical signal is blocked in the atrioventricular node or bundle of His due to a break in the electrical pathway. Heart block may be classified as first-, second-, or third-degree depending on severity.

put begins to fail, which means the heart gradually loses its ability to pump out normal amounts of blood to all body parts, due to an extremely slow heartbeat.

The most common causes of atrioventricular block include previous myocardial infarction, fibrosis (hardening) of the atrioventricular node, infective endocarditis (see page 113), calcification of the aortic or mitral valves (see Aortic and Mitral Valve Stenosis, page 116), and, rarely, congenital complete heart block (third-degree heart block that is present at birth).

Atrioventricular block can be diagnosed by a simple ECG, but more advanced testing may be necessary. Doctors can assess how well the vagus nerve is working, perform exercise testing, or administer certain drugs to determine how the heart responds. In some cases, electrophysiologic testing is the only means to provide a definitive diagnosis.

The mainstay of treatment in people who have symptomatic or severe heart block is pacemaker implantation. In some cases, atrioventricular block may occur only temporarily after myocardial infarction. Then, the need for pacing is temporary.

Less Serious Arrhythmias

While heart arrhythmias can be life-threatening, it is far more common for people to experience arrhythmias that are much less dangerous. Some of these may be treated to prevent symptoms from occurring. These types of arrhythmias are generally judged not to be as serious as others because they are unlikely to lead to cardiac arrest.

Supraventricular Tachycardia

Supraventricular tachycardia refers to a rapid heart rate originating in, or involving, the atria (supraventricular meaning "above the ventricles," thus, in the atria). Supraventricular tachycardias can cause heart rates of 140 to 240 beats per minute. In some instances, the heart rate can be slower and, in other instances, even faster than 240 beats per minute. While these tachycardias are not generally considered life-threatening, they can cause symptoms, and their treatment is usually based on the need to suppress these symptoms. Symptoms associated with these tachycardias include palpitations (see page 153), nervousness, lightheadedness, and syncope. Chest discomfort and shortness of breath can also be experienced during episodes of supraventricular tachycardia.

Supraventricular tachycardias are caused by abnormalities in the electrical pathways of the heart that result in a re-entry circuit, in which impulses are allowed to begin again (re-enter) repeatedly, rather than traveling along an appropriate pathway. These tachycardias may also be caused by abnormal electrical activity that results in electrical impulses being fired rapidly from somewhere other than the sinus node, where impulses normally begin (see Ectopic Atrial Heartbeats, below).

The diagnosis of supraventricular tachycardia is generally made with an ECG (see page 137) taken while symptoms are occurring. Treatment may involve the use of medications to control these rhythm disturbances or radiofrequency catheter ablation (see page 142), during which the abnormal pathways are identified and destroyed. The success rate of radiofrequency ablation is 90 to 95 percent.

Wolff-Parkinson-White Syndrome

A special type of supraventricular tachycardia, which is associated with an abnormal ECG even during normal rhythm, is the Wolf-

Ectopic Atrial Heartbeats

While many atrial tachycardias originate in the sinus node, some do not. Abnormal heartbeats that start in another part of the heart muscle are called ectopic, from the Greek word meaning "out of place." It is thought that some of these heartbeats originate around the bottom of the right atrium and the base of the pulmonary veins in the left atrium. This tachycardia cannot be initiated nor terminated by a pacemaker implanted in the atrium.

Parkinson-White (WPW) syndrome. The electrical abnormality of this particular disorder involves an additional electrical connection between the atrium and the ventricle other than the AV node. Normally, electrical impulses originating in the sinus node in the atria can travel to the ventricles only through the AV node. In people with WPW syndrome, at least one additional electrical connection, called an accessory pathway or bypass tract, between the atrium and the ventricle is present. Thus, the electrical impulses from the atrium can travel through two different pathways, causing the ECG to look abnormal during normal rhythm. This abnormality is known as ventricular pre-excitation.

Sometimes WPW syndrome is associated with other congenital abnormalities of the heart, such as Ebstein's anomaly (see below). WPW syndrome is a special case of a supraventricular tachycardia that can be more serious if other arrhythmias develop. If a person with WPW syndrome develops atrial fibrillation (see page 152) or atrial flutter (see page 155), the ventricular rate can become exceedingly fast because of the accessory pathway. This rapid ventricular rate may induce yet another arrhythmia, ventricular fibrillation (see page 138), a particularly serious arrhythmia that can lead to sudden death.

Diagnosis and Treatment of WPW Syndrome. People with WPW syndrome have characteristic changes in their ECG even during normal rhythm, most of the time. However, at times, the presence of the accessory pathway may be "concealed" on the ECG and its presence can only be detected during electrophysiological studies (see page 138). Tachycar-

Ebstein's Anomaly

Ebstein's anomaly is a congenital abnormality that causes several major defects in the heart. These include abnormalities in the tricuspid valve, ventricular septal defect (see page 222), a small right ventricle, pulmonic stenosis (see page 226), and pulmonary atresia (lack of an opening in the pulmonic valve). Approximately 50 percent of children born with Ebstein's anomaly have symptoms during infancy, which can include cyanosis (blue-tinted skin because of a lack of a oxygen), right-sided heart failure (see page 158), and rapid breathing. An estimated 10 percent of these children have Wolff-Parkinson-White syndrome (see page 150) and the arrhythmias associated with it.

Treatment depends on each child's specific array of anomalies and could include surgery or medication therapy for right-sided heart failure and arrhythmias.

dias associated with WPW that cause symptoms are most commonly treated with radiofrequency catheter ablation, but medications and surgical therapies are also occasionally used.

Atrial Fibrillation

Atrial fibrillation is a rapid rhythm of the upper chambers of the heart involving the presence of multiple electrical impulses traveling through the atria simultaneously. Thus, the electrical activation of the muscle at any one point can be extremely rapid (300 to 400 beats per minute) and irregular.

The prevalence of atrial fibrillation increases with age; it occurs in 0.5 percent of people aged 50 to 59 and 8.8 percent of people aged 80 to 89. Atrial fibrillation is rare during the first two decades of life. Some of the normal changes of aging that affect the heart muscle are thought to be at least partially responsible for causing atrial fibrillation.

Certain diseases and conditions can also cause atrial fibrillation, including:

■ Hypertension

■ Coronary artery disease (CAD; narrowing and hardening of the arteries that supply the heart. CAD mimics and hastens the normal aging process.)

■ Cardiomyopathy (disease of the myocardium)

■ Mitral valve disease (including stenosis and regurgitation, see pages 116 and 127)

■ Pericarditis (inflammation of the pericardium)

■ Thyrotoxicosis (a condition in which the body produces an excessive quantity of thyroid hormones)

■ Alcohol abuse

Atrial fibrillation remains the most common complication after open-heart surgery, occurring in about 20 to 40 percent of patients, and increasing the risk of stroke in this post-operative period.

In people who have atrial fibrillation, the most common symptom is palpitation (see Palpitations, page 153). Other common symptoms include lightheadedness, fatigue, and shortness of breath. Less common symptoms are angina and syncope. However, some people with atrial fibrillation do not have symptoms at all.

In the past, atrial fibrillation was divided into two categories: paroxysmal (a sudden, unpredictable onset that can end as quickly as it began and may or may not recur) and chronic (ongoing), but the terms were not standardized. Today, cardiologists refer to three types of atrial fibrillation, with the categories based on treatment:

Palpitations

Palpitations are forcible pulsations of the heart, causing an unpleasant awareness of the heartbeat. People who have experienced palpitations describe the feeling as a skipping, jumping, pounding, or racing of the heart. Palpitations can occur because a person has an underlying abnormal heart rhythm, but they can also occur when there is no underlying arrhythmia. Simple anxiety, drinking too much coffee, tobacco smoking, and overexertion may bring on palpitations. Any type of arrhythmia can also produce palpitations.

When the cause of palpitations is anxiety, stress, or some other lifestyle factor, treatment is aimed at modifying that factor. When palpitations are due to underlying arrhythmias, treatment focuses on the causative arrhythmia.

- Transient atrial fibrillation, a sudden onset that lasts less than 48 hours

- Persistent atrial fibrillation, a fibrillation episode that lasts more than 48 hours and that can return to a normal rhythm with either drug treatment or by electrical means (cardioversion)

- Permanent atrial fibrillation, or fibrillation that cannot be reversed by either medication or other means

Treatment

The goals of treatment for atrial fibrillation are to

- Prevent strokes

- Control heart rate and rhythm

- Prevent abnormal heart function

Prevent Strokes. When the atria are not pumping blood effectively, blood may be left in the atria after contraction. This blood may pool and clot, forming thrombi, or blood clots. If a piece of a thrombus breaks off and travels through the bloodstream, it may become lodged in an artery supplying the brain, resulting in stroke. Transesophageal echocardiography (see page 79) is helpful in identifying blood clots in the atria.

Preventing stroke associated with atrial fibrillation involves taking anticoagulants (blood thinners) prior to undergoing cardioversion or using medication to reverse atrial fibrillation. The risk of forming thrombi, or blood clots, in persistent atrial fibrillation is between 1 and 5 percent without the use of anticoagulants; the risk falls to under 1 percent with them.

Control Heart Rate and Rhythm. Several antiarrhythmic medications work effectively to control heart rate and rhythm. However, whenever doctors use drugs to control cardiac rhythm, the drug can have unexpected adverse affects on the heart's rhythm. Sometimes, in fact, doctors are hesitant to institute aggressive therapy to prevent atrial fibrillation simply because the drugs they used to control one abnormal rhythm could cause another.

In addition to medications, mode-switching pacemakers and radiofrequency ablation (see page 142) can serve as a means of rate control. Mode-switching pacemakers can switch from dual-chamber pacing to a single-chamber pacing pattern (see page 145). Mode-switching pacemakers used in combination with radiofrequency ablation of the AV node can be particularly helpful in treating paroxysmal (sudden or spasmodic) atrial fibrillation.

Cardiologists often use radiofrequency ablation to treat atrial fibrillation when medication therapy fails to control a rapid ventricular rate that can occur in conjunction with it, and sometimes when medications do not stop transient or persistent atrial fibrillation. Two types of radiofrequency ablation are performed for atrial fibrillation: In complete atrioventricular junctional catheter ablation, the electrophysiologist uses radiofrequency energy to destroy the atrioventricular node. The success rate is nearly 100 percent.

In the other procedure, atrioventricular nodal modification, the electrophysiologist uses radiofrequency ablation to modify the part of the atrioventricular node causing atrial fibrillation because its electrical circuit activates too frequently. This procedure is about 50 percent effective.

Focal (point of origin) sources of atrial fibrillation can also be treated with radiofrequency catheter ablation. This procedure is used both to identify and remove the areas that trigger the atrial fibrillation. These areas are usually located at the pulmonary veins and other venous junctions to the heart. Ablation of these sites can eliminate the atrial fibrillation or make resistant cases able to be treated with medications.

A surgical treatment alternative is the maze procedure. In this procedure, the surgeon makes multiple incisions in the atrium to form a path or maze through which the electrical impulses from the sinus node can travel to reach the atrioventricular node. This process can prevent atrial fibrillation.

Prevent Abnormal Heart Function. People who experience prolonged atrial fibrillation are at risk for atrial enlargement, or the atrium stretching out. When a chamber of the heart becomes enlarged, that chamber is less able to pump blood efficiently. Atrial enlargement also increases the risk of developing abnormal pathways on which the arrhythmia can continue. When this happens, the atrial fibrillation is less likely to stop on its own, and persistent atrial fibrillation is more likely to develop. Treating the arrhythmia with medications, ablation, or surgical interventions may help prevent atrial enlargement.

Atrial Flutter

Like atrial fibrillation, this tachycardia originates in the atria. It differs from atrial fibrillation because it tends to cause more regular atrial contractions, occurring usually at rates between 200 and 300 per minute. Doctors distinguish atrial flutter from atrial fibrillation on an ECG because atrial flutter typically produces "saw tooth" waves.

The incidence of atrial flutter is not known. Various studies have reported different figures: the incidence could be as high as one in every 81 people (about 1.2 percent) or as low as one in every 238 people (less than 0.5 percent). Doctors do know that nearly five times as many men have atrial flutter as do women. While atrial flutter can occur in people with abnormalities to their atria, it can also occur in people with normal atria. Like many arrhythmias, it occurs more commonly in the first weeks after open-heart surgery; approximately 10 percent of open-heart surgery patients experience this complication.

Doctors often call atrial flutter a "nuisance" arrhythmia. Its seriousness increases when it occurs in conjunction with atrial fibrillation: Some people alternate between periods of atrial flutter and atrial fibrillation. In addition, some people with atrial flutter develop a rapid ventricular rate. When people with atrial flutter have frequent periods of a rapid ventricular rate, their ventricle can dilate causing a condition called cardiomyopathy. Because an enlarged ventricle cannot pump blood as effectively as a normal ventricle, these people are at increased risk of developing congestive heart failure.

Symptoms, which typically develop in a person who has a rapid ventricular rate, include palpitations, lightheadedness, dizziness, shortness of breath, weakness, faintness, and sometimes syncope. If the ventricular rate becomes very rapid, a person may also experience angina (chest pain), especially if underlying coronary artery disease is present.

Cardiologists divide atrial flutter into type I and II, based on how fast the heart beats during an episode and how easy it is to stop the rapid rhythm. Type I flutter is slower and easier to interrupt, while type II is faster (as fast as 300 beats per minute) and more difficult to stop.

Atrial flutter commonly occurs after cardiac surgery, especially after procedures to repair congenital defects. Such surgeries may create a lesion, or scar, in a critical place in the heart's electrical circuitry. With atrial flutter, a scar allows the electrical impulse to re-enter, or start over again repeatedly, rather than to travel along an appropriate pathway. When the electrical signal re-enters, it creates the rapid twitching characteristic of atrial flutter.

Treatment strategies are similar to those of atrial fibrillation and are often instituted to correct the atrial fibrillation that alternates with flutter. Doctors may prescribe anticoagulant therapy to prevent the risk of stroke that occurs with atrial fibrillation. Radiofrequency ablation is useful for type I atrial flutter, with a success rate of over 90 percent.

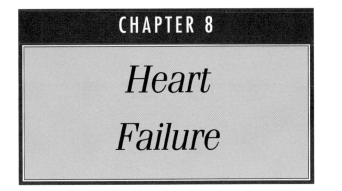

CHAPTER 8

Heart Failure

Introduction

The term "heart failure" can sound frightening. However, having heart failure does not mean that your heart has literally failed or that the outcome is dismal—the spectrum of heart failure is wide. What the diagnosis means is that although the myocardium, or heart muscle, continues to work, it cannot continue to pump efficiently enough to keep up with the demands of the body's organs for oxygen-rich blood.

In fact, heart failure is not a distinct disease but rather a description of what happens when the myocardium loses its ability to do its job in an efficient manner. Key aspects of heart failure are weaker contractions, cardiac remodeling (an enlarged misshapen heart), and an increase in blood volume, leading to an excess of fluid in the veins, organs, and tissues (congestive heart failure).

- *Weaker contractions.* When the heart's efficiency decreases, the strength of the heart's contractions diminish, reducing the amount of blood pumped out into the body's tissues. In addition, the myocardium may have trouble emptying out all of the blood it receives, causing the ventricles—the pumping chambers—to retain too much fluid and, as a result, to become enlarged.

- *Cardiac remodeling.* Whenever the heart's ability to function is impaired, the muscle must work at an accelerated pace in order to compensate for its diminished capability. As healthy cells take on the work of damaged ones, metabolism changes, and cells grow larger, or hypertrophy. Often, the entire heart becomes oversized, muscular, and misshapen and the valves become less competent and leak. When this happens, the heart is said to have remodeled itself. But even with these changes the heart is unable to pump blood efficiently and continues to deteriorate. Compared with a healthy heart muscle, which resembles a small, pink fist, the failing heart may appear gray, distorted, and enlarged. It can weigh twice as much as a healthy heart, perhaps a pound and a half.

■ *Increase in blood volume.* In addition, because heart failure means that less blood flows through the vascular system, the body tries to compensate by increasing blood volume. When the amount of blood that reaches the kidneys decreases, the adrenal glands are stimulated to secrete a hormone called aldosterone. This, in turn, prompts the body to retain water and sodium as a way of increasing volume. At the same time, the kidneys' ability to rid the body of sodium and water is inhibited.

■ *Congestive heart failure.* Consequently, fluid can build up in the body—hence the term "congestive heart failure." Because the failing heart pumps blood out with less force than is required, returning blood can back up and become congested in the veins and tissues. Weakness on the right side of the heart causes congestion in the legs, liver, and gastrointestinal tract, which causes edema, or swelling, in the lower legs, ankles, and abdomen, and loss of appetite. If the weakness is on the left side of the heart, fluid can collect in the lungs, causing breathing difficulties. This condition is called pulmonary edema. In many cases, the entire myocardium is weakened, and fluid can back up in the lungs as well as in the extremities.

However, with early diagnosis and treatment, the workload on the heart can be eased sufficiently to reduce symptoms and reverse heart failure. With timely and aggressive treatment, people with heart failure can live relatively active lives many years after the diagnosis is made.

Signs and Symptoms

Although patients with heart failure may have no symptoms at first, several problems can arise as the syndrome progresses. The signs and symptoms of heart failure generally fall into two categories: forward failure and backward failure.

The symptoms of forward failure are a product of poor cardiac output, the heart's inability to pump the blood with sufficient force to the body's tissues; they include weakness, fatigue, and a general sense of feeling unwell.

The symptoms of backward failure are a product of fluid congestion in the tissues; they include breathlessness, cough, and swelling in the feet, ankles, legs, or stomach. In congestive heart failure, the weakened

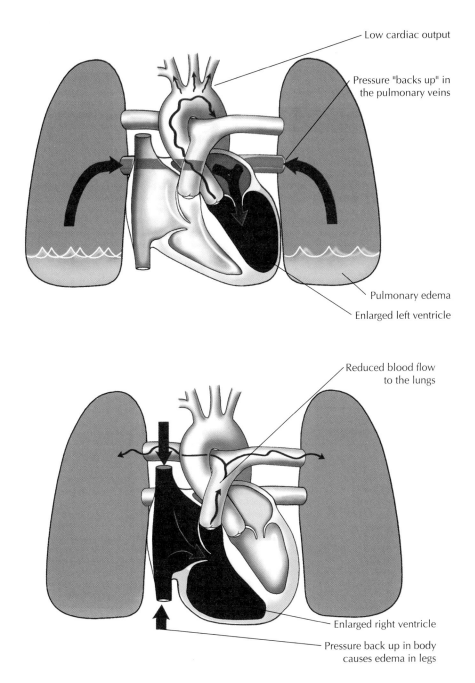

Low cardiac output

Pressure "backs up" in the pulmonary veins

Pulmonary edema

Enlarged left ventricle

Reduced blood flow to the lungs

Enlarged right ventricle

Pressure back up in body causes edema in legs

Congestive heart failure. When the right side of the heart becomes weakened, blood flow to the lungs is reduced and blood waiting to enter the right atrium from the veins of the body becomes backed up. This back up causes edema (swelling) in the lower extremities. Weakness of the left side of the heart means that blood returning from the lungs is backed up waiting to enter the left atrium. Pulmonary edema, or congestion in the lungs, and low cardiac output to the body results. In many cases, both right and left side congestive heart failure exist.

heart cannot keep fluids moving through the body, so fluid pools, especially in the lungs, causing breathing difficulties. Edema, or swelling, in the legs, ankles, and feet and ascites, or swelling in the abdomen, can also result. When fluid accumulates, weight gain can occur as well.

The stages of heart failure are classified as stage I, II, III, and IV. In the early stages of congestive heart failure, the most common signs and symptoms—breathlessness, weakness, fatigue, cough, and swelling—may not be noted. Over time, however, as the condition progresses, symptoms typically become more severe. A person suffering from heart failure may find that any exertion causes exhaustion and shortness of breath. Even routine activities can bring on feelings of weakness. Breathing may be labored, especially when lying down. When breathing is constricted, feelings of dread and anxiety may be experienced. In addition, sometimes people with congestive heart failure awaken from their sleep feeling as if they are being smothered.

By the time the condition progresses to its most serious form, stage IV, a person may become virtually housebound. Because fluid pools in the

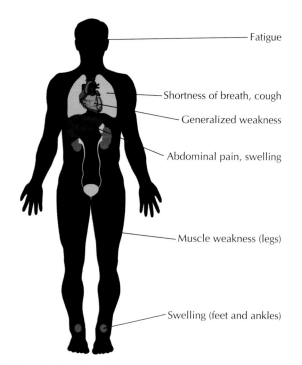

Symptoms of heart failure. Reduced cardiac output to the tissues of the body causes fatigue, generalized weakness, and shortness of breath. Congestion (fluid buildup) in the body and lungs causes swelling of the lower extremities and abdominal cavity and cough. (Adapted with permission from *Cleveland Clinic Heart Advisor*, Vol. 2, No. 5, May 1999, Torstar Publications Inc. All rights reserved.)

lungs when a person lies down, breathing may become more difficult during rest and sleep. Sleeping may be possible only in a sitting position or with the body propped up by pillows. Occasionally, blood and mucus are coughed up. In this advanced stage, the symptoms of heart failure often necessitate frequent visits to a hospital emergency room or extended hospital stays.

Heart failure is a serious, progressive condition. In the United States, an estimated 5 million people have been diagnosed with some form of heart failure, and the number of new cases has increased significantly in recent years—approximately 400,000 new cases are diagnosed each year. Approximately 2 million people have chronic congestive heart failure. In fact, heart failure is the only type of heart disease on the rise in the United States.

This increased incidence of heart failure is partly a reflection of the fact that, in general, people in the United States are living longer. Since the beginning of the twentieth century, longevity has increased by approximately 28 years. In 1994 there were 33.2 million Americans over the age of 65. This number is expected to more than double to 70.2 million in the year 2030. The number of people over the age of 75 is expected to triple during the first half of the twenty-first century.

The Aging Heart

Aging brings with it inevitable changes to the cardiovascular system. The heart's weight increases. The ventricular septum thickens, the ventricular chamber becomes smaller, and the left ventricle, the heart's major pumping chamber, becomes thicker and more muscular. The connective tissue in the myocardium becomes more rigid. The aorta, the major artery leading away from the heart, becomes progressively dilated and elongated.

These changes are affected by genetic factors and exacerbated by years of physical inactivity, poor diet, poorly controlled hypertension and diabetes, and smoking. Over time, they generally translate into a heart muscle that is less elastic and less flexible. Furthermore, as the aorta dilates and elongates, the pressure increases during systole (when blood is pumped out of the heart). This taxes the left ventricle as it works to propel blood out to the body's tissues.

In addition to inevitable age-related increase, the increased incidence of heart failure in the United States is a by-product of other medical success stories. Deaths from coronary artery disease (CAD) have declined in recent years. More people are surviving other forms of heart disease. Whenever the ability of the heart to function has been adversely affected by a previous heart disease, by other conditions, or by the aging process itself, the chances are greater that the heart will grow less efficient and show signs of failure.

Heart failure is most common in people over the age of 70. It is the leading cause of hospitalization among older people. Yet, a million of those who suffer from heart failure are younger than 60 years of age. In 1996, 43,837 Americans died of heart failure.

In addition, left untreated, heart failure can shave years off a person's life or diminish the quality of life considerably. Survival after a diagnosis of heart failure presents a mixed picture. Twenty percent of those diagnosed with heart failure die within a year, and 50 percent die within 5 years. Those who survive are six to nine times more likely to die suddenly from disturbances in heart rhythm brought on by heart failure than are those who do not have heart failure.

At the same time, the latest figures show that fewer people are dying from congestive heart failure in recent years. The decline in deaths from heart failure is related to effective strategies for preventing and treating the condition. Better and more timely treatment for people having heart attacks, for example, appears to prevent the loss of heart muscle that can lead to congestive heart failure. Also, more people are taking aggressive steps to improve their heart health in general.

Causes

Heart failure is not a distinct disease. Rather, it is a secondary condition that results when the myocardium has sustained injury or been weakened as a result of another, underlying disease or condition. The most common causes of heart failure are

- Coronary artery disease (CAD; narrowing of the arteries of the heart)
- Previous myocardial infarction (heart attack)
- Hypertension (high blood pressure)
- Valve disease
- Congenital heart disease
- Cardiomyopathy, a disease of the myocardium
- Endocarditis, an infection of the heart valves
- Myocarditis, an infection of the myocardium
- Diabetes

Coronary Artery Disease

Whenever blood flow to the heart is lessened because the arteries that supply blood to the myocardium have narrowed, the heart's function diminishes. While CAD usually begins at an early age, congestive heart failure occurs mostly in older people. In the United States, 8 out of 1,000 people over 70 years old are diagnosed with congestive heart failure each year. Most of these are women, probably because men are more likely to die from CAD before it advances to heart failure.

Conversely, when people lower their risk of CAD by controlling blood cholesterol levels, blood pressure, and diabetes and by exercising more frequently, adopting healthy eating habits, and not smoking, they substantially lower their risk of developing heart failure.

Previous Myocardial Infarction

Many people who would have died only a decade ago from an acute myocardial infarction (heart attack) survive today because of advances in treatment. The increased incidence of heart failure reflects the success of treatment for more acute heart problems. A past myocardial infarction creates scar tissue on the muscle that interferes with its normal functioning. People who survive myocardial infarctions are often left with hearts that have trouble keeping up with the body's demands.

Hypertension

Three-quarters of all people with heart failure have hypertension (high blood pressure), which means that the heart has to work harder to pump the blood throughout the body. Over time, this can weaken the heart. And because fewer than one in three people have their high blood pressure under control, hypertension-related congestive heart failure is on the rise.

On the other hand, increased public awareness of the importance of controlling hypertension, together with the availability of new hypertension medications that carry fewer side effects, means that more people are able and willing to control high blood pressure and thereby avert heart failure.

Valve Disease

Whenever the heart valves do not work properly, the heart has to work harder. In the past, rheumatic fever was the most common cause of valve disease. Antibiotics have all but relegated rheumatic fever to the past. Today, valve disease most commonly arises from congenital defects or age-related degeneration of the valves. Other causes include infective endocarditis (an infection of the lining of the the heart valves; see page 113), and calcification (a calcium buildup on the valves).

Congenital Heart Disease

Although most congenital heart defects are diagnosed and corrected early, usually in childhood, it is possible to have a congenital heart disease without being aware of it. When that is the case, serious muscle damage can be sustained over time. For more information on congenital heart disease, see Chapter 10, Pediatric and Congenital Heart Disease.

Cardiomyopathy

Cardiomyopathy is a degenerative disease of the myocardium. Most forms of cardiomyopathy are labeled "idiopathic," meaning the precise reason for its development cannot be determined. Cardiomyopathy can sometimes be linked to heredity, to excessive alcohol intake, and to viral infections. Primary cardiomyopathy is not a result of another condition such as hypertension, valve disease, artery diseases, or congenital heart defects. Secondary cardiomyopathy is a symptom of another identifiable condition, generally involving other organs as well as the heart.

There are three types of cardiomyopathy: dilated cardiomyopathy, hypertrophic cardiomyopathy, and restrictive cardiomyopathy.

Dilated Cardiomyopathy

Dilated cardiomyopathy is the most common type of cardiomyopathy. When the heart cavity becomes stretched and enlarged (cardiac dilation), the myocardium becomes weak and cannot pump adequately. Consequently, congestive heart failure and arrhythmias (disturbances in the heart's electrical impulses) can develop.

In cases involving significant cardiac dilation caused by cardiomyopathy, the leaflets of the mitral and tricuspid valves may not be able to close tightly enough. This can cause leaks, prompting a heart murmur.

Because blood flow naturally slows through an enlarged heart, thrombi (or blood clots) sometimes form. Sometimes, thrombi break free and these free-floating clots (or emboli) travel and become lodged in a small blood vessel elsewhere in the body. When thrombi adhere to the inner lining of the heart, they are called mural thrombi. Thrombi that form in the right ventricle occasionally break off and travel through the pulmonary circulation into the lung, forming pulmonary emboli.

If a thrombus detaches in the left side of the heart, it can be carried through the circulation to the brain, where it forms a cerebral embolus, which can cause a stroke. Thrombi also travel to form emboli in the kidneys, peripheral arteries, or coronary arteries. A person with cardiomyopathy may experience an embolus before any other symptoms appear.

When the primary symptom is the appearance of an embolus, anticoagulant (anticlotting) medication may be needed. Arrhythmias (disorders in the heart's rhythm) will sometimes be treated with antiarrhythmic drugs or implantable defibrillators (a device that delivers shock to the heart to help restore normal heart rhythm). Increased blood pressure is treated with vasodilating agents to relax the arteries. By lowering blood pressure, these medications decrease the workload on the left ventricle (see page 91).

In rare cases, a heart block (see page 148) develops because the heart's ability to conduct electrical excitation is impaired. When this happens, an artificial pacemaker may be needed (see page 145). For some people with progressive cardiomyopathy, a heart transplant may be considered. Alternative surgical procedures for this condition are also being developed.

Hypertrophic Cardiomyopathy

The second most common form of cardiomyopathy, hypertrophic cardio-myopathy, involves an abnormally large left ventricular muscle. In some cases in which the septum, the wall between the two ventricles, is also enlarged, the syndrome is known as hypertrophic obstructive cardiomy-opathy, asymmetric septal hypertrophy, or idiopathic hypertrophic subaortic stenosis. The thickened wall obstructs the blood flow from the left ventricle. Occasionally this will distort one leaflet of the mitral valve, resulting in leakage.

At the same time, a person may have an enlarged septum with no symptoms. In more than one-half of all cases, this form of the disease is hereditary: It is the most common cardiomyopathy in young adults. When the septum is not enlarged, the condition is called nonobstructive hypertrophic cardiomyopathy; the enlarged muscle usually does not interfere directly with blood flow.

The symptoms of hypertrophic cardiomyopathy include shortness of breath on exertion, dizziness, fainting, and angina pectoris (chest pain). As the blood flow from the left ventricle is obstructed, the heart is forced to increase its pace. An abnormal sound or heart murmur may develop, indicating a functional or structural problem. Some people experience cardiac arrhythmias (abnormal heart rhythms).

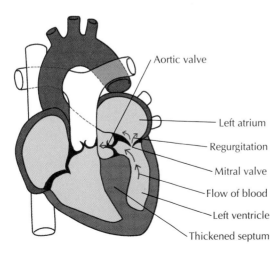

Aortic valve

Left atrium

Regurgitation

Mitral valve

Flow of blood

Left ventricle

Thickened septum

Hypertrophic obstructive car-diomyopathy. The left ventricle muscle and the wall of the sep-tum are enlarged. The enlarged septum causes an obstruction to blood flowing out of the left ventricle, reducing cardiac out-put to the body. The mitral valve may be unable to close tightly due to the enlarged septum causing regurgitation (leaking). (Adapted with permission from *Cleveland Clinic Heart Advisor*, Vol. 2, No. 5, May 1999, Torstar Publications, Inc. All rights reserved.)

Hypertrophic cardiomyopathy is usually treated with beta blockers (see page 171) or calcium-channel blockers (see page 92). If an arrhythmia develops, an antiarrhythmic drug may also be prescribed. Occasionally, surgery to correct the obstructive form may be recommended, especially if medication does not relieve the symptoms.

Restrictive Cardiomyopathy

Restrictive cardiomyopathy, in which the ventricle muscle becomes rigid, is the least common type of cardiomyopathy in the United States. When muscle loses flexibility, the blood does not flow smoothly into the ventricles. Almost always the result of another disease, restrictive cardiomyopathy produces exhaustion, swelling, and difficulty breathing on exertion. Symptoms are usually treated with diuretics (see page 170), but the cardiomyopathy itself is best treated, if possible, by correcting the underlying condition.

Infective Endocarditis

Endocarditis is a relatively rare but serious infection of the endocardium (lining of the heart) or heart valves (see also page 113). Whenever the infection and the resulting inflammation persist, the heart works less efficiently, putting it at risk of congestive heart failure.

Endocarditis occurs when bacteria in the bloodstream lodge on endothelial tissue (the inner surface of blood vessels) that has already been damaged. Endocarditis rarely occurs unless the heart tissue has already been injured by a congenital defect, disease, or previous treatment for heart disease. In the past, people who suffered from rheumatic heart disease (see page 118) were most at risk of infective endocarditis. With the decline in the incidence of rheumatic fever, children with congenital heart defects have become the most likely to contract endocarditis.

Yet any type of heart or valve defect places a person at any age at risk. People with a history of endocarditis or hypertrophic cardiomyopathy (see page 165) and people with replacement heart valves, aortopulmonary shunts, surgical patches, or permanent catheters are at increased risk of this infection.

Symptoms of endocarditis include an unexplained fever, loss of appetite, malaise, headache, and joint pain. Rapid diagnosis and treatment are essential. A medical examination will likely reveal a new heart murmur. A complete evaluation requires blood cultures and echocardiography (see page 168).

The prognosis is linked to prompt diagnosis and treatment, which as a rule involves antibiotics. In addition, because endocarditis can be contracted during certain dental or surgical procedures, doctors often recommend that people at high risk take antibiotics as a preventive measure before undergoing such procedures.

Myocarditis

Myocarditis is an inflammation of the myocardium, or heart muscle. It can be caused by a number of factors including a viral, bacterial, or fungal infection, toxic drug poisoning, or other diseases (such as rheumatic fever, diphtheria, or tuberculosis).

When the heart becomes inflamed, it is unable to pump blood efficiently. This can lead to congestive heart failure (see page 158), dilated cardiomyopathy (see page 164), and, in rare instances, sudden cardiac failure. In addition, certain bacterial infections can linger in the body for months or years, causing chronic inflammation, weakening the artery walls, and creating abrasions and blockages. As such, myocarditis can lead to acute myocardial ischemia (reduced oxygen to the heart muscle) and myocardial infarction (heart attack), even when there are no other signs of heart disease.

Myocarditis may develop after a flu-like illness or stomach virus. Symptoms of acute myocarditis resemble those of mild to moderate congestive heart failure, specifically left ventricular dysfunction—breathing difficulties, swelling, and exhaustion. In many cases, atrial or ventricular arrhythmias develop. Prompt diagnosis and treatment are important.

A complete evaluation includes blood tests, an electrocardiogram (ECG or EKG), and an echocardiogram (see page 168). A chest x-ray may show pulmonary edema, an accumulation of fluid in the lungs. In some cases, cardiac catheterization (see page 168) and endomyocardial biopsy (see page 169) are necessary to confirm a diagnosis of myocarditis. Myocarditis is usually treated with analgesics (pain relievers) or anti-inflammatory drugs. If myocarditis is due to a bacterial infection, antibiotics are also prescribed. Diuretics, digoxin, and angiotensin-converting enzyme (ACE) inhibitors are generally prescribed to facilitate blood flow and thereby relieve symptoms. Sometimes beta blockers are used as well. (see Medications, page 170)

Diabetes

Almost 16 million Americans have diabetes. This serious condition interferes with the body's ability to produce or respond to insulin, the hormone that allows cells to absorb sugar from the blood and use it for energy. Although the connection between CAD and diabetes has long been recognized, recent studies indicate that diabetes has a serious impact on the left ventricle, the heart's main pumping chamber, putting people with the disease at risk of congestive heart failure. Also, people with diabetes who have CAD are more likely than nondiabetics to develop heart failure after cardiac ischemia (reduced blood flow and consequently reduced oxygen to the heart). In addition, because diabetes can cause neuropathy (damage to nerve fibers), symptoms that would otherwise alert them to heart problems, in particular angina (chest pain), may not be so noticeable. It is therefore crucial that people with diabetes undergo regular cardiac evaluations and report any atypical symptoms, such as sweating, nausea, vomiting, shortness of breath, and fatigue, to their physicians at once.

Other Causes

Other factors that put the myocardium at risk are alcoholism, drug abuse (primarily cocaine and amphetamines), hyperthyroidism, chronic lung diseases such as emphysema, genetic disorders, rheumatic fever, chemotherapy for cancer, and viral and other infections.

Detection and Diagnosis

Prevention and early treatment are essential to limit the effects of heart failure. Because heart failure is a collection of symptoms rather than a disease, diagnosis and treatment can be challenging. Nevertheless, the sooner a diagnosis is made, the sooner treatment can begin. Timely treatment increases the chances that, although weakened, the heart muscle will be able to function more efficiently.

Once the signs and symptoms of congestive heart failure—swollen legs or ankles, difficulty breathing, weight gain due to fluid retention— are reported, the doctor begins a process not only to diagnose heart failure but also to discover its underlying cause. Improved technology has made it possible to detect even mild decreases in heart function early and therefore to treat them immediately and aggressively.

Beginning with a stethoscopic examination, the doctor listens for sounds that suggest congestive heart disease. Signs that could indicate kidney problems are noted, such as swollen veins in the neck, an enlarged liver, and edema (swelling) of the feet. Blood and urine tests are ordered, and other tests are likely to be recommended.

- *Electrocardiogram (ECG or EKG)* monitors heart rhythms and detects signs of damage from previous myocardial infarctions.

- *Chest x-ray* detects an enlarged or remodeled heart as well as congested lungs.

- *Echocardiography* uses ultrasound to detect myocardial or valve problems.

- *Cardiac catheterization,* in which a catheter (a thin plastic tube) is threaded through an artery or vein in the arm or leg and then into the heart, measures the pumping ability of the myocardium, checks for congenital cardiac defects, and determines coronary anatomy.

- *Magnetic resonance imaging (MRI)* uses powerful magnets to create computer-generated pictures of the myocardium. This diagnostic technique can identify residual damage from a myocardial infarction as well as congenital heart defects that may result in deteriorating heart function. In addition, MRI can diagnose myocardial diseases, especially those affecting the right ventricle.

- *Nuclear scanning tests,* involve injecting radioactive tracers into the blood that highlight the interior of the heart. Computer-generated images detail how efficiently the myocardium is supplied with blood and how well the heart's chambers are functioning. Some types of scans also identify any parts of the heart that are damaged by myocardial infarction.

- *Stress tests* use exercise or specific medications to stimulate the heart beyond normal activity, so that its level of functioning can be measured. A heart muscle that is deteriorating shows diminished capacity when stressed.

- *Pulmonary function tests* help diagnose and evaluate a number of lung diseases, including pulmonary edema. There are two general types of pulmonary function tests—ventilation tests and arterial blood gas studies.

  Ventilation tests, often performed in a doctor's office, outpatient clinic, or a hospital pulmonary-function laboratory, use a spirometer to measure lung function. Also called spirometry, from the Greek "to measure breathing," a ventilation test measures the volume and the flow rate of air moving in and out of the lungs. A person breathes into a tube connected to a spirometer. After inhaling deeply, the person exhales as quickly and forcefully as possible into the machine. Three readings are usually taken to provide an accurate measure.

  Arterial blood gas studies measure how well blood is filtered and oxygenated as it passes through the lungs. This blood test is done in an outpatient laboratory, a hospital, or a pulmonary function laboratory.

- *Cardiopulmonary exercise and metabolic testing* combine stress tests and pulmonary function tests to determine whether breathing difficulties are due to cardiac (heart) or pulmonary (lung) problems. This diagnostic procedure can be particularly helpful in identifying myocardial disease. Also, after a person has been diagnosed with heart failure, cardiopulmonary exercise and metabolic testing can be helpful in evaluating exercise capacity and response to therapy; this is especially important in people being considered for heart transplantation. During cardiopulmonary exercise testing, a person pedals a bicycle or walks on a treadmill as resistance increases. While on the bike or treadmill, the person breathes into and out of a tube connected to a spirometer. Metabolic testing offers a number of measurements taken during exercise, including heart rate, ECG, blood pressure, the amount of oxygen consumed, and the amount of carbon dioxide produced.

■ *Biopsy* involves the surgical removal of small pieces of tissue that are then examined under a microscope for signs of disease.

For more information on diagnostic testing, see Chapter 4, Diagnosing Heart Disease.

Treatment

A diagnosis of heart failure will necessitate lifestyle changes. A balance should be struck between rest, to conserve energy and avoid overtaxing the heart, and appropriate exercise, to ensure healthy circulation. A diet low in sodium and fat that allows a healthy weight to be achieved and maintained is essential to keeping the heart working as efficiently as possible.

In addition to such lifestyle modifications, specific medical treatment is usually needed to reduce symptoms and to help maintain a reasonable level of activity.

When the underlying condition is identified, it will be treated or, if possible, corrected.

Medications

A variety of medications are now available to help a weakened heart work more efficiently, reduce symptoms dramatically, and ease much of the limitations and distress caused by the syndrome. Some drugs actually improve survival rates for people with heart failure. Different drugs work in different ways, and medications are often prescribed in combination.

Diuretics

Diuretics, which have been used for several decades, help the kidneys rid the body of excess water and sodium, thereby decreasing blood volume and the heart's workload. This, in turn, reduces swelling throughout the body and helps eliminate fluid in the air spaces of the lungs. Diuretics prompt more frequent urination. They should only be used when congestive heart failure is a problem. Because potassium and magnesium can be lost as a result, dietary supplements of these minerals may be needed.

A 30-year-old diuretic, spironolactone (Aldactone), once routinely used in the treatment of heart failure, has recently proved effective in improving symptoms and reducing fatalities by nearly one-third when used in combination with other heart-failure medications. Spironolactone blocks production of the hormone aldosterone, which plays a key role in the development of heart failure.

Digitalis

Digitalis is the active ingredient in the purple foxglove plant. It has been used for hundreds of years to treat heart failure and is still prescribed.

Because digitalis causes the heart to beat more slowly and forcefully, it improves circulation and helps reduce the accumulation of fluid in the lungs and extremities. Often, digitalis and diuretics are prescribed together.

ACE Inhibitors

Angiotensin-converting enzyme (ACE) inhibitors are now believed to be the first line of treatment in most heart failure cases: Most heart failure patients are on these medications. ACE inhibitors help control symptoms and may slow the advance of the disease. These drugs block adverse effects of certain hormones that increase in response to heart failure and lighten the heart's load by dilating blood vessels and reducing the body's tendency to retain salt and water. Whenever blood vessels are relaxed, blood flows more smoothly, lightening the amount of work needed for the heart to pump blood out to the tissues and lowering blood pressure.

Developed during the 1980s, ACE inhibitors have become the keystone for treating heart failure. ACE inhibitors, such as captopril (Capoten) and enalapril (Vasotec), work to expand blood vessels and decrease resistance, facilitating blood flow. Specifically, these medications (also called vasodilators) block the production of a substance called angiotensin II, a powerful blood vessel constrictor. ACE inhibitors also seem to slow heart enlargement.

Beta Blockers

Until recently, beta blockers were not recommended for people with heart failure. However, new studies indicate that these drugs, which block stimulation by the hormone epinephrine (adrenaline), slow and stabilize heart rhythm and improve the function of the left ventricle. Beta blockers are often used in combination with diuretics, digoxin, and ACE inhibitors for patients with mild to moderate or severe congestive heart failure.

Carvedilol (Coreg) was the first beta blocker approved to treat congestive heart failure. It appears to slow the progression of heart failure significantly and improves life expectancy. Carvedilol exerts both beta-blocking and vasodilating effects. This medication is used for patients with mild to moderate congestive heart failure but not for those with severe, unstable heart failure, troublesome asthma, severe bradycardia (slow heartbeat) or electrical conduction disorders (see Chapter 7, Rhythm Disorders). It occasionally causes such side effects as dizziness, bradycardia, hypotension (low blood pressure), or signs of worsening heart failure.

Inotropic Drugs

In recent years, a number of drugs that work by increasing the force of heart muscle contractions and thereby facilitating the heart's pumping function have been tested to treat heart failure. These drugs are called inotropic drugs.

When heart failure is severe and chronic, intravenous (through a vein) treatment with inotropic drugs is often used during hospitalization. Specifically, intravenous dobutamine and nitroprusside infusions seem to improve the ability of the heart to fill with blood and then to pump blood back to the body's tissues. When given intravenously, dobutamine may improve heart function for weeks or even months.

Digoxin was previously classified as an inotropic drug, but it is now thought to work by other mechanisms than by affecting heart muscle contractions. It can be taken orally and has been found to decrease the need for hospitalization in more advanced cases of heart failure.

Hydralazine

Hydralazine (Apresoline) is used to treat heart failure. It lowers blood pressure and eases blood flow by relaxing the blood vessels. It is usually taken regularly, two to four times a day. Although uncommon, side effects can occur, including headache; rapid, irregular, or pounding heartbeat; numbness or tingling of the fingers or toes; loss of appetite; and diarrhea. More serious side effects include fever, joint or chest pain, sore throat, skin rash (especially on the face), unusual bleeding or bruising, weight gain, and swelling of the ankles. If these occur, contact your doctor immediately.

Nitrates

Nitrates are used to relax blood vessels, easing the demand on the heart muscle. Nitrates come in many forms, including small pills that are placed under the tongue, sprays that are atomized under the tongue, and patches that are applied to the skin. The most common side effect is headache, which can occur when the blood vessels in the head relax. Because nitrates cause blood pressure to drop, they can produce dizziness, flushing, and a pounding or racing heartbeat.

Angiotensin II Receptor-Blockers

A new class of medications, angiotensin II receptor-blocking drugs (ARBs), offers similar promise in treating congestive heart failure, without producing the coughing that sometimes occurs with ACE inhibitors. These medications include losartan (Cozaar), valsartan (Diovan), irbesartan (Avapro), candesartan (Atacand), and eprosartan (Teveten). Angiotension II causes the muscles of the arteries and capillaries to contract, thus increasing the resistance to blood flow and elevating blood pressure. ARBs block the effect of angiotensin II on blood vessel walls and in that way effectively lower blood pressure without lowering heart rate.

Electrolyte Deficiency and Medication Use

Some of the medications used most commonly to treat heart failure—specifically diuretics, which counteract water and sodium retention—cause increased urination. This causes loss of potassium and other minerals. Potassium, a dietary mineral and electrolyte, is needed to maintain a healthy water balance within the body's cells. In addition, potassium ensures that cellular enzymes work properly, and nerves respond appropriately to stimuli. Potassium also plays an important role in the muscles' ability to contract.

To combat potassium deficiency, doctors suggest a diet high in potassium, as long as the kidneys are functioning relatively normally. Foods high in potassium include bananas, cantaloupe, honeydew, prunes, grapefruit, oranges, tomato or prune juice, molasses, and potatoes. When dietary considerations are not enough to compensate for the deficiency, additional potassium may be prescribed in supplement form. ACE inhibitors, spironolactone, and ARBs (see page 172) can help increase potassium levels as well.

Left Ventricular Assist Devices

When the heart has become so damaged that medications cannot relieve the symptoms, a surgical approach—such as heart transplant—may be considered. Occasionally, heart failure can progress so quickly that heart function begins to deteriorate dangerously. Waiting for an appropriate replacement heart can pose the possibility of serious disability and perhaps fatality. A cardiologist may recommend the use of left ventricular assist devices (LVADs), essentially a partial artificial heart, as a way of prolonging life.

Currently used as a bridge to a heart transplant, these electrically powered pumps are implanted in the abdomen just below the heart. The blood is pumped from the left ventricle through a pipe and back out through another tube that feeds into the aorta. An LVAD is powered by a cable that passes through the wearer's skin. It is either plugged into an outlet or connected to a battery pack.

Since the cable runs through the skin, it carries a risk of infection. Also, pump failures can occur. Nevertheless, the use of LVADs has been life-saving for people with heart failure who are awaiting a heart transplant. In the future, these pumps may offer patients the option of using the pump on a long-term basis rather than as a bridge to transplant (see Cardiac Transplantation, page 175).

Surgery

Besides medication, surgery is an additional important treatment option for many people with heart failure. When congestive heart failure has been caused or exacerbated by a weak heart valve, repairing or replacing

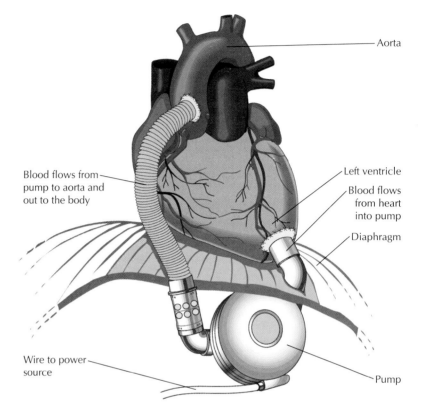

Left ventricular assist device (LVAD). While patients who need a heart transplant wait for a donor heart to be found, they may require an LVAD to be implanted to keep their heart functioning. This device assists the left ventricle in pumping blood out to the body. The LVAD is implanted in the abdomen just below the heart with a tube connecting to the left ventricle and another tube connecting to the aorta. Blood flows from the left ventricle through the tube and into the pump. The pump sends blood through the second tube and into the aorta for distribution throughout the body. (Adapted with permission from *Cleveland Clinic Heart Advisor*, Vol. 2, No. 6, June 1999, Torstar Publications Inc. All rights reserved.)

the damaged valves can be helpful (see page 122). When there is a leak between heart chambers or damaged cardiac tissue interferes with the heart's efficiency, surgery to repair heart tissues may be advised.

When appropriate, surgery is performed to repair left ventricular aneurysms, thin bulging spots of the heart that have formed, usually as a result of scarring from a myocardial infarction. Coronary artery bypass graft (CABG) surgery (see page 100) or sometimes balloon angioplasty (see page 96) can be used to prevent and treat heart failure caused by blocked arteries. Indeed, CABG is the most often performed surgical procedure to treat heart failure. However, when the heart has been severely damaged or its efficiency severely limited, the best option may be heart transplant.

Cardiac Transplantation

For people with serious and irreversible heart failure, exchanging a diseased heart for a healthy donor heart can offer the promise not only of survival but also of returning to a relatively normal life.

The first human heart transplant was performed in December 1967. Since then, the procedure has become an established treatment for advanced heart disease. Each year, approximately 2,300 heart transplants are performed in the United States. About 75 percent of heart transplant patients are male, 85 percent are white, 51 percent are aged 50 to 64, and 20 percent are aged 35 to 49.

Cardiac transplantation is considered for an otherwise healthy patient whose heart is failing and for whom other types of therapy have not been successful in relieving symptoms and reversing the progressive deterioration in heart function. Candidates for cardiac transplantation are generally bedridden and require intravenous inotropic drugs in order to remain in stable condition.

Contraindications to Cardiac Transplantation.

Because there is a critical shortage of donor organs, cardiac transplantation is generally limited to those patients who are both most disabled by heart failure and most likely to benefit from a new heart. There are certain conditions—called comorbid conditions, or contraindications—that tend to negatively affect both the survival and health of the patient after transplantation, and patients who have any of these conditions are often not considered as transplant candidates. For example, the existence of certain diseases (such as an active form of cancer) may be a contraindication. During the process of evaluating a person's suitability for transplantation, the doctor considers the patient's risk of death without a heart transplant and weighs that against the presence and severity of other potential contraindications to cardiac transplantation.

The following is a list of major contraindications:

- *Age,* over 55, especially if accompanied by other contraindications.

- *Pulmonary vascular hypertension:* Long-standing heart failure can cause significant pulmonary vascular hypertension (increased pressure in the pulmonary artery), a condition that can cause serious complications within the first year after cardiac transplantation.

- *Lung disease:* Severe chronic obstructive pulmonary disease (diseases that obstruct the flow of air in the lungs) can make a patient particularly prone to pulmonary infections after a heart transplant and may also necessitate the use of a ventilator after the surgery.

- *Kidney or liver failure:* Both conditions can interfere with the success of a heart transplant.

- *Diseases of the peripheral (noncardiac) blood vessels:* Symptoms of vascular disease (see Chapter 9, Diseases of the Blood Vessels) may become more severe after a heart transplant and the risk of stroke may increase. Patients who have already had a stroke may find it difficult to follow the rigorous medical routine that follows a transplant and to engage in rehabilitation after cardiac transplantation.

- *Infection:* Cardiac transplantation is delayed until an active infection is adequately treated, because the immunosuppressive medication given for a transplant can increase the severity of the infection.

- *Cancer:* The presence of a recent or active cancer is a contraindication to a transplant, but people who have recovered from cancer can be considered as transplant candidates.

- *Stomach ulcers:* Patients with active stomach ulcers may experience bleeding during the surgery or during recovery, and ulcers are usually treated while a recipient is awaiting transplantation.

- *Diabetes:* In the past, diabetes was considered a strong contraindication to cardiac transplantation, but recently, transplants in patients who have diabetes that has not damaged other organs (such as the kidneys, nerves, and eyes) has proven successful.

- *Obesity:* When a person is obese, it is more difficult to match up the donor heart according to size. In addition, obesity may create complications because of some of the postoperative medications needed. Therefore, obese patients with heart failure are usually put on a strict weight-loss program to improve heart failure and reduce postoperative risk.

- *Psychiatric disorders:* People with some mental illnesses may be less willing or able to comply with the rigorous medical follow-up that is required after a transplant.

- *Substance abuse:* In all likelihood, tobacco use before cardiac transplantation will continue after transplantation, and smoking increases the fatality and complication rates of the surgery. A history of alcohol and drug abuse may indicate an unwillingness to modify such behavior and therefore puts the patient at risk for serious complications following transplantation.

The Procedure. Cardiac transplantation involves replacing a diseased heart or heart and lungs with a healthy donor organ or organs. The donor organ is completely removed from someone who has died, then kept cool in a special solution as it is transported, sometimes across the country. (See how Organ Donors Are Located, page 180.)

During the operation, the patient is placed on a cardiopulmonary bypass machine, or a heart-lung machine, which allows surgeons to bypass the blood flow around the heart and lungs. As blood is circulated through this device, carbon dioxide is removed, and oxygen is infused. The heart is then removed, or amputated, leaving only the back walls of the atria—the heart's upper chambers. The backs of the atria on the

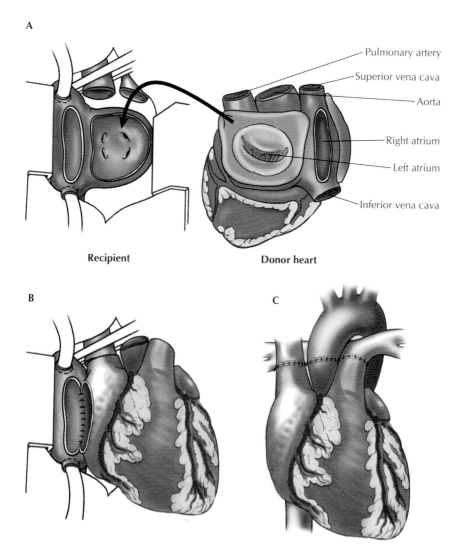

Heart transplantation. (A) The diseased heart is removed leaving only the back walls of the left and right atria. The backs of the atria on the donor heart are opened. (B) The donor heart is sewn in, atria to atria. (C) The great vessels, the aorta, the pulmonary artery, and the superior and inferior venae cavae, are attached and blood flow to the heart is resumed.

replacement heart are opened, and the donor heart is sewn, atria to atria, into the chest cavity.

Once the new organ is in place, the blood vessels are reconnected, allowing blood to flow back through the heart and lungs. The blood warms up the heart, and, in response, the muscle begins to pulsate. Many times, the new heart is started with an electrical shock. Before removing a patient from the heart-lung machine, the surgeons examine the heart's chambers and each connected blood vessel for leaks. Most patients are able to walk around a few days after surgery. Assuming there are no signs that the body is rejecting the new organ, the patient is able to return home within several weeks.

During the surgery, the nerves leading to the heart are cut. Therefore, the transplanted heart beats faster (about 100 to 110 beats per minute) than a normal heart does (70 beats per minute). The new heart does not hasten its pace as quickly or readily in response to exercise and activity. Although transplanted hearts are not completely normal, they function with a remarkable degree of power and efficiency.

Results and Complications. How well a patient fares after surgery depends on many factors, including age, general health, and response to the transplant. Recent figures show that the chances of surviving the initial rigors of the operation are greater than 95 percent and that 70 to 75 percent of heart transplant patients live at least 5 years after surgery. Nearly 85 percent of patients return to work or to their normal activities. Many are able to swim, cycle, run, and engage in other sports. Some heart transplant patients have even competed successfully as professional athletes.

The most daunting obstacle to successful transplantation has been the body's rejection of the donor organ. In 1983, the drug cyclosporine was introduced to suppress the rejection response. The use of this and even newer medications, which must be taken for life, has dramatically decreased heart rejection. As a result, survival rates after transplantation have risen significantly. However, because these drugs suppress the immune system, the use of these medications has increased the risk of infection after heart transplant (see page 180).

The availability of donor organs is a serious obstacle to making transplantation a more widely used treatment. The need for donor hearts far exceeds the supply. Today approximately 4 million people are candidates for transplantation, but currently only about 2,500 operations are performed annually in the United States. Hospitals and national organizations are working to enhance public awareness of this shortage in order to increase organ donations. In addition, ways of improving organ distribution are being explored. The use of LVADs (see page 173) is another option when donor hearts are not available.

Cardiac transplant surgery is, as a rule, the last resort for treating severe heart failure. Whereas the success rate of cardiac transplantation has improved significantly since the procedure was first introduced, the shortage of donor organs and cost of the operation make it impractical except in the most serious cases.

Rejection.   Rejection entails a complicated natural process by which the body's immune system detects the presence of a foreign object and works to expel it. The immune system protects the body from any substance or object that seems to threaten its health and integrity. Leukocytes (white blood cells) travel throughout the body, detecting and attacking foreign substances that could be infectious or toxic.

Rejection is the process by which these cells identify and react to the transplanted heart as a foreign object. If the immune process is left unchecked, leukocytes move to rid the body of the new organ, eating away at the tissue and eventually destroying the replacement heart.

In order to prevent rejection, immunosuppressant drugs are an essential part of treatment. Medications such as cyclosporine, azathioprine, prednisone, and several others suppress the immune system's responses so that the immune system does not damage the new organ. Because rejec-

Chimeric Technology

With the introduction of cyclosporine, the immunosuppressant used most commonly to treat organ rejection, the success rate for heart transplantation has increased significantly. Nevertheless, addressing possible immune incompatibility between the donor heart and the person receiving the heart remains a considerable challenge in transplantation. The only way to avoid rejection is by depressing the immune system for the lifetime of the organ. The use of immunosuppressants can be expensive and can cause serious side effects.

However, a new procedure called chimeric technology may enhance both long-term survival and the quality of life after heart transplantation. Bone marrow is taken along with the replacement heart from the organ donor. The heart is sent directly to the hospital for transplantation. The bone marrow is sent to a laboratory, where it is specially processed.

Meanwhile, the organ recipient receives a dose of irradiation and drugs to restrain his own marrow cells. The processed donor marrow cells are then infused intravenously the day after surgery. Once the cells "take," new blood cells are produced, establishing an immune tolerance to the donor organ. In other words, chimeric technology seems to stimulate the immune system to tolerate the transplanted organ without the use of immunosuppressant medications by making the transplant recipient's bone marrow more closely resemble the donor marrow.

How Donor Organs Are Located

Cardiac transplantation is an operation in which a defective heart is replaced with a healthy one. The healthy heart comes from a person who has died of other causes. By making provisions to donate a heart, a person who has died gives another person the chance to live.

Donor organs are located and matched through the United Network for Organ Sharing (UNOS). Replacement hearts and heart-lungs become available when an individual shows no signs of life. Although brain dead, the body is kept alive by a machine. Most hearts come from individuals who die before age 45, usually as a result of an automobile accident, stroke, gunshot wound, suicide, or head injury.

Today, there is a serious shortage of organs available for transplantation. Because most people do not make arrangements for donating their organs after death, only a fraction of suitable organs become available for donation. About 6,000 people are waiting for a heart or heart-lung transplant at any given time, and a person may wait months for a transplant. More than 25 percent of those people awaiting transplants do not live long enough to receive one.

tion can occur at any time after transplantation, a strict regimen of immunosuppressive drugs must be followed for the rest of the person's life.

After the operation, the doctor routinely monitors for signs that the body is rejecting the new heart. Biopsies of the myocardium are usually performed every week for the first 3 to 6 weeks after surgery, every 3 months for the first year, and then once a year. Small pieces of tissue of the transplanted organ are removed and analyzed. If microscopic examination shows damaged cells appear, the doctor readjusts the dose or perhaps changes the type of immunosuppressive medication.

Infection. The dose of the immunosuppressive medication is balanced to protect the transplanted organ without shutting down the immune system. Without an active immune system, an individual is vulnerable to severe infections. Therefore, medications to ward off infection are also part of the treatment regimen. Avoiding situations where risk of infection is high becomes important.

Other Complications. Coronary artery disease (CAD), or blockage in the arteries that supply blood to the heart, develops in almost one-half of the patients who receive heart transplants. Early on, CAD is a problem in less than one-fifth of patients. However, because sensation is most often dulled with a transplanted heart, the chest pain felt by people with CAD who do not have a heart transplant may not be felt by people with transplanted hearts. Without this early warning signal, coronary blockage can develop undetected, increasing the chance of myocardial infarction.

In addition, when taken over time, immunosuppressant medications can cause kidney damage, hypertension, osteoporosis, and, in rare cases, lymphoma, a cancer that affects the immune system.

At the same time, most people find that cardiac transplantation provides relief of most of their old symptoms and allows them a new opportunity to actively engage in and enjoy their lives.

Other Surgical Treatments

To close the widening gap between people suffering from serious, life-threatening congestive heart failure and the limited number of cardiac transplantations, doctors and researchers are developing promising alternative treatments.

Ventriculectomy. Ventriculectomy, also referred to as the Batista procedure, involves slicing parts of the myocardium to reduce the size of the left ventricle. When the heart has become large and muscular, reducing the left ventricle remodels the heart to a more normal shape and size. This decreases the pressure in the heart and increases overall efficiency. Ventriculectomy may be effective for people suffering from dilated cardiomyopathy, in which the heart cavity becomes stretched and enlarged.

Cardiomyoplasty. Cardiomyoplasty is an experimental surgical procedure that takes muscles from the back or abdomen and wraps them around an ailing heart. Contractions in the additional muscle are stimulated by a pacemaker-like implant, boosting the heart's pumping activity. The long-term benefits and risks remain to be determined, and this procedure is used only rarely.

Infarct Exclusion. This evolving operation reconstructs the left ventricle of the failing heart after myocardial infarction. Surgeons place a "purse-string" suture inside the base of the left ventricular scar to reshape a portion of the dilated myocardium. The results have been promising. Although most people who undergo this procedure are candidates for cardiac transplantation, after surgery most were able to resume active lives and were not relisted for transplantation.

What the Future Holds

A larger percentage of the American population than ever before is entering middle and old age. More people are surviving relatively serious heart conditions thanks to advances in medical treatment. The issues of the aging heart will inevitably capture increased attention and resources in medical and scientific communities.

Indeed, with heart failure affecting a growing number of Americans, many medical centers around the country are establishing clinics specially designed to treat it. Medical and pharmaceutical laboratories are seeking ways to prevent, or at least delay, its progression. New therapies, including new drugs, surgical procedures, and mechanical devices, are being tested and developed. Even in cases where the condition cannot be reversed, many new treatments aim at prolonging life and improving its quality.

As more is learned about the cellular and molecular changes that occur during the progressive deterioration of the heart, better drug treatments will likely become available.

Beyond drug treatments, scientists are developing ways to use a patient's own tissue to regenerate healthy heart muscle. For patients with significantly scarred hearts, it may soon be possible to transform marrow cells into myocardial cells and thus transform a diseased heart into a healthy one.

In terms of heart transplant, hospitals and organizations nationwide are developing better systems for locating and distributing organs to patients who need them. Scientists are exploring more effective immunosuppressant medications with fewer long-term side effects to combat rejection. In addition, easier, less invasive ways of monitoring rejection of the donor heart are on the horizon to replace the biopsies that are now used.

Because the shortage of donor organs seems likely to continue, other sources for transplantable hearts are being developed. Xenotransplantation—using hearts from animals—is promising, particularly genetically engineered pig hearts. Small, totally implantable mechanical assist devices that do not require any wires passing through the skin would greatly reduce the risk of infection and make these devices more feasible for long-term use.

CHAPTER 9

Diseases of the Blood Vessels

Introduction

The vascular system—the elaborate network of arteries and veins through which blood flows to deliver oxygen and nutrients to the body's tissues and organs—is made up of two distinct and interconnected circulatory networks: pulmonary circulation and systemic circulation. Pulmonary circulation, involving a rather short bundle of vessels, delivers blood from the heart to the lungs, where the blood is purified and oxygenated. Deoxygenated blood returning to the heart from the veins of the body enters the right atrium. From the right atrium, blood is pumped to the right ventricle and then into the pulmonary artery, which forks into each lung and branches into arteries. The arteries then branch into capillaries, which absorb oxygen. The red oxygenated blood returns to the heart through four pulmonary veins, two from each lung. The oxygen-rich blood then enters the left atrium and then the left ventricle.

Systemic circulation is the vascular network that supplies blood to the other parts of the body. This labyrinth of arteries and veins begins at the aorta (the main artery leading away from the heart), which receives oxygenated blood from the left ventricle. The arterial system branches off into ever-smaller vessels, from arteries to arterioles to capillaries. After the blood in the capillaries distributes oxygen and collects carbon dioxide and other waste products from the tissues, it travels back to the heart through small venules and then through the larger veins. As part of the blood's circuitous journey, it passes through the liver and kidneys, where cellular waste products are removed or processed.

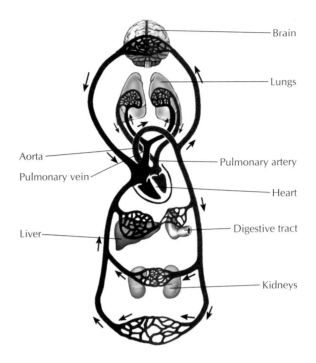

Aorta

Pulmonary vein

Liver

Brain

Lungs

Pulmonary artery

Heart

Digestive tract

Kidneys

The vascular system. In systemic circulation, the arteries (beginning at the aorta; see right side of illustration) carry oxygen-rich blood to the body's tissues. The arteries branch off into smaller capillaries, where the oxygen and nutrients of the blood are distributed to the body's tissues and carbon dioxide and waste are picked up. The capillaries then become veins (see left side of illustration), which carry oxygen-poor blood back to the heart (waste products are first delivered to the liver and kidneys for processing or removal). In pulmonary circulation, deoxygenated blood that has returned to the heart is sent through the pulmonary veins to the lungs for reoxygenation. The blood, now oxygenated, returns to the heart through the pulmonary arteries. The oxygenated blood is then pumped out through the aorta beginning systemic circulation again.

Now bluish-red deoxygenated blood from the upper portion of the body enters the right atrium through the superior vena cava. Blood from the lower portion of the body enters through the inferior vena cava.

In order for the blood to make this journey efficiently and effectively, the circulatory system relies on clear passage and vessel elasticity. Although the quantity of blood within the body remains relatively constant—approximately 7 percent of body weight—just where the blood concentrates and how forcefully it moves vary.

For example, when a person is eating, the blood supply to the stomach increases in order to aid in digestion. During rigorous physical activity, more oxygen, and therefore more blood, is directed toward the affected muscles. When the body is cold, blood concentrates in the inner vessels in order to conserve heat; when the body is warm, blood rushes to the skin, through which heat is dispelled. Because healthy blood vessels are strong, elastic, and smooth, blood flows through them readily, and changes in its volume and pressure are easily accommodated.

Diseases of the Arteries

A wide variety of diseases and conditions can affect the vascular system. The specific diseases that affect arteries and veins are related to the differences in structure and function between them.

Arteriosclerosis of the Extremities and Cerebral Circulation

As a person ages, arteries naturally grow thicker, stiffer, and less pliant, and calcium deposits form along the walls. Other factors, including hypertension (high blood pressure), high cholesterol, diabetes, smoking, obesity, and stress, can damage delicate blood vessels. This progressive hardening of the arteries is called arteriosclerosis.

Arteriosclerosis—popularly called "hardening of the arteries"—is the most common cause of chronic disease of the circulatory system. Usually, the effects of arteriosclerosis can be felt in the arteries that nourish the extremities—the legs, feet, arms, and hands. Occasionally, it also affects the cerebrovascular arteries in the neck and head that nourish the brain. (For information on diseases of the coronary arteries—arteries that supply the myocardium, or heart muscle, with oxygenated blood—see Chapter 5, Coronary Artery Disease.)

As arteriosclerosis advances, occlusions or blockages coupled with increasing rigidity in the arteries can impede blood flow. If blood is prevented from reaching the tissues and organs for a long enough period of time, they become deprived of the nutrients and oxygen they need for healthy functioning.

Most people affected by vascular disease are over the age of 65. As a higher percentage of the population in the United States has become older, the incidence of arterial disease has progressively increased. Studies indicate that up to 5 percent of men and 2.5 percent of women over the age of 60 have symptoms of vascular disease. Men are at least three times more likely than women to have silent vascular disease, or vascular disease that becomes apparent only with diagnostic tests.

Signs and Symptoms

The symptoms of arteriosclerosis vary in type and severity, depending on how much of the circulatory system is involved. In addition, the severity of the symptoms is contingent on the degree to which the collateral circulation—a distinct alternative vascular network—is available. The collateral vessels work as a natural emergency bypass for the blood supply—the blood is routed around the blockage. This emergency system can succeed in reducing symptoms, but it will not eliminate them.

During the early stages of arteriosclerosis, there are often no symptoms. When there are symptoms, they tend to be seen merely as a nuisance. Although the symptoms may be only mildly annoying—leg pain or cramps, edema (swelling) around the ankle, and cold, painful sensations in the hands or feet—they can be warning signs of more serious systemic heart disease.

The most common symptom of arteriosclerosis is intermittent claudication—severe pain, usually in the calf muscles, felt most intensely while walking and subsiding when at rest. Intermittent claudication makes walking difficult and painful.

Signs that the blockage is more severe include pain in the buttocks or thighs, as well as leg pain that occurs during rest. At its worst, a serious and prolonged lack of blood to the tissue can cause critical ischemia (oxygen deprivation) in the leg, foot, and toes, showing up as ulcerations (sores that do not heal) and gangrene (death of tissue and subsequent bacterial invasion). These are indications that the tissue has been seriously damaged.

In approximately one-half of all cases, symptoms of intermittent claudication remain stable or abate, presumably due to the development of collateral blood flow. In approximately 15 to 20 percent of cases, intermittent claudication progresses to critical leg ischemia (ulcers and gangrene).

When arteriosclerosis affects the cerebrovascular system (the blood vessels supplying the brain), the most serious symptoms are ministrokes called transient ischemic attacks (TIAs) and stroke (see page 194).

Implications of Arteriosclerotic Disease

Arteriosclerosis is usually first felt in the lower extremities—the feet and legs. Consequently, lower-extremity arterial disease should be viewed as more than just a pain in the legs. Instead, disease of these arteries is often a telltale sign of more diffuse and significant arterial disease. People who have arterial disease—even if it does not cause overt symptoms—are at higher risk of stroke, myocardial infarction (heart attack), and cardiovascular death.

Arteriosclerosis versus Atherosclerosis

Healthy arteries are sturdy, pliable, and elastic. Because their linings are smooth, blood flows freely. With age, the blood vessels thicken, harden, and lose elasticity, and calcification (the formation of calcium deposits along the vessel walls) is more likely to occur. Other factors, such as smoking, hypertension, consistently high blood cholesterol levels, diabetes, obesity, and stress, can weaken the vessels and make them rigid. The process by which the arteries gradually harden is called arteriosclerosis.

One particularly damaging form of arteriosclerosis is called atherosclerosis, a progressive condition that occurs when the intima (the innermost lining of the arteries) become thick and uneven. As the artery walls become rough, specialized white blood cells become entrapped, creating clusters and attracting oxidized low-density lipoprotein (LDL) cholesterol. Fatty streaks form that thicken the artery lining and absorb calcium deposits, cellular waste, and fibrin (a protein formed during blood clotting), creating scablike deposits called plaque.

The collateral circulation offers some natural protection from both atherosclerosis and arteriosclerosis by providing detours around the narrowed or blocked sections of the arteries. Nevertheless, if the arteries narrow sufficiently, arterial circulation becomes impaired, and a person will most likely feel it in the legs or feet. Furthermore, these conditions can make a person more vulnerable to stroke (see page 194) and myocardial infarction (heart attack), especially if atherosclerotic plaque clots form and break off. Atherosclerosis is the most common cause of stroke and coronary artery disease.

■ At least 28 percent of people with arterial disease in the lower limbs also have coronary artery disease (CAD; see Chapter 5).

■ People with intermittent claudication are two to three times likelier to develop serious heart disease.

■ As many as 75 percent of people with severe lower-extremity arterial disease will have a fatal myocardial infarction or stroke.

■ Within 5 years of the diagnosis, 20 percent of people with intermittent claudication will have a nonfatal myocardial infarction or stroke.

If arteriosclerotic disease is diagnosed early, it can be effectively addressed, generally by modifying diet and lifestyle and by engaging in exercise as prescribed. These important changes can significantly lower a person's risk of more serious cardiovascular disease.

Causes and Prevention

Although the precise cause of arteriosclerosis is unknown, many factors appear to contribute to the condition. Some of these factors cannot be modified, such as age, gender, and race. However, other factors that increase a person's likelihood of developing arteriosclerosis, such as smoking, sedentary lifestyle, high-fat diet, uncontrolled diabetes, hypertension, and hyperlipidemia (high levels of cholesterol and triglycerides in the blood), can be actively addressed. Adopting healthier habits can reduce the impact of arteriosclerosis and, in some instances, actually reverse the disease process. Regular exercise, a diet low in saturated fatty acids, controlling hypertension and diabetes, and managing stress can translate into healthier, smoother, more elastic blood vessels.

Age.   The incidence of vascular disease increases with age. The risk of vascular disease in the lower extremities increases almost fivefold for men older than 50. It may well be that lower-extremity arterial disease will become more common as life expectancy increases in the general population. Increasing age also raises the risk of stroke—for every decade after age 55, the risk of stroke more than doubles. However, people who maintain healthier habits are more likely to counteract much of the impact of aging on the vascular system.

Gender.   Men over age 50 are 2.5 times more likely to experience intermittent claudication than are women of the same age. However, after the age of 70, the prevalence of the condition becomes the same for men and women. In addition, men, particularly those under age 65, have a greater risk of stroke than women.

Race.   Because black men and women, on average, develop hypertension at a younger age than whites, they are more likely to develop serious atherosclerotic conditions. Although CAD is less likely to develop in black men than in white men, black men are at higher risk of stroke related to hypertension and diabetes. Black women, especially those who are obese, are at higher risk of vascular disease than are white women. Blacks are almost twice as likely to have a nonfatal stroke and 1.5 times more likely to die as a result of a stroke than are whites.

Diabetes.   There is a strong connection between diabetes mellitus and the development of arterial disease, including stroke. According to some studies, as many as 25 percent of patients who undergo surgery to replace diseased vessels in the leg and feet have diabetes. Furthermore, people with diabetes are seven times as likely to undergo amputation of an extremity than are people who do not have the disease.

By controlling diabetes, a person can limit the damage inflicted by the disease on the blood vessels. In addition, because many people with diabetes are overweight, maintaining a healthy weight limits the negative impact of obesity on both the condition itself and the vascular system.

Hypertension.   Hypertension is constant, abnormally high blood pressure within the vascular system. This condition damages the smooth delicate blood vessels. Left untreated, hypertension leads to an increased risk of arteriosclerosis and related stroke. The likelihood of developing arterial disease as a result of hypertension is almost twice as high for women as it is for men. However, once hypertension is brought under control, through either diet and exercise or medication, the vascular complications are significantly reduced.

Hyperlipidemia.   Almost half of the people who have arterial disease also have hyperlipidemia, or high levels of cholesterol and triglycerides in the blood. Whenever blood cholesterol levels are consistently high, fatty plaque builds up along the arterial walls, specifically at places that are already weakened. This buildup causes the blood vessels to narrow. In addition, the greater the plaque buildup, the more likely that thrombi (blood clots) will form, which can create blockages. Evidence suggests that once hyperlipidemia is brought under control through diet or medication, the progression of arteriosclerosis slows dramatically.

Smoking.   Cigarette smoking is a serious risk factor for cardiovascular disease. Smoking makes the heart work harder as it pumps blood to the body's tissues and organs. Carbon monoxide, a toxic gas found in cigarette smoke, damages the lining of the blood vessels; nicotine, another component of cigarette smoke, causes vessels to constrict. In addition, because smoking increases fibrinogen levels, which increase the blood's tendency to clot, people who smoke are at increased risk of thrombosis (formation of blood clots).

Studies show that cigarette smoking nearly doubles the risk of ischemic stroke. For women who take high-dose oral contraceptives, smoking significantly increases the risk of stroke. Although people who smoke cigars or pipes seem to have a higher risk of death from CAD, and possibly stroke, the risk is not quite as great as for cigarette smokers, perhaps because cigarette smokers are more likely to inhale the smoke.

Studies also indicate that passive or second-hand smoking is a significant health hazard. Estimates approximate that exposure to second-hand smoke accounts for 37,000 to 40,000 cardiovascular deaths each year.

Once a person stops smoking, the risk of developing arteriosclerotic-related circulatory disease, and possibly stroke, immediately decreases. People with intermittent claudication are especially urged to stop smoking at once.

Diagnosis and Detection

The symptoms of vascular disease vary. Although a stroke is a clear medical emergency requiring immediate medical attention, many of the symptoms of vascular disorders—leg cramps, tingling, or cold feet or hands—are merely troublesome. Nevertheless, it is important to discuss even minor discomfort with your doctor, especially if you have any other risk factors, because these symptoms can signal more serious cardiovascular problems.

Your doctor will perform a physical examination, including checking your pulse and measuring pressure around the leg and foot if you report pain in these areas. If blockages in the arteries are suspected, you may be tested for diabetes. When coupled with diabetes, arterial disease tends to be more severe and widespread.

The most commonly used diagnostic tests include blood pressure monitoring, exercise stress tests, ultrasound, and angiogram. For more information on these and other dignostic tests, see Chapter 4, Diagnosing Heart Disease.

Blood Pressure Monitoring.   As arteries progressively narrow, there is a fall in systolic blood pressure, the force with which the blood is pumped away from the heart. A precise reading of pressure can indicate the extent of disease. Sensors, such as continuous-wave (CW) Doppler, which uses ultrasound to locate blockages in the arteries, can measure systolic pressures in the toes, ankles, calves, and upper thighs.

Exercise Stress Test.   Exercise stress tests are particularly helpful in assessing intermittent claudication. In particular, measuring the blood pressure in the ankle provides a good indication of the extent of arteriosclerosis. Measurements are made while you are wearing ankle pressure cuffs and are walking on a treadmill. Once the walk is completed or if pain develops, you lie down and pressure at the ankle is measured again.

Ultrasound.   Ultrasound—high-frequency sound waves—can generate pictures of the arteries and indicate the degree to which they have narrowed and the fluidity with which blood courses through the vessels.

Angiogram.   Angiograms are especially useful in evaluating the degree of arterial narrowing from atherosclerosis both in the arteries leading to the brain—which are near the skin's surface—and in the lower limbs. During angiography, a contrast medium (dye) is injected into the bloodstream through a catheter (a long, thin tube, which can be inserted into a vein and moved through the body). X-rays or moving images of the arteries are then generated. Angiography can detail size and shape of the arteries anywhere in the body as well as the location of any arterial occlusions or abnormalities.

Treatment and Results

In many cases, lifestyle modifications are all that are needed to halt the arteriosclerotic process. In fact, of all the people who are diagnosed with arteriosclerosis, only 20 to 30 percent have symptoms that progress after 10 years to the point of requiring medical intervention. Nevertheless, symptoms such as intermittent claudication should be taken seriously, as they are generally signs of systemic atherosclerosis and could foretell a myocardial infarction or stroke.

Typically, therapy for arteriosclerosis is aimed in two directions. First, treatment is geared toward reducing symptoms in the affected area and halting the progression of vascular blockage. Depending on the severity of the condition, treatment ranges from such nonsurgical measures as exercise, risk factor modification, and medication to such surgical interventions as angioplasty, stent insertion, bypass grafting, and amputation.

Second, therapy aims at preventing more serious atherosclerosis-related cardiovascular complications such as stroke and myocardial infarction. For this, the most effective treatment appears to be the daily use of aspirin.

Exercise Therapy. Regular exercise, coupled with modifying certain risk factors—particularly stopping smoking—has long been the mainstay of therapy for atherosclerosis. Studies suggest that exercise is the most consistently effective medical treatment for this vascular disease. As long as intermittent claudication is not disabling, adopting healthier practices may prove sufficient in limiting, and perhaps reversing, the effects of the arteriosclerosis. Studies show that appropriate exercise or activities, such as walking, leg exercises, and treadmill exercise, done three to four times weekly can relieve chronic leg pain within 3 months.

Medication. For the most part, arteriosclerosis and its effects on the extremities and cerebral circulation respond best to simple, if not always easy, measures. By modifying their lifestyle habits to include a healthy diet and exercise, and by controlling risk factors such as high blood cholesterol levels, diabetes, and hypertension, many people are able to avoid more aggressive medical intervention.

However, when high cholesterol, hyperlipidemia, and hypertension are factors, and they cannot be controlled sufficiently through diet and exercise, appropriate medications may be prescribed. Although these medications do not work to relieve symptoms such as leg cramps and pain, they lower the risk of more serious arteriosclerotic events, such as myocardial infarction and stroke.

Antithrombolytic agents or blood-clotting modifiers are often used to thin the blood, improving blood flow. Daily use of aspirin may work sufficiently to prevent clotting, reducing intermittent claudication. In addition, aspirin decreases the risk of related cardiovascular events, such as stroke, myocardial infarction, and tissue damage. Usually, aspirin (in a dose a doctor recommends) is taken daily for extended periods, often for life. Ticlopidine (Ticlid), a prescription blood-clotting modifier, is an alternative for people who cannot take aspirin. It seems especially effective for people who have had a stroke or who have medical problems that can lead to a stroke.

Invasive Treatments. While most symptoms of arteriosclerosis-related vascular disease can be addressed through exercise and lifestyle modification, in some instances more invasive interventions are needed. This is especially true when pain, specifically intermittent claudication, becomes persistent and debilitating or when nonhealing ulcers, infection, or gangrene develop on the leg or foot, indicating tissue damage. Angioplasty and bypass surgery are two therapeutic options.

Balloon Angioplasty. In balloon angioplasty—or percutaneous transluminal angioplasty (PTA)—a tiny balloon is carried through the artery on the tip of a catheter and placed across the blockage. The balloon is then inflated for several minutes. As it expands, the atherosclerotic plaque is compressed and pushed aside, clearing the affected artery. However, because arteries can reclose even after a successful angioplastic procedure, vascular stenting may provide a more durable opening (see below). (For more information on balloon angioplasty, see page 96.)

Bypass Surgery. Bypass surgery does not cure the arteriosclerotic process, but it does work to correct some of the damage done. Revascularization, a surgical procedure in which the congested section of the artery is replaced or bypassed, is performed when there is an immediate chance that the limb will be lost. Either a synthetic conduit or a vein taken from another part of the body is used to bypass the blocked section of the artery. Studies show that surgical revascularization can prevent loss of tissue in 85 to 90 percent of cases. (For more information on bypass surgery, see page 100.)

Stents. Because neither angioplasty nor bypass surgery addresses the underlying disease process, there is always the chance that the opened vessel or new arterial graft will begin to narrow over time. To prevent this, stents—collapsible metallic wire mesh tubes—can be inserted after balloon angioplasty to prop open the artery.

During angioplasty, the stent is positioned over a balloon catheter and transported to the blockage. As the balloon inflates, the coil expands and locks into place, establishing a permanent support within the artery. Stents prevent the artery from renarrowing and, in so doing, substantially reduce the need for subsequent bypass surgery.

Even with conventional stents, however, arteries can renarrow. But the incidence is only 10 to 15 percent as compared to 25 to 35 percent with balloon angioplasty.

Arterial Embolism

Many times, when atherosclerotic plaque accumulates, a thrombus (blood clot) forms along the artery wall. Occasionally, a piece of undissolved plaque or thrombus breaks free from the artery wall and is carried through the circulatory system until it becomes lodged elsewhere. A free-floating thrombus is called an embolus. When an artery is blocked by an embolus, restricting blood flow, the blockage is called an embolism.

Signs and Symptoms

When an embolus or a group of emboli wedges in the artery of a leg or arm, blood flow is slowed, causing inflammation, pain, and numbness in the area. A person can experience intermittent leg cramps and cold, painful sensations in the hands or feet. If the condition is not monitored and treated promptly, gangrene can develop in the arm or leg tissue below the obstruction. Gangrene is a serious condition in which tissue in the arm or leg dies from lack of oxygen. When a thrombus travels through the bloodstream and lodges in one of the arteries leading to the brain, it is called a cerebral embolism, which can result in stroke.

Detection and Diagnosis

Timely and accurate diagnosis of an embolism is especially important because tissue below the obstruction can die if the embolus is not removed or dissolved. If an embolus is suspected, the diagnostic process will include one or more tests:

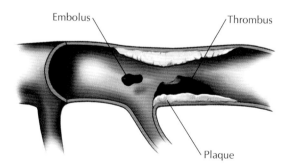

Embolus   Thrombus

Plaque

Because atherosclerotic plaque damages arterial walls, a thrombus, or blood clot, may form at the site of the plaque buildup. When a piece of a thrombus breaks off, it is called an embolus. An embolus may lodge in a narrowed artery, blocking blood flow; this is called an arterial embolism. Depending on where the blockage occurs, a stroke or myocardial infarction (heart attack) may result.

- Angiogram, an x-ray that uses tracer dyes, to indicate the location of the embolus (see page 190)

- Ultrasound, which uses sound waves to create computer images, to identify variations in blood flow (see page 190)

- CT scan, which uses x-rays to create textured computer images (see page 73)

Treatment

In order to prevent an embolism from causing permanent or extensive damage in the leg or the brain, blood flow must be restored within a few hours. This can be accomplished through the use of either medications or surgery.

Medication. In most cases, a thrombolytic (blood clot–dissolving) agent is injected directly into the affected artery to dissolve the embolism. In a process called intra-arterial thrombolysis, a catheter is passed into the artery. A thrombolytic agent, such as streptokinase, urokinase, or tissue-plasminogen activator (t-PA), is infused while angiography documents the progress of clot dissolution. It can take as long as 48 hours for the clot to dissolve completely. A related technique involves using pulse-spray in which the thrombolytic agent is delivered in high-pressure injections through a catheter.

Surgery. If the health of the limb is at immediate risk or if a stroke seems imminent, surgery may be performed to remove the embolus from the artery. In most cases, balloon angioplasty is performed, although in some cases lasers are used to open blocked arteries. Blocked or damaged arteries also can be removed or bypassed with an artificial shunt. After any of these procedures, anticoagulant medication such as aspirin, warfarin (Coumadin), or dipyridamole (Persantine) may be prescribed to guard against the development of future emboli.

Stroke

Although stroke, a condition that affects the brain, may appear to have little to do with heart disease, the truth is that the head and heart are closely related. Both stroke and myocardial infarction are serious symptoms of cardiovascular disease. A myocardial infarction is centered within the heart, a stroke within the brain. In fact, a stroke can be considered a "brain attack."

Like the heart, as well as all other organs in the body, the brain needs oxygenated blood to survive. The term "stroke" describes a series or variety of events that occurs when the blood supply to a part of the brain is dramatically interrupted.

Symptoms of Stroke

Without exception, stroke is a serious medical emergency. If you experience any of the classic warning signs of stroke, do not ignore them, thinking they will pass. Call 911 or go to the emergency room immediately.

- Sudden paralysis, numbness, or weakness in one side of the face or body
- Sudden partial or complete blindness or double or blurred vision
- Inability to speak or make sense
- Sudden loss of physical coordination or balance
- Sudden intense headache

For additional symptoms of stroke, see page 196.

Just as angina occurs when blood to the heart is temporarily blocked, ministrokes called transient ischemic attacks (TIAs) occur when blood to the brain is obstructed for a short time. Symptoms of TIAs are the same as those of stroke, but they tend to be briefer, lasting anywhere from several minutes to an hour. As angina can be a warning sign of an impending heart attack, so ministrokes can be a warning sign that the stroke is about to occur.

Types of Strokes

There are three types of stroke: cerebral thrombosis, cerebral embolism, and cerebral hemorrhage.

- *Cerebral thrombosis,* the most common form of stroke, is ordinarily a product of atherosclerosis. Like a coronary thrombosis (a myocardial infarction prompted by a blockage in the coronary artery, a cerebral thrombosis involves a thrombus that has grown so large within an artery in the neck or brain that it blocks blood flow (see also carotid artery disease, page 197).

- *Cerebral embolism* occurs when a piece of plaque or thrombus (an embolus) breaks free from the lining of a blood vessel and travels through the bloodstream to lodge in one of the arteries leading to the brain. Cerebral embolisms are most often caused by CAD or valvular disease.

- *Cerebral hemorrhage* occurs when an artery in or near the brain bursts. As blood floods tissue, pressure on the brain and blood loss

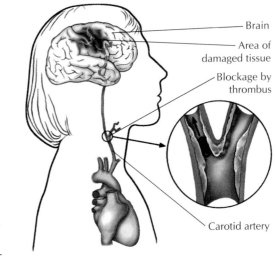

Brain

Area of
damaged tissue

Blockage by
thrombus

Stroke. When a thrombus
(blood clot) forms in the
carotid artery impeding blood
flow to the brain, a stroke may
result. A stroke occurs when
lack of blood to the brain
causes permanent damage to a
portion of brain tissue.

Carotid artery

bring on symptoms. Usually, a cerebral hemorrhage is caused by an injury to the head or an aneurysm, a blood-filled sac that has ballooned out from a weak spot in an arterial wall (see page 198).

Symptoms

Symptoms of a stroke include the following:

- Sudden weakness or numbness in the face, arm, or leg on one side of the body
- Abrupt deterioration of speech, vision, or sensation
- Dimness or impaired vision in one eye
- Loss or near-loss of consciousness
- Confusion
- Severe and persistent headache
- Sudden memory loss
- Unexplained dizziness
- Sudden falls

Emergency symptoms include any of the above symptoms that occur with startling abruptness, a sudden loss of consciousness, or complete or partial paralysis that cannot be traced to an injury.

Symptoms of transient ischemic attacks (TIAs) usually last only a few minutes. These include the following:

- Sensations of weakness

- Tingling or numbness

- Blind spots or blurred vision

- Loss of balance

- Poor coordination

Frequently due to atherosclerosis, TIAs precede a serious stroke by days, weeks, or months.

Typically, stroke-related symptoms either come and go or progress gradually over a period of days. When the stroke is caused by a thrombus—a stationary blood clot—symptoms usually develop gradually. The symptoms are typically more abrupt and more serious when a stroke is caused by an embolus that has traveled through the bloodstream and lodged in the cerebral artery.

Risk Factors

The chances of having a stroke rise with age, for people of any age who smoke, and for women who take high-dose oral contraceptives, especially if they smoke. Hypertension and diabetes, especially when uncontrolled, increase the risk of stroke significantly (see also pages 188 to 190).

Additional risk factors for stroke include

- *Carotid artery disease:* The carotid arteries, which supply the brain with oxygenated blood, can be damaged by atherosclerosis. Carotid arteries narrowed by atherosclerosis can lead to a stroke when the blockage is great enough to prevent blood flow or if an embolus (blood clot) lodges in the narrowed artery. If the carotid artery is blocked, the doctor may hear a bruit (an abnormal sound in the neck) when he listens with a stethoscope. Treatments are available to prevent carotid artery disease from leading to stroke, including carotid endarterectomy and carotid artery angioplasty and stenting.
  - *Carotid endarterectomy* is a surgical procedure in which an incision is made in the neck, the carotid artery is opened, and the atherosclerotic plaque is removed; it is the traditional surgical treatment for carotid artery disease. Endarterectomy carries a number of risks, however, and is not suitable for all patients.
  - *Carotid artery angioplasty and stenting* is a less invasive treatment—similar to what is used for coronary artery disease (CAD) and in other noncoronary arteries—and is showing promise for carotid artery disease.

- *Heart disease:* People with heart disease have more than two times the risk of stroke as people without heart disease. Heart conditions that can particularly lead to stroke are atrial fibrillation (rapid, uncoordinated beating of the atria, the heart's upper chambers), valve disorders, and myocardial infarction. These disorders are all associated with the formation of emboli, which can travel to the carotid and cerebral arteries. Medications to thin the blood and keep it from clotting are often given to people with these heart conditions.

■ *Transient ischemic attacks (TIAs) or a previous stroke:* These events are strongly related to the risk of having a stroke.

Diagnosis

In order to determine whether a stroke has occurred or is about to occur, a doctor will identify the type and location of the stroke through a series of diagnostic tests, including an angiogram, an x-ray using a tracing liquid that highlights blood circulation and computed tomography (CT) or magnetic resonance imaging (MRI), both of which use computerized scanners to create diagnostic images.

Treatment

Once a stroke has occurred and has led to brain damage, medications cannot correct the damage to the brain. However, the clot-dissolving agent t-PA (see page 194), if given within 3 hours after the onset of a stroke caused by a blockage, can prevent brain damage. T-PA can cause bleeding, however, and must not be used if the stroke is caused by a cerebral hemorrhage.

People who have had a TIA, a previous stroke, or a condition that could lead to a stroke may be given anticoagulant medications (such as aspirin or warfarin) to prevent the formation of clots and to minimize the chance of future strokes.

Rehabilitation has been successful in helping people to relearn movement and functional skills that a stroke has caused them to lose. As a result, there is much potential for recovery after a stroke.

Aneurysm

An aneurysm is an abnormal distention or bulging of the lining of a blood vessel wall. Aneurysms usually form in places where the wall has been weakened or damaged; pressure within the blood vessel causes the wall to thin and balloon out. There are two types of aneurysm:

■ Degenerative aneurysms, which develop because arteriosclerosis has damaged the blood vessel

■ Dissecting aneurysms, which originate in a lesion or tear in the vessel wall

Although aneurysms can form in any blood vessel, they occur most commonly in the aorta (aortic aneurysm), the main blood vessel leading away from the heart; in the abdominal area below the kidneys (abdominal aneurysm); and in the chest cavity (thoracic aneurysm).

In most cases, a small aneurysm poses no threat. However, because aneurysms attract arteriosclerotic plaque, the chance is increased that a thrombus will form and break off, creating an embolism. In addition, an aneurysm can grow large enough to press on organs and cause pain. The greatest risk, though, lies in the possibility that, as the aneurysm grows, the wall will rupture, flooding nearby tissue with blood. In some cases, the aneurysm can disrupt blood flow.

The larger the aneurysm, the greater the risk that it will burst. While aneurysms are not always life-threatening, a sudden rupture, especially in the aorta or the heart wall, can be fatal. If an aneurysm has formed in the artery leading to the brain, surgery may be advised to remove it. In the event of cerebral hemorrhage, where blood has flooded into the tissues, surgery may also be indicated.

Symptoms

With many aneurysms, there are no symptoms. The most common symptom of aneurysm is pain in the area. Dissecting aneurysms in particular can cause significant pain, which is often difficult to distinguish from the pain associated with an acute myocardial infarction. With abdominal aneurysms, the pain may be felt in the midstomach or low back. With thoracic aneurysms, the pain may radiate from behind the sternum (breastbone) to the back. There may also be breathing difficulties, hoarseness, coughing, and tightness upon swallowing.

The larger the aneurysm becomes, the more likely it is to burst. Depending on the location of the aneurysm, rupture can cause shock, loss of consciousness, stroke, or myocardial infarction.

Causes and Prevention

An aneurysm typically balloons out of the wall of an artery where the wall has become weakened as a result of disease, injury, or congenital abnormality. In the case of a degenerative aneurysm, hypertension or atherosclerosis has usually damaged the wall.

■ *Hypertension:* This condition subjects delicate blood vessels to rigorous pounding. Over time, this thrashing takes its toll and weakens the vessel walls. As a result, aneurysms are more likely to develop, and plaque more likely to accumulate. Hypertension can also lead to aortic dissection—a split in the aortic wall—that makes it vulnerable to rupture. It is essential to control hypertension; your doctor will check your blood pressure regularly and may suggest that you monitor your blood pressure at home (see page 61). Your doctor may

Dissecting Aneurysms

Dissecting aneurysms usually develop in the aorta and its main branches and are found most often in middle-aged black men who have hypertension. In a dissecting aneurysm, blood flows through a tear in the artery's inner layer. The blood flowing between the layers of the artery wall causes the layers to separate; the splitting of the wall can lead to blockages to blood flow and bursting of the arterial wall.

Although it is not always clear what is the cause of a dissecting aneurysm, some contributing factors are

- Marfan syndrome—about 20 to 40 percent of people with Marfan syndrome (a genetic disorder of connective tissue that causes abnormalities of the eyes, long bones, and circulatory system) develop dissecting aneurysms.

- Aging—the normal aging process itself makes the aorta more vulnerable to injury.

- Hypertension—among the people in whom aortic dissection occurs, at least 70 percent have hypertension.

- Pregnancy—this seems to be a contributing factor, presumably because it causes an increase in blood pressure. Except when pregnancy is a factor, aortic dissection rarely occurs in people younger than 40 years of age.

- Congenital conditions—congenital bicuspid aortic valve, a weakness in the structure of the aortic valve, seem to be present in about 20 percent of cases.

prescribe antihypertensive drugs to lower blood pressure and to limit the damage that can be sustained otherwise.

- *Atherosclerosis:* The damage to the arterial wall from atherosclerosis makes it vulnerable to the development of an aneurysm. For more information about atherosclerosis, see page 187.

Detection and Diagnosis

Any significant delay in diagnosis increases the chances that the aneurysm will rupture or dissect. Therefore, timely diagnosis is important. At the same time, aneurysms are not easily diagnosed, especially because they can exist without symptoms. Although pain may occur, it is usually inconsistent. Nevertheless, once an aneurysm is detected,

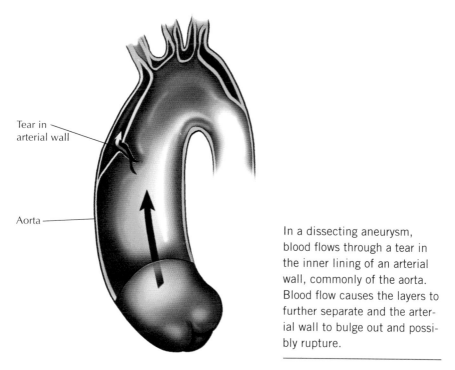

Tear in arterial wall

Aorta

In a dissecting aneurysm, blood flows through a tear in the inner lining of an arterial wall, commonly of the aorta. Blood flow causes the layers to further separate and the arterial wall to bulge out and possibly rupture.

however small, it must be monitored, as it can grow and become unstable, increasing the chances of an abrupt rupture.

People with atherosclerosis or hypertension are usually screened regularly for aneurysms. With an abdominal aneurysm, the doctor may feel a pulsating lump in the middle of the stomach during a physical examinaton. With a thoracic aneurysm, a murmur in the aortic valve may be audible through a stethoscopic examination.

X-rays, aortography (an x-ray of the aorta, after injecting a contrast dye), or imaging techniques such as echocardiography (page 71), MRI (page 69), or CT (page 73) are the most reliable diagnostic tests. Any of these can indicate the size and location of the aneurysm. Transesophageal echocardiography (TEE; see page 79) is an efficient method of making the diagnosis in the thoracic aorta.

Treatment and Results

As long as an aneurysm is small and the symptoms are minor, doctors will monitor it over time. Periodically, the doctor may use ultrasound or a CT scan to check for any change in size. Medications are usually not prescribed.

However, when an aneurysm is large, between 5 and 6 cm, or there are symptoms, antihypertensive agents may be used to control blood pressure. Surgery may be necessary to remove the section of the artery

Surgery to correct aortic aneurysm. When an arterial wall becomes weakened or damaged, pressure within the vessel may cause the area to balloon out into a blood-filled sac called an aneurysm. In some cases, surgery to remove the section of the artery that balloons out may be necessary. The section is replaced using an artificial graft.

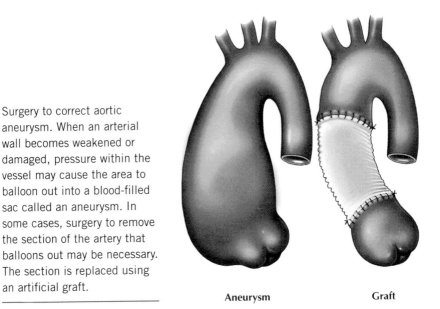

Aneurysm   **Graft**

that balloons out. A patch or artificial aortic graft is then sewn in place. In cases where the aneurysm is close to the aortic valve, valve replacement may be recommended (see page 122).

When the surgery involves an abdominal aneurysm, the risk of mortality is 3 to 5 percent; when it involves a thoracic aneurysm, it is somewhat higher. In order to repair a thoracic aortic aneurysm, open-heart surgery may be necessary.

In rare instances, stroke and paraplegia—paralysis of the lower half of the body—can occur as a result of aortic surgery. Strokes occur when a cerebral embolism or atherosclerotic debris blocks a major artery during aortic surgery. If circulation to the spinal cord is interrupted, paraplegia can occur. However, a number of maneuvers can reduce the incidence of these complications. For example, in a technique called retrograde cerebral perfusion, an anticoagulant fluid prevents blood clotting in the brain.

Although repairing an aortic aneurysm surgically is complicated and carries some risk, neglecting an aneurysm presents an even higher risk. Some 60 percent of people who undergo surgery for aneurysms survive longer than 5 years; only 20 percent of those who are not surgically treated survive that long.

Diseases of the Veins

The veins are the vessels that bring oxygen-depleted blood back to the heart. Venous circulation consists of two sets of vessels: subcutaneous or superficial veins (those just below the skin) and deep veins, both of which can connect frequently to each other.

Veins have three layers: inner, middle, and outer. More numerous than arteries, they also have a larger capacity and thinner, less elastic walls. In addition, they have valves that prevent backup as the blood is propelled toward the heart. Veins are subject to a number of conditions that disrupt circulation, the most common of which is thrombophlebitis.

Thrombophlebitis

When a thrombus forms in a vein and blocks the circulation of blood back to the heart, the condition is called thrombophlebitis or phlebitis. Phlebitis, the inflammation of a vein, causes swelling, pain, tenderness, and redness, most commonly in the legs, less frequently in the arms. It most commonly affects superficial veins and is slightly more common in women than in men.

Thrombophlebitis is often a result of trauma—an injury that crushes the vein, a medical procedure that pierces the vein, or a medication that irritates the vein. It can also occur in conjunction with infection. The clotting in superficial thrombophlebitis is usually visible under the skin.

Doctors can usually diagnose superficial thrombophlebitis just by looking at the area. Although it may cause some discomfort, superficial thrombophlebitis is seldom associated with serious complications, and it usually clears up within a week or two. In most cases of superficial thrombophlebitis, doctors monitor the condition, rather than treating it. Elevating the area, applying heat, and perhaps taking anti-inflammatory medications such as aspirin are enough to relieve pain and swelling. If an infection is involved, antibiotics are prescribed.

Deep-Vein Thrombosis

Deep-vein thrombosis, also called phlebothrombosis, is a thrombus in a vein without inflammation. It often develops after an extended period of inactivity, mostly affecting people who are bedridden after an accident, surgery, or some other medical condition. This type of thrombosis usually develops deep within the vein of the calf, although it can develop in other places in the leg or pelvis. Rarely, veins in the shoulder can be affected. While in most cases deep-vein thrombosis brings only minor discomfort, a permanent blockage can develop and in rare instances a pulmonary embolism (an embolus that travels to the lungs) occurs.

In order to confirm the presence of deep-vein thrombosis, x-rays with a radioactive tracer are needed. In some cases, Doppler tests are used. These tests detect turbulence around the blockage through ultrasound images. Blood tests may be ordered to rule out infection.

To treat deep-vein thrombosis, a doctor may administer an anticoagulant medication, such as heparin, to dissolve the thrombus. After the thrombus has been dissolved, oral anticoagulants such as aspirin or warfarin (Coumadin) may be recommended to prevent the formation of new

Varicose Veins

Veins may become stretched and swollen. Usually occurring in the legs, varicose veins are unsightly and may be painful. They may also result from damage to the valves in the veins.

Treatment may involve staying off the feet and wearing support stocking or elastic bandages. Surgery may be performed for uncomplicated varicose veins that produce symptoms, which may include soreness and itchiness. In severe cases, blood flow is disturbed. The varicose veins are removed, and the remaining veins quickly enlarge and take over their function.

thrombi. People who have thrombosis are urged to stay active and to continue walking. They are discouraged from sitting for long periods of time, as that position presses on the veins in the legs and pelvis.

If, as happens occasionally, the thrombus breaks loose and travels to the lung, surgery to insert a filter or tie off the vein may be performed, and anticoagulant medication is administered.

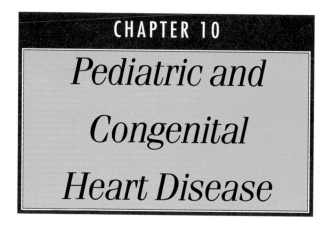

CHAPTER 10

Pediatric and Congenital Heart Disease

Introduction

Congenital heart disorders, which form while the fetus is developing in the uterus, affect 8 to 10 of every 1,000 children and are the most frequent congenital malformations in newborns. Congenital heart defects can produce symptoms at birth, during childhood, and sometimes not until adulthood. These birth defects are the result of an interaction of genetic and environmental factors.

Geneticists estimate that single mutant, or abnormal, genes account for about 3 percent of congenital heart diseases, and 5 percent are due to more complex chromosomal abnormalities. Another 3 percent are the result of known environmental factors, including rubella (German measles) and fetal alcohol syndrome. The remainder are the result of random or multifactorial effects.

At the present time, approximately 500,000 people in the United States have grown into adulthood with congenital heart disease, and about 20,000 more people with some form of congenital heart disease reach adulthood each year. Advances in treating heart disease have yielded many treatment options for both children and adults with congenital heart problems, allowing most of them to lead normal lives.

Congenital heart disease occurs when the heart or blood vessels connected to it do not develop normally before birth. Most congenital heart defects involve either an obstruction to blood flow or an abnormal routing of blood through the heart chambers. The structural defect may occur in the heart wall, the heart's main blood vessels, the heart valves, or a combination of these structures.

Signs and Symptoms

A congenital heart problem may be diagnosed before birth, immediately after birth, or during childhood; some are not diagnosed until adolescence or early adulthood, when the defect becomes severe enough to cause symptoms.

Newborn infants with certain types of congenital heart disease, such as transposition of the great vessels (page 214) and tetralogy of Fallot (page 211), may have cyanosis, or blue-tinted skin. Cyanosis indicates that not enough oxygenated blood is circulating throughout the body; it is sometimes associated with clubbing of the hands and feet. When an infant has clubbing, the ends of the fingers and toes enlarge and bend inward. Other symptoms in infants that signal a heart defect include eating difficulties, lack of sucking strength, poor growth, and rapid, labored breathing.

Symptoms in older children and adults include shortness of breath with exertion. Some congenital defects cause no symptoms but are discovered when a doctor listens to the heart during a routine physical examination or during a checkup for another problem.

Diagnosis: Exams and Tests

All congenital heart disorders are diagnosed through the same set of exams and tests.

The sounds made by a congenital heart defect are often so distinctive that a doctor can identify the disorder by listening to the heart with a stethoscope. The tests that help confirm the diagnosis and provide more detailed information about the condition are described below. Some of these tests may be performed before a child is born. For more information on diagnostic techniques see Chapter 4, Diagnosing Heart Disease.

Prenatal Ultrasound

Some congenital heart defects can be diagnosed before birth. An ultrasound exam, also called a sonogram, uses sound waves to create images of the developing fetus in the uterus. It is the most commonly used noninvasive test (a test that does not require breaking the skin or inserting instruments inside the body).

Ultrasound is so exact that it can identify several abnormalities in the developing infant before birth including some valve defects; irregularities in the size, shape, and position of the main blood vessels leading into and out of the heart; and the size and condition of the heart walls.

By diagnosing heart defects before a child is born, parents and doctors can plan for the appropriate medical and surgical care to be available at the time of delivery and thus improve the newborn's chances of survival.

Echocardiogram

This form of ultrasound provides the most important information about congenital defects because it shows the heart in action as well as the size and shape of the blood vessels, heart walls, and valves. An echocardiogram is repeated as the child grows to follow the development of the heart as well as the possible progression of a congenital heart abnormality.

There are two main techniques of performing the echocardiogram: transthoracic echocardiography, in which the ultrasound probe is placed on the outside of the chest wall, and transesophageal echocardiography, described below.

Transesophageal Echocardiography

A specialized form of ultrasound, transesophageal echocardiography (TEE) utilizes an ultrasound probe inserted into the esophagus. This eliminates some of the tissue layers through which ultrasound waves must pass, thereby creating a clearer image of the heart. TEE provides specific anatomic information for posterior abnormalities (those that are behind the heart) and anterior abnormalities (those that are directly in front of the heart) that cannot be gained from transthoracic echocardiography. TEE provides better images of structures within the heart than does magnetic resonance imaging (MRI; see page 208) and provides good images of problems such as atrial septal defects (see page 223). It is commonly used to evaluate adults with congenital malformations, and it may enable doctors to avoid invasive techniques such as cardiac catheterization and angiography (see below).

Intravascular Ultrasound

Intravascular ultrasound (IVUS) is an advanced ultrasound technique that utilizes a catheter (a long, hollow tube) fitted with a miniaturized ultrasound probe. The catheter is inserted into a blood vessel in the groin and advanced to the heart, where it is inserted directly into the wall of a coronary blood vessel. IVUS allows doctors to view the full circumference of the vessel and is used to supplement information gained from coronary angiography (see below).

Cardiac Catheterization

The use of cardiac catheterization in congenital heart disease has undergone a major evolution over the past 20 years. Previously, this direct view inside the heart via a tiny catheter inserted into a vein (usually in the groin) and moved up to the heart was used primarily for diagnosis. The emphasis has shifted to its use in interventional procedures, as in the treatment of congenital disorders. Cardiac catheterization is used to open narrowed arteries and insert stents, or small metal "ladders" that hold open arteries after such procedures (see page 97).

Coronary Angiography

In coronary angiography, doctors inject dye directly into the coronary arteries and then take x-rays and video films of them. In younger children with congenital malformations who have myocardial ischemia (insufficient blood flow to the heart muscle), coronary angiography is useful in finding dysfunctional coronary arteries. Adults over the age of 40 scheduled for heart surgery to repair some aspect of their congenital malformation often first undergo angiography to check for the presence of coronary artery disease (CAD). This aids surgeons in planning the best treatment strategy for CAD in adults with congenital heart disease.

Chest X-ray

A chest x-ray shows the position of the heart in the chest and its relationship to the lungs. Chest x-ray images for each congenital anomaly are very distinctive.

Electrocardiogram

Some congenital anomalies cause distinctive changes in the heart's electrical rhythm. During an electrocardiogram (ECG or EKG), a technician places electrodes, or conducting pads, on the chest, arms, and legs, and the heart's rhythm is recorded on graph paper.

Magnetic Resonance Imaging

Cardiac MRI provides good views of structures outside of the heart; unlike x-rays, it produces clear images of soft tissues. Doctors use MRI to supplement ultrasound information in people who have defects in the aorta and other coronary blood vessels.

Positron Emission Tomography

Positron emission tomography (PET) is unique in that it shows the metabolic (chemical) functioning of tissues and organs, unlike other imaging techniques, which show only structure. PET creates images that measure blood flow and show the rate at which body chemicals are metabolized by the heart tissues as they work. Certain heart abnormalities characteristically use up specific chemicals at specific rates.

Treatment

General Guidelines

Some congenital heart defects are mild and do not become much more serious over a person's lifetime and therefore do not require treatment.

Other congenital heart disorders can be treated effectively with medication or an increasing number of other nonsurgical interventions, called transcatheter procedures, which are performed using cardiac catheterization (see page 207 and below).

Many congenital heart defects still require surgery as the primary treatment. Timing of surgery is important, since some defects require at least some repair immediately at birth. Others may not require surgery until the child grows into school age or adolescence and sometimes not until adulthood. In some cases, heart transplantation is a viable alternative to reparative surgery (see Heart Transplantation, page 228).

The treatment of some disorders may entail a series of operations throughout infancy, childhood, and adulthood. Problems that are mild in childhood may become more serious over time; an adult may require repair of a congenital defect that did not cause trouble or need treatment earlier in life (see Changing Practices in Reoperations for Congenital Heart Anomalies, page 227). People with congenital defects will generally be monitored by a specialist throughout their lives.

In addition, children and adults with congenital heart defects, corrected or uncorrected, are at greater risk for acquiring the heart infection endocarditis and will need to be given antibiotics before certain dental and surgical procedures to prevent acquiring this infection (see Infective Endocarditis, page 113).

Transcatheter Procedures

Transcatheter procedures are surgical procedures performed through a tiny catheter that is inserted into a vein (usually) in the groin and moved up to the heart. Both balloon angioplasty (see page 96) and stent placement (see page 97) to open narrowed arteries as well as the repair of a variety of heart defects can be performed with this technique.

There are many advantages to using transcatheter procedures. With these procedures the risks of open-heart surgery, as well as chest scars, can be avoided. Many children can undergo catheterization procedures as outpatients and return to their normal activities in a day or two.

Most children undergoing these treatments do not require general anesthesia but only sedation and local anesthesia. The success rate of transcatheter procedures is higher when intravascular ultrasound and transesophageal echocardiography (see page 207) are used during the procedure. These diagnostic tools give doctors immediate feedback about the procedure they have just performed and allow them to make revisions immediately if necessary.

Choosing a Doctor and Hospital

When choosing a doctor and hospital for treatment of congenital heart problems, parents (or adults with congenital defects) should ask several questions (see Questions to Ask the Doctor and Hospital, below). One of the most important elements of treatment is finding a doctor specializing in pediatric and congenital heart disease. Parents may wish to obtain the names of several doctors and hospitals with the most experience in repairing congenital heart defects to get a second opinion.

A second opinion can help determine whether a recommended procedure is the most appropriate treatment for the problem at this time. Sometimes delaying surgery until a child is older is the best choice. A pediatric cardiologist or surgeon with experience in treating different congenital heart diseases and performing complex heart surgeries can

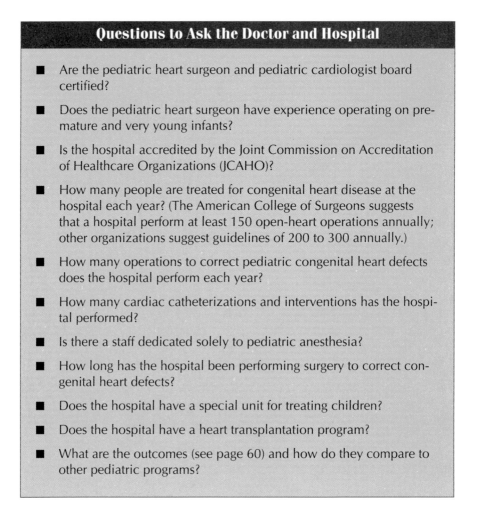

Questions to Ask the Doctor and Hospital

- Are the pediatric heart surgeon and pediatric cardiologist board certified?

- Does the pediatric heart surgeon have experience operating on premature and very young infants?

- Is the hospital accredited by the Joint Commission on Accreditation of Healthcare Organizations (JCAHO)?

- How many people are treated for congenital heart disease at the hospital each year? (The American College of Surgeons suggests that a hospital perform at least 150 open-heart operations annually; other organizations suggest guidelines of 200 to 300 annually.)

- How many operations to correct pediatric congenital heart defects does the hospital perform each year?

- How many cardiac catheterizations and interventions has the hospital performed?

- Is there a staff dedicated solely to pediatric anesthesia?

- How long has the hospital been performing surgery to correct congenital heart defects?

- Does the hospital have a special unit for treating children?

- Does the hospital have a heart transplantation program?

- What are the outcomes (see page 60) and how do they compare to other pediatric programs?

recommend the most effective treatment or combination of treatments for a particular heart defect.

Tetralogy of Fallot

Description

Four main structural abnormalities occur in tetralogy of Fallot (TOF), the most common congenital cause of cyanotic or "blue" babies. The two most serious of these defects are the ventricular septal defect and pulmonary stenosis; the other two abnormalities are abnormal placement of the aorta and right ventricular hypertrophy, or enlargement of the right ventricle.

In ventricular septal defect, there is an opening in the ventricular septum, the wall of the heart that normally provides a solid separation between the ventricles. The defect creates an abnormal blood flow called shunting. In pulmonary stenosis, blood flow through the pulmonary artery, the artery that carries blood from the right atrium to the lungs, is obstructed to some degree at or near the pulmonic valve.

Both ventricular septal defect and pulmonary stenosis must be corrected because they threaten life by decreasing blood flow to the lungs. As a result, blood is not properly oxygenated in the lungs before it is sent into the general circulation, which is why TOF is the most common cause of cyanosis at birth. When there is at least some degree of blood flow to the lungs, babies might not be blue at birth, but the cyanosis may become noticeable by approximately 6 months of age as the baby grows and the limited blood flow cannot keep up with the child's growth needs.

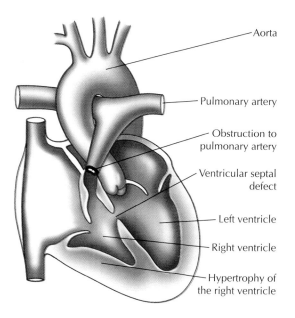

Aorta

Pulmonary artery

Obstruction to pulmonary artery

Ventricular septal defect

Left ventricle

Right ventricle

Hypertrophy of the right ventricle

Tetralogy of Fallot. This congenital heart disorder is characterized by four anomalies: ventricular septal defect (a hole in the wall dividing the ventricles), pulmonary stenosis (obstruction of the pulmonary artery), hypertrophy (thickening) of the right ventricle, and abnormal placement of the aorta (not seen).

Other symptoms and signs include shortness of breath, delayed growth and development, clubbing, and polycythemia (too many red blood cells).

Beginning at approximately 2 months of age, children with TOF often have attacks of hypoxia, a reduction of oxygen supply, which often are brought on by infection or an increase in activity. During a hypoxic attack, children are irritable, cyanotic, and have a rapid heart rate. These attacks, which may occur several times each day, last from a few minutes to a few hours.

Treatment and Results

The first surgical repair for TOF often occurs at birth. The surgeon creates a shunt, or new passage, to improve blood flow to the lungs, thus ensuring oxygen delivery to tissues throughout the body. The shunt serves as a temporary solution, and more extensive procedures to correct the defects are performed after the child has grown and developed further. The precise timing of surgical repair depends on each child's rate of growth and development, but research has confirmed that surgical repair is most successful when completed by age 5 years. Further benefit may be realized when all surgical repairs are completed in the first year of life. Early repair minimizes the damage to vital organs that can occur when tissues do not get enough oxygen. Early surgery may stop heart enlargement, which can occur when defects are not repaired, causing the heart to work harder and the heart muscle to stretch.

Surgeons generally close the ventricular septal defect in one operation and correct the pulmonary stenosis by performing a separate opera-

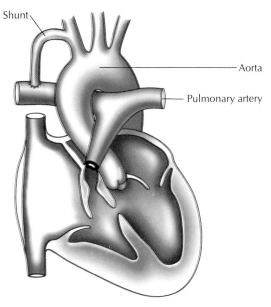

Initial surgical repair of tetralogy of Fallot. The surgeon creates a shunt to bypass the obstructed pulmonary artery and improve blood flow to the lungs. The shunt is only a temporary repair; more surgical procedures will be necessary to correct the defects.

Long-Term Survival After Surgical Repair of TOF

Research on approximately 1,000 children who have undergone complete TOF repair and been followed for at least 10 years shows that 90 to 95 percent of these children survived and have good heart function. Other studies indicate that at 30 years of age, the survival rate is about 86 percent.

tion to remove all obstruction to blood flow to the lungs. Sometimes, the procedures are done at the same time.

Experience has taught pediatric heart surgeons that repairing the defects with the child's own heart tissue—native tissue, or tissue transferred from other parts of the heart (generally the pericardium, the tissue lining the heart)—yields a far better result than using artificial tissue (such as polyester or plastic) or human tissue grafts.

Native tissue is also optimal because it grows as the other heart structures grow and as the child does; in contrast, non-native tissue fails to grow or even shrinks as the child grows. As a result, when native tissue is used, children have fewer and less serious complications caused by unequal growth. In particular, use of native tissue greatly minimizes the chances of residual pulmonary stenosis (an obstruction in blood flow through the pulmonary artery), which often occurs when non-native tissue is used.

Some children with less serious disease can undergo repair of pulmonary stenosis in a nonsurgical procedure called transcatheter balloon valvuloplasty. In this procedure, a catheter fitted with a balloon on its tip is inserted into a vein in the groin and advanced to the blocked area. The balloon is inflated to open the area of blocked blood flow.

Long-Term Follow-Up

Children with repaired TOF should be monitored throughout their lives by cardiologists who specialize in following children with congenital heart defects into adulthood. These specialists watch for the most common problems that can happen in this group of people, which include the following:

- Residual pulmonary stenosis, or some degree of blood-flow obstruction in the pulmonary artery, which occurs in about 25 percent of people with corrected TOF. Treatment is individualized according to each person's condition.

- Residual ventricular septal defects, or small holes in the wall between the ventricles, which occur in up to 20 percent of people with surgically corrected TOF. Generally, these small holes are fairly insignificant. Treatment is individualized and depends on whether there are accompanying abnormal heart rhythms.

Transposition of the Great Vessels

Description

In babies born with transposition of the great vessels, the positions of the heart's two main arteries (called the great vessels), the aorta and the pulmonary artery, are reversed. The pulmonary artery normally carries oxygen-poor blood to the lungs, where it is reoxygenated, and the aorta distributes oxygen-rich blood to every cell of the body.

It is easy to understand why such a reversal has serious consequences: It causes oxygenated blood to recycle through the lungs, never reaching oxygen-starved tissues throughout the body. This is why transposition is the second most common cause of cyanosis in newborn babies. This defect is so severe that 90 percent of babies born with it do not survive beyond the first year of life without reparative surgery.

Some babies are born with an additional defect—a patent ductus arteriosus (a still-open fetal blood vessel) or an atrial or ventricular septal defect (see page 220)—which allows some oxygen-rich blood to circulate through the body. Babies with transposition who are born without this additional defect require an emergency nonsurgical catheter procedure

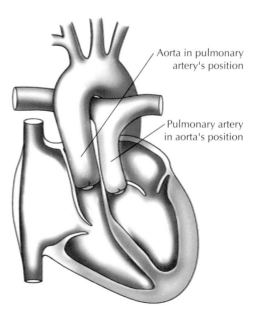

Aorta in pulmonary artery's position

Pulmonary artery in aorta's position

Transposition of the great vessels. In this congenital heart defect, the positions of the aorta and pulmonary artery are reversed.

very soon after birth to keep them alive until they are stable enough to have reparative surgery. Pediatric cardiologists perform this intervention, called balloon atrial septostomy. The doctor inserts a catheter tipped with a balloon into a vein in the groin and advances it to the left atrium. The doctor then triggers the release of the balloon and pulls the catheter back to the right atrium, which creates a temporary passageway that redirects blood flow so that blood is sent to the lungs for oxygenation. After this life-saving procedure, oxygen-rich blood is delivered to the body tissues, at least temporarily until the baby can undergo a full reparative surgery.

Treatment and Results

Surgical repair has the greatest success if performed by or before the time an infant reaches 2 weeks of age. When necessary—if an infant is not strong enough to undergo surgery during the first 2 weeks of life—surgeons can perform the operation later. Studies have not yet defined the upper age limit of safe surgical repair, and children and their unique heart abnormalities are evaluated on a case-by-case basis.

The most effective surgical repair of transposition of the great vessels is the arterial switch procedure. In this complex and technically difficult operation, pediatric cardiac surgeons essentially re-create a normal heart by relocating the aorta and the pulmonary artery to their intended positions. This reroutes systemic and pulmonary venous blood flow as nature intended it, so that deoxygenated blood is sent to the lungs through the pulmonary artery for oxygenation, and oxygenated blood is channeled to

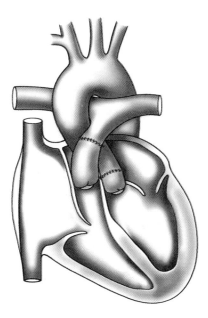

Arterial switch procedure to correct transposition of the great vessels. The aorta and pulmonary artery are relocated to their correct positions.

the aorta and out into the general circulation. Whenever possible, surgeons use native tissue from the atrium or the pericardium during the arterial switch procedure. If they cannot access enough native tissue, they use prosthetic tissue.

Before the arterial switch procedure became commonly used in the 1980s, procedures to correct transposition involved rerouting the blood within the heart to the correct arteries (*atrial* switch procedure); the arteries themselves were not moved. These operations led to complications, the most serious of which resulted in right ventricular dysfunction (as the weaker right ventricle was used to pump oxygenated blood throughout the body), and are now rarely used. Some adults who had undergone these procedures as children require additional surgeries to correct these complications. Although the arterial switch procedure carries its own set of complications, long-term complications appear to be less severe than for the earlier corrective procedures.

Hypoplastic Left Heart Syndrome

Description

In hypoplastic left heart syndrome (HLHS), the left side of the heart does not develop normally during fetal growth. Infants with this disorder are born with a very small left ventricle and underdeveloped aorta, which severely limits the heart's ability to pump blood throughout the body. Babies born with HLHS may seem normal at birth but most will

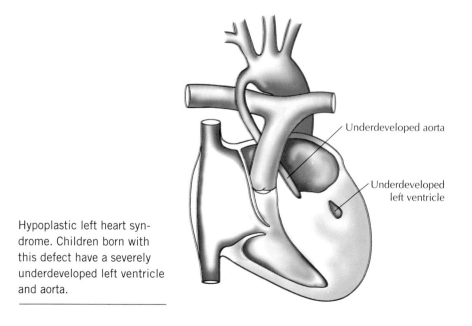

Hypoplastic left heart syndrome. Children born with this defect have a severely underdeveloped left ventricle and aorta.

Underdeveloped aorta

Underdeveloped left ventricle

require medical attention within the first few days of life to survive. HLHS is a rare but serious condition and remains the largest single cause of death from heart disease in children during the first week of life.

Treatment and Results

Parents of babies born with this condition have two medical options: a three-stage surgical repair or heart transplantation. Because pediatric hearts are not always available for donation and transplantation involves its own set of complications, the three-stage surgical repair is often the best option. The goal of these procedures is to rechannel the blood so that the right ventricle serves as a pump to circulate oxygenated blood throughout the body. The first, and most risky, stage of the repair, called the Norwood procedure, currently has about a 70 percent survival rate. Recent surgical advances to the Norwood procedure have greatly improved survival of infants with HLHS.

Formerly, during stage I of the repair, surgeons used either synthetic or non-native (nonheart) human tissue to reconstruct the aorta. Both types of graft are prone to calcification, a process that hardens the tissue, which was one factor contributing to the high failure rate of the traditional procedure. Non-native and synthetic grafts also do not grow at the same rate as the baby's heart, which causes complications. A separate problem that occurred with the traditional stage I, or Norwood, procedure was brain damage caused by the extended length of time required to perform the operation, during which the infant's heart had to be stopped and placed on cardiopulmonary bypass (a device used to oxygenate the blood and sustain circulation during open-heart surgery). At best, the traditional Norwood procedure required infants to be without normal circulation for an average of 55 minutes.

Multiple advances now allow the use of better grafts and also decrease operating time significantly. In the modified Norwood procedure, pediatric heart surgeons avoid the use of nongrowing patch grafts by using the baby's own tissue from other areas of the heart (native tissue). Not only are the native grafts superior, but using them decreases operating time significantly, which means a shorter time that the child is without normal circulation. While the procedure is too new to have allowed doctors to collect data on a large group of children who have been treated, pediatric surgeons think that this reduced operating time will lower the current rate of brain damage, which is estimated at 6 percent.

Stage II repair is generally performed at about 6 months of age and stage III repair, the Fontan procedure, is usually performed when the child is between ages 2 and 3 years old. Timing of the operations is crucial and carefully determined by the results of tests monitoring the child's heart function and overall growth and development. Survival rates

---

Long-Term Survival After Surgical Repair of HLHS

Children born with HLHS formerly did not survive. But recent advances in surgical treatment have greatly improved current survival rates. In a study of children who underwent a three-stage surgical repair for HLHS, survival at 5 years was 70 percent for those considered to be at standard risk. Most of the fatalities occurred in the first month of life; children who died later were primarily of a higher-risk group, such as those with additional complications. Five-year survival rates for surgical repair of HLHS are similar to those for heart transplantation.

---

for children undergoing stage II and stage III repair are significantly higher than for stage I.

Following surgical repair or heart transplantation, children will need monitoring and heart medication throughout their lives.

Coarctation of the Aorta

Description

Coarctation, or narrowing, of the aorta is a common congenital heart defect, accounting for approximately 8 percent of all congenital heart

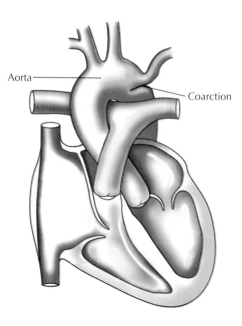

Coarctation (narrowing) of the aorta. The narrowed segment can be removed surgically and the two remaining ends joined together.

defects and second in prevalence only to ventricular septal defect (see page 222). Because it is relatively common and can have serious consequences, all babies are checked at birth for signs of coarctation.

This initial test simply involves measuring blood pressures and pulses at multiple pressure points. When significant differences are found, doctors perform additional tests (usually MRI; see page 208) to check for the presence of coarctation of the aorta.

In coarctation, there is severe stricture or narrowing at some point of the arch of the aorta. The aorta, the main blood vessel exiting the heart, arches at its peak before branching out to carry blood to the rest of the body. In about 95 percent of cases, coarctation occurs just beyond the left subclavian artery, the artery that occurs approximately at shoulder level.

Because of the stricture, the blood pressure in the arms is lower than it is in the legs, which causes a series of symptoms. Infants with this condition have shortness of breath, difficulty in feeding, and failure to thrive. Often, they have a relatively rare symptom in infants, pitting edema—a severe form of edema, or fluid retention, which causes pits to form when a finger is pressed gently into the edematous area, such as that on the leg. Pitting edema indicates a severe degree of heart failure in these infants.

Approximately one-fourth of babies with coarctation are diagnosed within the first week of life and another fourth within the next 3 weeks, with most in varying stages of severe forms of heart failure. Approximately 20 percent of infants with coarctation have only this condition, while the remainder have one or more other associated defects, including (in order of decreasing frequency):

■ Ventricular septal defect (see page 222)

■ Atrial septal defect (see page 223)

■ Aortic stenosis (see page 225)

■ Mitral stenosis (see page 227)

■ Mitral regurgitation (see page 227)

■ Transposition of the great vessels (see page 214)

When the coarctation occurs by itself, approximately three times as many boys have the condition than do girls. However, when multiple congenital heart malformations are involved, the incidence ratio is nearly equal for boys and girls.

Diagnostic Techniques

Defining the exact location, length, and severity of the narrowing in coarctation of the aorta is important to planning the most appropriate treatment. MRI, with its high degree of sensitivity, is particularly useful in identifying these characteristics of the coarctation. MRI allows a complete and detailed view of the thoracic aorta (the portion of the aorta in the chest) and the abdominal aorta (the portion in the abdomen). It also helps detect the other abnormalities that can occur with coarctation, such as a patent ductus arteriosus (a fetal blood vessel that, during the first two months after birth, should transform into a fibrous cord; when it does not, it may require surgical removal).

MRI is often done in conjunction with cineangiography, a diagnostic technique that provides a series of moving pictures of the heart in its various cycles. Cineangiography allows doctors to measure pressure inside the heart and also to detect basic changes in the heart's hemodynamic function (the heart pumping ability) that can result from coarctation. Identifying all these is critical to diagnosis and planning treatment.

Treatment and Results

Surgery is almost always conducted to repair coarctation. The narrowed segment of the aorta is removed and the two remaining ends are joined. Most children with coarctation need surgery within the first few weeks of life. If surgery must be delayed for any reason, some children can be stabilized with oxygen, antihypertensive (blood-pressure-lowering) medications, diuretics, and antiarrhythmic (rhythm normalizing) medications.

Repeat MRIs are useful in monitoring children who have had surgical repair of coarctation. In some children, the repaired aorta does not grow normally. It may develop with some degree of narrowing, although not as severe as the original coarctation. When narrowing occurs, a pediatric cardiologist dilates the area in a nonsurgical procedure called balloon angioplasty (see page 96).

The other common complication that develops is an aneurysm, a fluid-filled sac formed when the wall of the aorta narrows at the place where the surgery was conducted. Aneurysms are generally repaired surgically.

Atrial and Ventricular Septal Defects

The atrial septum is the wall separating the atria, the two upper chambers of the heart; the ventricular septum divides the ventricles, the two lower chambers. The septa are normally solid, but defects occur in them, causing shunts, or openings. These openings are also called communication defects.

Atrial and ventricular septal defects are among the most common congenital heart defects. Of children with congenital heart malformation, ventricular septal defects, many of which repair themselves, affect as many as 30 to 50 percent, while atrial septal defects occur in about 7 percent. Septal defects can occur alone or in conjunction with other congenital defects.

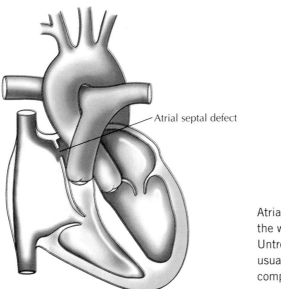

Atrial septal defect

Atrial septal defect—hole in the wall separating the atria. Untreated atrial septal defects usually do not lead to medical complications until adulthood.

While there is a wide range of severity in both defects, ventricular septal defects are more likely to cause symptoms and problems, although half of these are considered minor. The occurrence of problems has to do with the pressures inside the various parts of the heart. The pressures inside the atria are fairly equal; thus when there is a hole between them, pressure

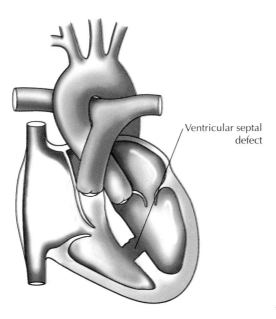

Ventricular septal defect

Ventricular septal defect—hole in the wall separating the ventricles. Larger openings can lead to cyanosis (blue-tinted skin) because the tissues of the body do not receive enough oxygenated blood.

problems are not generally an issue. However, pressure in the left ventricle is much higher than that in the right, so the pressure difference between them is significant. When a hole develops between the two ventricles, a disturbance in pressure is more likely to become a problem.

Ventricular Septal Defects

Description

Ventricular septal defects are more common than atrial septal defects; isolated ventricular septal defect, in which the defect occurs without any other heart defect, is the most common congenital heart defect. Approximately 65 percent of all ventricular septal defects are isolated. Two classification schemes distinguish ventricular septal defects from each other: where they occur and how they affect heart function. Ventricular septal defects are further divided into four types depending on where the defect occurs on the septum and size of the defect (large or small).

Defects that are about the same size as the opening of the aortic valve are considered large; those smaller than the aortic valve opening are classified as small. Most ventricular shunts are small and cause few symptoms, although nearly all produce a heart murmur. The smaller the shunt, the louder the murmur, because blood flows through it under greater pressure than through a larger shunt.

Less severe ventricular shunts may cause no symptoms in infants or sometimes what doctors call nonspecific symptoms. Nonspecific symptoms are those that are hard to pinpoint to any specific problem because they can occur with several different conditions; nonspecific symptoms include not feeding vigorously and not growing properly. As the child grows, the shunt may begin to cause shortness of breath, easy fatigue, and lack of stamina. Very minor shunts may not cause any symptoms at all, even in adulthood.

Larger ventricular shunts may cause the pressure between the two ventricles to equalize, which is how the severity of ventricular septal defect is classified. The most severe defects result in the most serious disturbance in pressure between the two ventricles. These are called group IV defects and affect about 10 percent of people with ventricular septal defects.

The more severe the defect, the more likely it is to cause cyanosis because the tissues are not properly oxygenated. People who develop group IV ventricular septal defects generally develop Eisenmenger's syndrome (see page 223).

Treatment and Results

Approximately half of all ventricular septal defects are small and up to 75 percent close spontaneously as the infant grows. About 5 to 10 percent of moderate to large ventricular septal defects undergo some degree of

Eisenmenger's Syndrome

About 10 percent of people with ventricular septal defects develop Eisenmenger's syndrome, which generally results in death by the age of 40. Because the shunt is so severe, the pressures in the pulmonary arteries are abnormally elevated, a condition called pulmonary hypertension.

Over time, the high pressures inside the pulmonary arteries cause them to hypertrophy, or thicken, creating an irreversible process in which pulmonary hypertension and hypertrophy inside the pulmonary artery both increase in severity. This combination of problems results in right-heart failure. Because the right side of the heart works so hard to compensate for these abnormalities, its muscle eventually stretches out and fails to work properly. There is no treatment for pulmonary hypertension.

spontaneous closure. Whether defects close spontaneously may also depend on where on the septum they occur. In general, spontaneous closure is most likely to occur during the first year of life, and 90 percent of shunts that close on their own do so by age 10; spontaneous closure in adulthood is rare.

When a ventricular septal defect does not close spontaneously and causes symptoms (cyanosis, shortness of breath, and pressure problems between the two ventricles), it must be closed surgically. Echocardiograms (see page 207) assess the size of the shunt and the function of the heart; surgical timing is based on these results and whether the child is growing normally. In most cases, ventricular shunt closure can be accomplished through a small incision on the side of the chest.

Surgical repair of ventricular shunts is very successful. While up to 20 percent of people who have undergone surgical repair may develop a residual shunt, or a new opening, only about 5 percent will need a second repair, although all children and adults with a residual shunt need to be followed closely.

Atrial Septal Defects

Description

Atrial septal defects account for about 7 percent of all congenital heart defects. They occur twice as commonly in girls as in boys. The overwhelming majority of atrial shunts occur spontaneously without a known cause, but some are due to a genetic anomaly that also causes congenital defects of the upper extremities. There are several types of atrial septal defects, which vary according to the size and location of the shunt.

The majority of babies born with atrial shunts have no symptoms, and generally there is no heart murmur because of the nearly equal pressures in the two atria. Often, an atrial septal defect is not detected until adulthood, when it produces symptoms. Babies who have symptoms may have shortness of breath, failure to thrive, and difficulty in feeding. Echocardiograms reveal the nature of the defect and help doctors decide when and if surgery is necessary to close the shunt.

Most people with an untreated atrial septal defect do not have symptoms until some time after the third decade of life. By the time these people reach their 50s, 70 percent have symptoms serious enough to impair their ability to lead a normal life, including shortness of breath, fainting, palpitations, and inability to exercise without fatigue.

Untreated atrial septal defects commonly lead to particular medical conditions in adults, the most common of which is pulmonary hypertension (high blood pressure in the pulmonary arteries). Pulmonary hypertension eventually affects as many as 15 to 20 percent of adults with untreated atrial septal defects. This complication rarely occurs before age 20 but is found in 50 percent of untreated adults by the time they reach age 40.

As with ventricular septal defect, about 5 to 10 percent of people with atrial septal defect eventually develop Eisenmenger's syndrome (see page 223). Other possible complications include right-sided heart failure, atrial fibrillation (page 151), atrial flutter (page 154), and stroke.

Treatment and Results

When an atrial septal defect is discovered in adults, surgery may still be a viable option. Surgical repair performed before age 25 is a low-risk procedure with an operative mortality rate (the rate of death associated with surgery and the immediate postoperative period) of just 1 to 3 percent. In addition to age, pulmonary pressure is an important predictor of long-term wellness and lack of complications. People most likely to benefit from atrial septal closure have a systolic pressure in the main pulmonary artery of less than 40 mm Hg. People under age 25 who undergo atrial shunt closure and have systolic pulmonary pressure less than 40 mm Hg have a long-term mortality similar to people without atrial septal defect.

When atrial septal defect closure is performed in people over age 40, survival rate and exercise capacity are improved, but the procedure does not prevent the risk of complications, including arrhythmias (heart rhythm disorders) and stroke. One arrhythmia, atrial fibrillation, occurs in 50 to 60 percent of people over age 40 with atrial septal defect, whether or not they have had a surgical repair.

Blood clots can occur in people with atrial septal defect, whether or not it has been surgically treated. Some 5 to 10 percent of people with atrial septal defects eventually develop blood clots, especially when they also have atrial arrhythmias. When the heart does not beat appropriately, blood has a moment to pool unnaturally, which can cause it to clot. Anti-coagulation medications are often prescribed to prevent clotting.

Congenital Valve Defects

The heart has four main valves:

- The mitral valve, between the left atrium and ventricle
- The tricuspid valve, between the right atrium and ventricle
- The aortic valve, between the left ventricle and the aorta
- The pulmonic (also called pulmonary) valve, between the right ventricle and the pulmonary artery

These intricate leaflets of tissue forcefully and efficiently open and shut to control blood flow into, within, and out of the heart.

Any of the heart's four valves can have a congenital defect. The most common valvular defects are aortic stenosis, pulmonic stenosis, tricuspid atresia, and anomalies of the mitral valve.

Aortic Stenosis

Normally, the aortic valve has three leaflets of tissue forming the valve; about 85 percent of children who have congenital aortic stenosis have bicuspid aortic valve—one with two leaflets of tissue. In another 14 percent of children with aortic stenosis, the tissue fails to differentiate into leaflets at all, resulting in a drop-shaped opening. In both cases, the stenosis, or obstruction, is due to an abnormal thickening of leaflet tissue. The thickening inhibits the valve from opening and closing properly to control blood flow; this is called a lack of valve mobility.

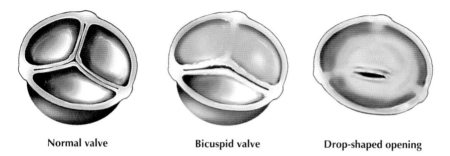

Normal valve   **Bicuspid valve**   **Drop-shaped opening**

Congenital defects of the aortic valve. In bicuspid valve, the valve has two, instead of the normal three, leaflets. A valve that does not develop any leaflets has a drop-shaped opening.

In infants born with congenital aortic stenosis, the degree of symptoms depends on how severe the aortic stenosis was during fetal development. At its mildest, aortic stenosis is characterized by almost normal heart function; the only finding may be a heart murmur. In these children, aortic stenosis is often a progressive disease: As they grow, the abnormal valve cannot keep pace with the increasing work demands of the heart.

Often, the condition worsens with rapid growth spurts, when the heart's workload is dramatically increased. Treatment includes surgical repair or replacement (see page 122).

Some infants with congenital aortic stenosis are born with more severe problems because stenosis during gestational development was more severe and the pressure in the developing left ventricle was abnormally high. At birth, these infants tend to have severely impaired functioning of the left ventricle and, as a result, left-sided heart failure.

Pulmonic Stenosis

The severity of pulmonic stenosis depends on the stage of congenital development at which it occurs; the earlier a defect occurs in gestation, the more severe it generally is. If there is a severe narrowing in the valve opening during fetal development, the pressure in the right ventricle can become very high. When pressures are high, the muscle forming the right ventricle hypertrophies, or thickens. In some cases, the muscular hypertrophy is so severe that the size of the right ventricle is greatly reduced.

Even infants born with moderately severe pulmonic stenosis may have no symptoms at birth; the condition is only detected because of the presence of a heart murmur. An electrocardiogram shows characteristic abnormalities, and a chest x-ray often shows an enlarged heart muscle. Despite the abnormalities, right ventricular function may be normal in some of these infants. In its more severe form, pulmonic stenosis may cause infants to be cyanotic because the right ventricle does not function properly and not enough blood is returning to the lungs for oxygenation.

Treatment is based on the severity of the condition, the presence of other congenital defects, and the infant's general health; most children with congenital pulmonic stenosis undergo pulmonary valvotomy, a surgical procedure during which the valve opening is enlarged. Doctors measure the blood pressures in the right side of the heart to help them time surgery.

Depending on the severity of the pulmonic stenosis and the child's general health, the condition may be repaired by balloon valvuloplasty, a nonsurgical procedure. A catheter fitted with a balloon on the tip is advanced to the narrowed valve and then inflated. The inflation of the balloon creates a larger opening in the valve.

Tricuspid Atresia and Regurgitation

Congenital defects may cause atresia, or the lack of an opening, in the tricuspid valve. Isolated congenital tricuspid atresia is rare. More commonly, the tricuspid valve does not suffer total atresia but is slightly underdeveloped; this often occurs when the right ventricle underdevelops congenitally. In both forms, infants are generally quite ill at birth, with severe cyanosis. In other cases, generally in conjunction with other defects, the tricuspid valve may have some degree of insufficiency and develop regurgitation, in which the valve cannot properly control blood flow, and some blood flows backward through the valve.

Congenital Mitral Valve Problems

Congenital defects of the mitral valve can cause stenosis, regurgitation, or atresia. While all are relatively rare, they are generally the most severe congenital valvular problems.

- *Congenital mitral stenosis* (narrowing of the mitral valve) causes severe symptoms in early infancy, including pulmonary edema (an accumulation of fluid in the lungs) and pulmonary hypertension that causes severe congestive heart failure (see page 158). It is often associated with other anomalies in the left side of the heart.

- *Mitral regurgitation* (improperly controlled blood flow; some blood flows backward through the valve) is also often associated with other congenital malformations or as the result of correcting other malformations. For example, when transposition of the great vessels is surgically repaired (see page 214), the mitral valve can be adversely affected and mitral regurgitation can occur.

- *Mitral atresia* (or lack of an opening in the mitral valve) is exceedingly rare but may be associated with other congenital anomalies. When mitral atresia does occur, it often causes pulmonary venous obstruction, in which blood flow through the pulmonary veins, which return oxygenated blood from the lungs to the heart, is greatly reduced.

Because each of these conditions is rare and often associated with other conditions, their repair is highly individualized and timed according to the need for other surgical procedures.

Changing Practices in Reoperations for Congenital Heart Anomalies

Children with congenital heart anomalies may need a second or even a third operation to rerepair the original defect or to accommodate the child's growth. Twenty years ago, pediatric cardiac surgeons tended to delay reoperation until the child experienced persistent cyanosis or growth delay because reoperations were so risky. Many times, surgeons waited until a child's life was in danger.

For example, in children with tetralogy of Fallot, complications of the right ventricle and the tricuspid valve often developed before surgeons intervened again. Today, surgeons monitor children carefully, looking for changes in right ventricular dimension and early signs of tricuspid incompetence. Rather than waiting for overt problems, surgeons now intervene early if there is movement toward either of these problems.

Today, reoperations are performed much sooner, before there is irreversible damage to the heart muscle or growth delay. Advances in pediatric surgical techniques have significantly lowered the risks in reoperation, which are now no higher than in the initial operation.

Cardiac specialists continually improve and refine treatments for each congenital cardiac anomaly, including those for subsequent operations. Improvements in diagnostic techniques help pediatric cardiologists and cardiac surgeons periodically reassess a child's cardiac status and carefully time a second procedure. In many cases, the necessity and timing of reoperation can be estimated by the nature of the original congenital problem.

Children and adults with congenital anomalies who have undergone cardiac surgery are monitored three to four times annually by echocardiography to assess cardiac function and growth until their condition stabilizes, which means there is little continuing change in the congenital anomaly and heart function. After that, monitoring is generally performed yearly throughout a person's lifetime.

The ability to perform surgery successfully on very small infants and children is due to several advances in pediatric heart surgery. One is the increasing availability of pediatric-sized instruments. Greater success is also realized because of new and better techniques of performing cardiopulmonary bypass (see page 217) in children. Also, during the initial operation, the pediatric surgeon may plan for reoperations by modifying initial surgical techniques, including how and where the initial incision is made.

Heart Transplantation

Heart transplantation is a viable option for infants and children of all ages when congenital defects cannot be repaired. Infants and younger children are typically candidates for a heart transplant when complex, irreparable congenital defects exist.

However, the scarcity of donor hearts, particularly those of appropriate size, make heart transplantation more difficult in infants and children than it is in adults. Because the wait for an appropriate heart can be longer for a child than for an adult, pediatric cardiac centers have developed techniques to support the child until transplantation is available.

One advanced life-support technique is called extracorporeal membrane oxygenation. Doctors implant a pump into the patient, which forces the blood to circulate; the pump is attached to a membrane containing an oxygen supply. Older children may be candidates for left-ventricular assist devices, larger mechanical pumps that are more like an artificial heart than the extracorporeal membrane, that keep the heart beating until a new heart is found.

Transplant is not only a more technically challenging operation in children than it is in adults, but it also requires that parents consider life-long issues, such as the side effects of antirejection drugs, which can affect appearance and physical development during puberty.

A child who has undergone a heart transplant benefits from a post-surgical medical team that includes pediatric cardiologists who specialize in taking care of children after transplant, specially trained nurses, social workers, and family counselors versed in managing both the medical and psychological issues relevant to transplant, especially during puberty and adolescence.

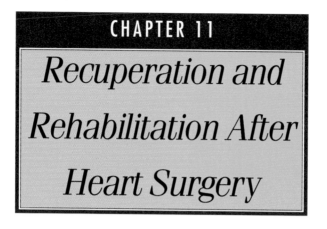

CHAPTER 11

Recuperation and Rehabilitation After Heart Surgery

Introduction

A t many hospitals that perform heart surgery, people who are about to undergo surgery are asked to visit a preoperative testing and education department. There, they learn from cardiac nurses what to expect when they awake from surgery and for the remaining days they will spend in the hospital. Just as important, the nurses provide instruction regarding self-care during the recuperation time at home.

Why is postsurgical care taught before surgery rather than just before the person goes home? Often after surgery, people are less alert because of having had anesthesia and because they take analgesics, or pain medications. Both dull the senses and the ability to comprehend details, such as instructions about caring for wounds, taking medications, modifying the diet, and activity guidelines.

The nurses who do this type of teaching recommend that family members who will visit in the hospital and be at home with the person who has had heart surgery, especially those who will assist in caring for their relative, be present for this presurgical teaching. This instruction is also especially useful in helping them understand what to expect when they see their loved one after surgery and when they take that person home.

The caretakers can serve another role: They are the ones who recall more of the details relevant to recuperation in the postsurgical period, when the patient is drowsy because of the lingering effects of anesthesia and analgesics.

The Stages of Recuperation

The first 6 weeks after heart surgery are a crucial period for recuperation. After 6 weeks, incisions are generally healed, and the patient is ready to resume previous activities. These first 6 weeks can be divided into four main stages of recuperation:

- The first 24 to 48 hours, when patients who have undergone heart surgery remain in the cardiovascular intensive care unit (ICU).

- The next 3 to 5 days, when the patient remains in the hospital after leaving the ICU.

- The first 5 weeks at home.

- The period beginning 6 weeks after surgery.

The First 24 to 48 Hours after Surgery

If you undergo heart surgery, you will probably have little recollection of the first 1 to 2 days after the procedure when you will still be heavily sedated from the anesthesia you received during surgery—a drowsiness compounded by the analgesics administered to keep you comfortable. Family members, however, will be acutely aware of this stage of recuperation and may find it the most dramatic because of the many different tubes and wires that are attached to you after surgery, as well as the various monitors necessary to track vital information regarding the heart and other vital body organs. Understanding the purpose of this plethora of medical equipment will alleviate some of the uncertainty and anxiety that may arise upon seeing this technologic maze.

After heart surgery, the doctors monitor you carefully, making sure that your heart and respiratory system are functioning optimally after surgery. The first 24 to 48 hours are an especially critical time to monitor heart and lung function, as the heart has essentially undergone a major trauma during surgery. Among the monitoring equipment used during this first stage of recovery are:

- *Heart monitor:* The heart monitor is attached to a continuous electrocardiogram (ECG or EKG). Conducting leads, or wires, are attached at several places on the chest through adhesive patches, and then to a monitor that continuously records the heart rhythm and rate.

    In addition to the monitor in your room, there is a monitor at a monitoring station in the ICU. There, specially trained nurses watch over all monitors continuously, checking for any problem with how fast the heart is beating and the pattern in which it beats.

The monitors in the monitoring station are programmed to set off an alarm when abnormalities occur. The monitoring nurses immediately alert the nurse caring for you so that immediate action can be taken to correct abnormalities. Doctors in the ICU are ready to diagnose problems and prescribe medications necessary to correct rhythm and rate problems that often occur during the early postoperative period.

Knowing about this system of monitoring helps you, the patient, and family members to be assured that your heart function is carefully scrutinized every second during the first and most critical hours of recuperation after surgery.

- *Arterial pressure line:* A catheter inserted into an artery in one of the arms monitors the pressure in the arteries. This provides important information about how the heart is working after surgery.

- *Heart pressure:* A catheter is inserted into a vein in the neck: This intravenous line is threaded directly into the heart to monitor pressures inside the heart, providing another piece of information about how well the heart is working.

In addition to the monitoring equipment, you are "connected" to several other tubes in the first days of recovery. These tubes probably include the following:

- *One or two intravenous (IV) lines:* These IVs are necessary to deliver fluid to prevent dehydration, because during the first days after surgery, you are generally not allowed to eat or drink and must have enough fluid to prevent dehydration. The IVs also deliver medications. Because many intravenous medications may be necessary immediately after heart surgery, cardiac surgeons prefer to have at least two lines available so that more than one medication can be administered at any time.

- *Foley catheter:* This small pliable tube is placed into the bladder through the urethra, the body orifice through which urine is eliminated. The catheter is connected to a bag that collects urine. This eliminates the need to leave the bed to empty the bladder during the first days, when complete bed rest is essential.

- *Chest tubes:* Small tubes are placed on the incision line and sewn in place when surgeons suture (stitch) the incision line. These tubes allow blood and fluid that would otherwise collect at the surgical site to drain from the body. Because the blood is collected and carefully measured, these tubes also help doctors and nurses monitor the amount of blood loss after surgery.

During these first 24 to 48 hours after surgery, you will need complete rest. Although it is important for family members to visit and provide soothing and calming supportive comments, family members should realize ahead of time that you are not fully alert and may not remember many of the events that are taking place. Because rest is so important, and also because so many nurses, doctors, and other health-care professionals are present in the ICU, visiting time during this stage of recovery is generally greatly restricted.

In most cases recovering patients do not eat in the ICU. At this stage doctors might allow you to suck on ice chips and sometimes to take sips of water. This allows the body, especially the intestinal tract, to "wake up" after anesthesia. Since nausea is common after anesthesia, withholding food and liquids protects you from vomiting, which can be a strain.

Before you leave the ICU, your doctor tries to remove as many tubes and wires as possible. The arterial pressure monitoring line and the neck catheter must be removed before you leave the ICU. Often the chest tubes, the Foley catheter, and one IV line are removed at this time. One IV line is generally left in place when you leave the ICU, as are the leads for monitoring the heart rate and rhythm.

Leaving the ICU: The Next 3 to 5 Days

After leaving the ICU, people who have undergone heart surgery generally go to a "step-down unit" for the second stage of recovery. This means the level of monitoring is less intensive than that in the ICU but more than that on a regular hospital floor. Most people remain attached to a heart monitor, although now it is a portable version. The leads are connected to a battery-operated portable monitor about the size of a transistor radio, which transmits the heart rate and rhythm to a monitoring station continuously staffed by specially trained nurses.

The goals of this stage of recovery are to get you moving, eating, and performing your own personal hygiene and to make sure your heart rate and rhythm are normal as you engage in these activities. In the first day or two while in this step-down unit, you will receive your first food. You will probably begin with clear liquids (broth, gelatin, juice) and then progress to "full liquids" (cream soups, pudding, milk). This will allow your intestinal tract to become reaccustomed to food.

Within a day or two, you will receive regular food as tolerated. Often, though, appetite is poor during this time. You may still be experiencing pain, which decreases appetite. The effects of analgesia may make you nauseated, suppressing your appetite. During this time, you will be concentrating on taking in small amounts of food, which is so necessary for healing after heart surgery.

Most step-down units provide phase I cardiac rehabilitation. Specially trained exercise physiologists will work with you at this stage of your recovery to get you out of bed and keep you moving on a regular basis. Although this may be painful and difficult, it is important for many reasons. Getting out of bed and moving as soon as possible after surgery helps prevent complications of any type of surgery but, especially after heart surgery, there is a need to prevent thrombosis, or the formation of blood clots. Moving will help prevent this complication.

Getting out of bed and walking also helps the heart start working again, which speeds its return to normal functioning. Finally, getting up and using the muscles limits the amount of strength lost by muscles. Lying in bed causes muscles to lose strength very quickly. When this happens, people find it more difficult to recover from surgery.

It is normal for people at this stage of recovery to experience pain from the surgical incision. This is especially true when the breast bone or ribs have been cut to allow the surgeon access to the heart. Pain experts recommend that people take pain medication on schedule at this stage of recuperation, rather than waiting for the pain to become unbearable. If you were to wait until the pain becomes severe before you take a dose of pain medication, you would find it more difficult to control the pain.

Many heart surgery centers offer opportunities for patients and their families to learn about diet, wound care, activity recommendations, and psychosocial issues of heart surgery in this second stage of recovery. Although you may be too fatigued to sit through classes or comprehend this information, these classes will be particularly helpful for your family.

Your family should realize that you might not act quite like yourself during this stage of recovery. You will probably be exceptionally fatigued. This is a result of the surgical anesthetics (as most people feel the effects of anesthesia for several days after surgery) and sleep deprivation, as you will most likely leave the ICU suffering from lack of sleep. ICU conditions often do not allow a good night's sleep. ICUs are often noisy, with monitors continuously sounding, and bright most of the day and the night; also, nurses and doctors are constantly at the bedside to provide the necessary intensive monitoring.

The physical stress of surgery is very draining. Knowing all this, it is easy to understand why you might be out of sorts, cranky—just not yourself during this stage of recovery. Rather than call attention to it, family members should encourage you to rest and limit visiting time so you can do so.

Before leaving the hospital, doctors will make sure your heart rate and rhythm are normal and that you are able to eat a full meal. In addition, they will make sure that oral pain medication can effectively control the pain that you will still feel when you return home.

At Home During the Next 5 Weeks

During the next 5 weeks at home, you will gradually return to your former routine and lifestyle. You should plan on progressing a little more each day. The goal is to assume all care for yourself during this time, in comfortable stages.

One of the most important strategies during this time is to get up, bathe (which might be modified until the incision is sufficiently healed), and get dressed every morning. Although you will rest a significant portion of the day the first week after returning home, getting dressed is important to establish an attitude of progress and to gradually gain more strength and independence for yourself.

Heart surgeons generally recommend that once you return home, you should walk around for 5 minutes, five times a day, spread out over the normal course of a day. This is essential to regain strength and will also prevent thromboses. It will also help strengthen your heart and help you to regain normal functioning. Walking should be slowly paced (with the pace gradually increasing) and never rushed. If at any time you become fatigued or short of breath—both of which are common during the first weeks after heart surgery—simply stop and begin a period of rest.

By the third week after surgery, most of this shortness of breath and fatigue should be gone, especially if you are faithful to your five daily (albeit brief) walks. By the time you have reached the 6-week mark from the day of surgery, you should be walking a total of a mile per day, divided into 3 to 5 walks. This may vary depending on your age and whether you have had previous heart surgeries, as well as your general physical condition.

Good nutrition, although always important, is especially critical during this time. Your body is particularly demanding of good nutrition for two reasons: It has just undergone a major trial, and the incision as well as the heart muscle itself must heal. See Nutrients Essential to Healing after Surgery, page 237.

Wound Care

Wound care is a very important part of this stage of recovery. Some people who have undergone heart surgery have their sutures or staples removed before leaving the hospital. Others do not (they either return to the doctor's office for removal or a home-care nurse removes them). Both before and after the sutures or staples are removed, wound care is essential. Before leaving the hospital, the nurse will teach you how to care for the wound, which includes the following:

■ *What type of bathing is allowed.* The nurse will inform you when it is safe to get the incision wet in the shower. Before that, sponge bathing is recommended. See Bathing after Heart Surgery, page 238.

■ *How and how often to dress or bandage the wound.* You may be able to care for the wound yourself, or you may need the assistance of a home-care nurse. You should discuss this with your doctor before you leave the hospital. You can arrange for the appropriate

Nutrients Essential to Healing After Surgery

- *Protein.* Protein is needed to make new tissue and repair injured tissue, both important in closing the wound. It also is an ingredient in making white blood cells, which help fight infection. Skimping on protein delays healing and decreases resistance to infection, one of the most common complications of surgery and a main reason that wounds are slow to heal.

- *Vitamin A.* Vitamin A boosts the production of fibroblasts, cells that form the body's connective tissue that closes the wound. It also forms leukocytes (white blood cells) to fight infection. Foods high in vitamin A include sweet potatoes, carrots, evaporated skim milk, apricot nectar, liver, ricotta cheese, cantaloupe, tomatoes, squash, and spinach.

- *Vitamin C.* Vitamin C helps speed healing by encouraging the body's production of fibroblasts and leukocytes. Foods rich in vitamin C include orange juice, tomatoes, kiwis, papaya, strawberries, spinach, sweet potatoes, and cantaloupe.

- *B vitamins.* At least three B vitamins help prevent wound infections: pyridoxine (B_6), thiamin (B_1), and riboflavin (B_2). These vitamins also help the body use protein and calories more efficiently. Pyridoxine-rich foods include chicken, fish, pork, eggs, liver, oats, soybeans, and bananas; thiamin-rich foods include liver, unrefined whole grains, legumes, and brewer's yeast. Foods rich in riboflavin include meat, fish, poultry, eggs, dairy products, broccoli, asparagus, turnip greens, and spinach.

- *Minerals.* Magnesium, iron, copper, and zinc play many roles in wound healing. All are necessary in making the protein that builds new cells to close wounds. Iron and copper carry oxygen to the wound, another essential ingredient in wound healing.
    - Magnesium-rich foods include unprocessed whole grains, legumes, nuts and seeds, avocados, and bananas.
    - Iron-rich foods include lean meats, legumes, whole grains, nuts and seeds, and green leafy vegetables.
    - Copper-rich foods include shellfish, liver, whole grains, nuts and seeds, and legumes.
    - Zinc-rich foods include seafood, meats, whole grains, and legumes.

- *Essential Fatty Acids.* Some dietary fat is always necessary, and essential fatty acids are crucial to healing. The body is unable to make essential fatty acids, which are needed for the formation of cell membranes and also to boost the immune system to help prevent infection. Most people eat a minimum of 25 grams of fat daily (and generally, around 40 to 60 grams); even 25 grams is enough to supply the necessary amounts of essential fatty acids.

Bathing After Heart Surgery

You will probably be allowed to shower when the incision is healing and dry. The following guidelines are recommended in the first weeks when the incision is still healing and you are still feeling weak:

- Place soapy water on your hand or washcloth and gently wash the incision(s) up and down. Until the scabs are gone and the skin is completely healed, do not rub the incision with a washcloth.

- When showers and baths are permitted, they should be limited to 10 minutes. The water temperature should be warm—not hot or cold. Extreme water temperatures can cause faintness.

type of care and bandaging material to be delivered to your home by a hospital supply company.

- *How to monitor the wound for signs of infection.* Redness, warmth, and drainage from the wound signal infection and so does fever. These signs warrant a call to the doctor.

- *What to place on the wound.* You should not apply any ointments, oils, or salves unless the doctor or nurse specifically advises doing so.

Helping the Sternum Heal

It takes about 6 to 8 weeks for the sternum (breastbone) to heal. During this time, you will be able to do light household chores, such as laundry, shopping, cooking, light gardening, dusting, and washing dishes—as your energy allows. Remember not to stand in one place for longer than 15 minutes.

Although it is all right to perform activities above shoulder level—such as reaching for an object or brushing your hair—do not hold your arms above shoulder level for a longer period of time.

Lifting heavy objects is restricted—do not lift anything that weighs more than 20 pounds. Avoid any activities that require pushing or pulling heavy objects, such as shoveling snow or mowing the lawn.

Check with your doctors to confirm which activities are allowed and which are not.

Medication Schedule

Establishing a medication schedule and being vigilant about it will help you toward a speedy recovery. Although you may have been on one set of medications before surgery, this will probably change after surgery. Once you return home, you should only take those medications that are prescribed when you are discharged from the hospital. Carefully review the entire list of medications with your doctor before leaving the hospital. Remember, you may feel so much better after heart surgery that you may think that you do not need to take all your prescribed medications. This is a dangerous mistake, as it could prevent your heart from functioning properly. Stick to the prescribed medications even if you are feeling well—so that you will continue to do well. Talk it over with your doctor at your checkup.

Taking pain medication at home will help you get up and get going. If you are in pain, you probably will not want to get up, but failure to do so will delay healing and regaining strength. It is better to take pain medication as needed to be comfortable and allow movement. Gradually, you will find that you can reduce the dose and the frequency.

Often, the last dose to be stopped is the one you take at bedtime. This is because it is normal to be more aware of pain in the quiet of the night. Just as taking pain medicine is important to get moving in the early days of this stage of recovery, it is also important to make sure you get a good night's sleep in the later stages of recovery. Sleep allows the body to heal.

Controlling Leg Swelling

Leg swelling is quite common in this stage of recovery. This is especially true in people who have had vein grafts taken from their legs. Veins in the legs return blood to the heart. If veins have been removed from the legs for use as bypass grafts, blood may be slower in returning to the heart. This can cause some fluid to accumulate in the ankles and lower legs. Swelling can be controlled by

- Elevating the feet higher than the heart when resting, which should be done on the bed or couch with several pillows under the legs at least three times per day for 1 hour

- Not crossing the legs

- Walking daily—walking helps promote circulation, which eliminates swelling

- Wearing support stockings as recommended by the doctor

Mental Functioning and Sleep Problems

Some people become frustrated during this stage of recovery because they feel they are not as sharp mentally as they were before surgery. These cognitive changes are normal after heart surgery. The entire body, including the brain, was seriously stressed during surgery, especially if the surgery involved stopping the heart and circulating the blood through a heart-lung machine. Just as muscle strength returns, so does normal cognitive functioning. Patience is needed to avoid the frustration that can accompany this side effect of surgery. You should not force yourself to work or perform mentally stressful tasks, such as balancing a checkbook, in the first couple of weeks after surgery.

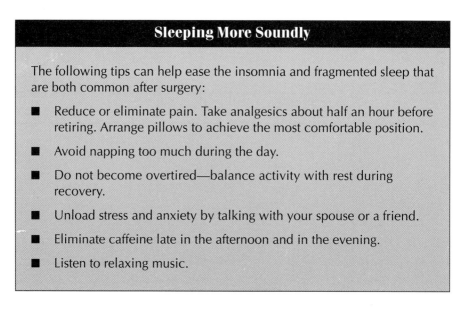

Sleeping More Soundly

The following tips can help ease the insomnia and fragmented sleep that are both common after surgery:

- Reduce or eliminate pain. Take analgesics about half an hour before retiring. Arrange pillows to achieve the most comfortable position.

- Avoid napping too much during the day.

- Do not become overtired—balance activity with rest during recovery.

- Unload stress and anxiety by talking with your spouse or a friend.

- Eliminate caffeine late in the afternoon and in the evening.

- Listen to relaxing music.

Sleep problems are also common during this stage of recovery. Insomnia and fragmented sleep are both common; they both occur for several reasons: the lingering effects of anesthesia, the discomfort related to healing, changes in the daily routine, and stress from the personal concerns brought on by having had surgery. See Sleeping More Soundly, above, for guidelines on improving sleep, and consult your doctor if sleeping soundly remains a problem.

Sexual Relations

During this third stage of recovery, you may wonder about having sexual relations. Discuss with your surgeon and cardiologist when a return to sexual activity is safe. Doctors generally gauge this on your physical ability. The amount of energy required to have sexual intercourse with a spouse or regular partner is similar to climbing about one or two flights of stairs or walking about half a mile at a brisk pace. If you cannot perform these activities without developing angina (chest pain) or shortness of breath or becoming overtired, you will need additional recovery time before resuming sexual activity.

Some things you should keep in mind as you return to sexual activity:

- Anxiety on the part of either you or your partner may interfere with sexual arousal and performance.

- Medications may also interfere with sexual arousal and performance.

- A sexual relationship has both physical and emotional aspects.

- Plan sex when you are rested and physically comfortable.

- For the first 6 to 8 weeks after surgery, use positions which limit pressure or weight on the breastbone or tension on the arms and chest.

- Partners should be caring, honest, and loving with each other, speaking openly and frankly.

Recovery After 6 Weeks

By 6 weeks after surgery, incisions are usually entirely healed and most people have assumed their former routine. If you worked outside the home before surgery, you will probably be able to return to work, at least on a part-time basis.

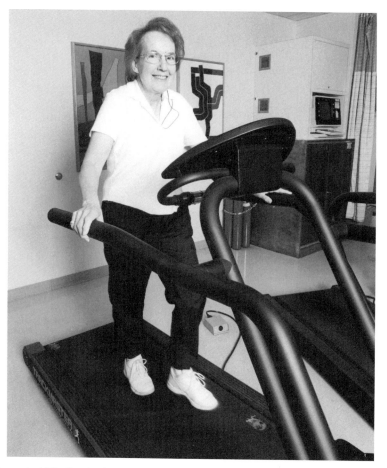

Cardiac rehabilitation includes cardiovascular monitoring while exercising on a treadmill or exercise bicycle.

Phase II cardiac rehabilitation, or a monitored and guided form of exercise, is strongly recommended beginning at 6 to 8 weeks after surgery. Specially trained nurses and exercise physiologists monitor blood pressure and pulse rate as you exercise on treadmills and exercise bicycles.

During the first weeks of rehabilitation, you will probably be connected to a portable heart monitor that tracks heart rate and rhythm, yielding important information about how much exercise you can tolerate safely, especially as you progress in your exercise program. Depending on the heart's condition, you will undergo intermittent or continuous heart monitoring for the remainder of the rehabilitation program.

Experts recommend continuing in a cardiac rehabilitation program for approximately 12 weeks after heart surgery. During the initial weeks, you will most likely attend these monitored exercise sessions three times weekly. The number will drop to twice weekly and then to weekly sessions. This weaning is encouraged, as it is designed to help you learn to incorporate exercise into your own life.

Some people choose to enter a phase III rehabilitation program, which is essentially a maintenance program that can continue indefinitely. This is a guided exercise program monitored by a team of specially trained cardiac nurses and exercise physiologists. Other people develop a phase III, or lifelong, exercise program on their own.

Living with Heart Disease

It is normal to feel depressed, angry, frustrated, and afraid after heart surgery. Depression is one of the most common emotions to affect people who have undergone heart surgery, even if they have never been depressed in the past. For example, you may not know what to expect or be unable to do simple tasks without becoming overtired. Once you resume your regular activities, the negative feelings you had experienced initially should gradually go away.

It is natural to be frightened and anxious about your heart, which has traditionally been regarded not only as a vital organ, but also as the center of the entire individual. An injury—which includes surgery—may be perceived as a threat to the whole person, body and soul. Heart experts say that the necessity of making lifestyle changes in several areas simultaneously after heart surgery places a heavier emotional burden on a person than might be felt with other diseases.

There are excellent strategies to relieve the emotional blues as well as the fear and anxiety. These include the following:

- Getting dressed first thing in the morning, every day
- Getting out of the house and walking daily

■ Resuming enjoyable and favorite hobbies and social activities

■ Sharing feelings with a spouse, friend, religious leader, or mental health professional

■ Enjoying a visit with friends

■ Sleeping soundly

■ Joining a support group, such as Mended Hearts, a group for people who have had heart surgery and their families

■ Attending a cardiac rehabilitation program; research shows that people who join and regularly attend a monitored exercise program are less likely to be depressed and anxious. The same is true for their family members.

Knowing that feelings of anxiety, fear, and depression are normal should be helpful in relieving them. If you experience these common feelings, do not hesitate to discuss them with your doctor or with a mental health professional. Staff in the cardiac rehabilitation program are an excellent sounding board for these feelings. In fact, many rehabilitation programs include sessions in which you can feel free to discuss these feelings, as well as techniques that will help empower you to handle them.

Compliance

Doctors prescribe medications and many lifestyle changes for people who have had heart surgery. These lifestyle changes include dietary changes, exercising, and stopping smoking. In some cases, the doctor may also prescribe a regular schedule of testing, such as blood tests for people who have had a heart transplant (to monitor for rejection) or echocardiograms to check for heart function in people who have had a heart transplant or surgery to correct congestive heart failure.

Anyone who has had heart surgery is advised to adhere to a regular schedule of checkups. Based on extensive experience, your doctor knows that these factors will give you the best possible chance of recovering fully and leading a normal life. Although you may carefully adhere to this advice and these schedules during the first weeks or months after surgery, you may find yourself becoming somewhat lax as time goes on and you feel better.

Cardiologists cannot emphasize strongly enough the importance of compliance to medications, diet, and lifestyle changes. Long-term compliance ensures the success of recovery and a return to the most normal life possible. Understanding the reasons for taking medications, exercising, and having recommended tests with help with compliance. Always ask any questions about recommended treatments so that you understand them clearly. Moreover, family members can be helpful in encouraging compliance of treatment regimens. For more information on adapting your household to being "heart healthy," see Chapter 12, New Approaches for a Heart-Healthy Household.

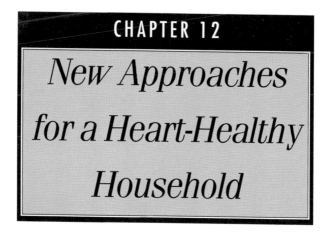

CHAPTER 12

New Approaches for a Heart-Healthy Household

Introduction

With a diagnosis of heart disease comes numerous recommendations for making lifestyle changes, especially with regard to diet, exercise, and stopping smoking. Doctors give this advice with greater urgency when a person has suffered the consequences of heart disease, such as a heart attack (myocardial infarction) or angina (chest pain), that necessitated a procedure to restore blood flow to the heart.

The second half of the title of this chapter—*heart-healthy household*—emphasizes an important point. Although only one person in a household may have heart disease necessitating lifestyle changes, it is much easier for that member of the family to achieve success if the entire household embraces the changes that are needed.

Trying to cook and serve two sets of meals—one heart-healthy version for the person with heart disease and another for the rest of the family—is a setup for failure for several reasons: first, the extra work involved in preparing two meals; second, the feelings of deprivation that are more likely to surface at the dinner table if the rest of the family is eating what was a favorite meal; and third, the perception of a lack of emotional support. This could cause the person with heart disease to feel isolated from the rest of the family, which is detrimental to the entire family.

Heart disease need not isolate a family member. In fact, it can actually bring the family together by involving everyone in heart-healthy eating and activities. Another positive benefit for the whole family to adopt a healthy lifestyle is the tremendous power of prevention. Practicing heart-healthy habits can prevent a spouse and children from developing heart disease, which is the ultimate goal of preventive medicine.

Revising Meal Plans, Shopping, and Cooking

Dietary change is one of the most important strategies to reduce cholesterol and lower blood pressure, both potent risk factors for coronary artery disease. Changes in diet are also a key aspect of therapy for people with congestive heart failure.

Feeding your heart well involves far more than simply knowing the goals of nutrition therapy outlined in Chapter 2, Keeping the Heart Healthy. Translating this theory into everyday practice—how to fill your plate—involves several steps, including limiting dietary cholesterol and eating more fruits, whole grains, and legumes (see Six Nutrition Goals to Reduce Coronary Artery Disease Risks, page 247).

A 1996 survey found that two-thirds of respondents believed that eating healthier means eating food that does not taste good. Dissolve this misconception with an exercise that creates the appropriate image of healthy food. Close your eyes and create the image of a New England peak-of-fall day. With your mind's-eye paintbrush, splash together every shade of yellow, red, burnt orange, crimson, amber, brown, and green in the natural world, each color bursting into the next to create the ultimate still-life portrait.

Now imagine the complex process nature orchestrated to produce that scene. Keep your eyes closed and turn that still-life portrait into a fiesta of nature's wonders. Imagine sampling these gorgeous treasures one at a time: sweet papaya, succulent ruby red tomatoes, robust

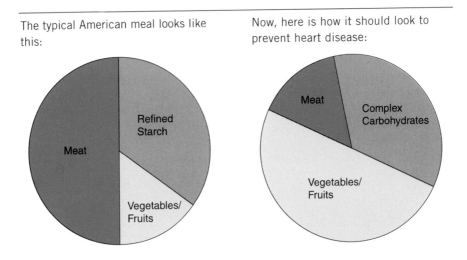

The typical American meal looks like this:

Now, here is how it should look to prevent heart disease:

> ## Six Nutrition Goals to Reduce Coronary Artery Disease Risks
>
> 1. Eat more vegetables, fruits, whole grains, and legumes.
>
> 2. Choose fat calories wisely.
>
> 3. Eat a variety, and just the right amount, of protein foods. For example, the latest scientific knowledge about soy has led to the advice to eat about 25 to 40 grams of soy protein daily. Accomplishing this involves knowing the protein content of soy foods, where to buy these items, and how to prepare them (see page 253).
>
> 4. Limit dietary cholesterol.
>
> 5. Use complex carbohydrates for energy, and limit the intake of simple carbohydrates.
>
> 6. De-emphasize sodium and increase intake of potassium, magnesium, and calcium.

whole wheat bread with a whirl of rich peanut butter, juice-filled tangerines, dulcet grapes, soft deep green watercress, nutty brown rice. These images should create a feeling of satisfaction rather than deprivation.

Six Nutrition Goals to Reduce Coronary Artery Disease Risks

Eat More Vegetables, Fruits, Whole Grains, and Legumes

To take in good amounts of the phytochemicals, minerals, B vitamins, vitamin C, fiber, and antioxidants that protect against heart disease and lower blood pressure, include the following on a daily basis (see also Serving Sizes, page 248):

■ *3 to 5 servings of fruits:* Maximize the benefit of fruit by choosing at least 3 different colors and 2 to 3 different textures daily: blue blueberries, red watermelon, green apples, orange citrus. Select a different 3 to 5 fruit servings for the next day.

■ *5 to 6 servings of vegetables:* Gain the most nutrition from vegetables by choosing at least 3 different colors and 2 to 3 different textures daily: stalky green broccoli, leafy dark-green romaine lettuce, dark-orange winter squash, red bell peppers, strong-flavored white onions. Pick a different 5 to 6 vegetable servings tomorrow.

Serving Sizes

- *One vegetable serving* = $^1/_2$ cup cooked or 1 cup raw

- *One fruit serving* = $^1/_2$ cup berries, 1 cup melon chunks, 1 piece whole fruit (such as 1 orange or 1 apple), $^1/_2$ cup canned fruit (canned in juice)

- *One grain serving* = 1 slice bread, $^1/_2$ small bagel ($^1/_3$ bakery bagel), $^1/_2$ cup cooked grain (such as rice or quinoa), $^1/_2$ cup pasta, $^1/_2$ cup hot whole-grain cereal, $^1/_2$ to 1 cup cold cereal (read label for the equivalent of 70 to 80 calories)

- *One legume serving* = $^1/_2$ cup cooked beans or peas (such as split peas or black beans), 6 ounces tofu (soybean curd), 4 ounces tempeh (fermented, textured, soybean product)

- *5 to 10 whole-grain servings (depending on your calorie needs):* Use at least 7 grains per week; for example, barley on Monday, brown rice on Tuesday, oatmeal on Wednesday, flaxseed on Thursday, bulgur wheat on Friday, quinoa on Saturday, and rye bread on Sunday.

- *At least 1 serving of legumes:* Plan lunchtime protein with legumes, such as split-pea soup, garbanzo beans on salad, and fat-free refried beans rolled into a flour tortilla.

Choose Fat Calories Wisely

Two strategies help limit fat to 15 to 25 percent of total calories and to a better type of fat: subtract and substitute (see also Chapter 2, Keeping the Heart Healthy; also see Fat Gram Percentages Per Calorie Level, page 249). Limit added fats whenever possible; when they cannot be avoided, choose fats highest in monounsaturated fatty acids (see page 29). This includes olive oil, canola oil, nuts, natural peanut butter, and olives.

The American Heart Association recommends that everyone limit total fat intake to 30 percent of calories or less; however, cardiologists who treat coronary artery disease recommend that people at high risk of, and those diagnosed with, heart disease limit fat further. Similarly, while the American Heart Association recommends limiting saturated fat grams to less than 10 percent of calories, prevention specialists advise a lower level—5 percent of calories—for high-risk people and those diagnosed with heart disease. The following table translates these guidelines into fat grams.

Fat Gram Percentages Per Calorie Level

Calorie Level	Total Fat Grams*	Saturated Fat Grams†
1,200	20 to 40	6.5 to 13
1,500	25 to 50	8.5 to 17
1,800	30 to 60	10 to 20
2,000	33 to 67	11 to 22
2,200	37 to 73	12 to 24
2,500	42 to 83	14 to 28
3,000	50 to 100	17 to 33

*The lower end limits fat to 15% of calories; the higher end to 30% of calories.
†The lower end limits saturated fat grams to 5% of calories; the higher end to 10% of calories.

Eat A Variety, and Just the Right Amount, of Protein Foods

Commonly eaten protein foods, meats and dairy products, are among the main culprits in increasing the risk of heart disease. Reduce this nutritional risk factor by balancing animal, fish, and vegetable sources of protein. Plan at least two vegetable-protein dinners each week (black bean burgers, tofu stir-fry); at least two fish dinner meals weekly (especially fish high in omega-3 fatty acids, such as salmon and tuna); and one to two skinless poultry meals weekly (a meal is 2 to 3 ounces of cooked poultry). Limit red meat to one meal weekly (2 to 3 ounces of pork, beef, veal, cheese; although cheese is not a meat, its nutritional profile is similar to that of red meat).

Following this simple guide greatly reduces saturated fat, cholesterol, and total fats and at the same time boosts the phytochemicals, fiber, vitamins, and minerals needed to fight heart disease.

Limit Dietary Cholesterol

Dietary cholesterol is found only in foods of animal origin, because cholesterol must be manufactured in the liver. To limit cholesterol to 200 milligrams daily, restrict the intake of egg yolks to 2 to 3 weekly and red meat and poultry to 2 to 3 ounces twice weekly.

Use Complex Carbohydrates for Energy; Limit the Intake of Simple Carbohydrates

Eat half of your daily calories as complex carbohydrates: whole grains, vegetables, fruits, and legumes. Limit simple carbohydrates (regular soda, sweets, and fat-free foods such as pretzels and coffee cakes) to just 5 percent of calories (for example, if you eat about 1,800 calories daily, one 8-ounce glass of regular soda would take up this 5 percent of calories).

Low-fat and fat-free foods that are high in calories may cause more problems than they solve. By focusing on their reduced-fat content, many people may ignore the fact that these foods are high in calories. Research indicates that Americans are gaining weight on reduced-fat foods, and the consumption of high-calorie, low-fat or fat-free foods should be limited.

De-Emphasize Sodium and Increase Intake of Potassium, Magnesium, and Calcium

The best way to decrease dietary sodium is to reduce the number of convenience, processed, and fast foods that you eat. The American Heart Association recommends that all Americans restrict the amount of dietary sodium to 2,400 milligrams daily, which is the equivalent of about 1 teaspoon of table salt. While shaking salt onto food does add sodium, most people get the majority of their sodium from convenience, processed, and fast foods. A frozen TV dinner, for example, can have as much as 2,000 milligrams of sodium.

Increasing foods high in potassium, magnesium, and calcium is just as important—if more important—than reducing dietary sodium (see below). The only additional action necessary to take in enough of these heart-saving minerals is including 2 to 4 servings of nonfat milk, yogurt, or fortified soy milk daily.

Healthier Shopping

It is no wonder that consumers report being confused in the grocery store. According to the Food Marketing Institute, the average grocery store has 30,000 items, and every grocery store does not have the same 30,000 items. This means that consumers can encounter thousands more products by shopping in several different stores. The following suggestions can ease the confusion of purchasing items for a healthier heart:

Sodium and Congestive Heart Failure

People diagnosed with congestive heart failure generally must follow a diet with stricter sodium restriction than do people with other types of heart disease. Because the recommended amount of sodium varies from individual to individual, people with congestive heart failure should discuss this level with their doctors.

1. Linger in the produce aisle; in fact, spend most of your time there, choosing carefully and trying new kinds of produce. Fill about half your grocery cart with produce, following the guidelines on page 247 about choosing fruits and vegetables. The only questionable choices are coconuts and avocados, which are very high in fat and calories and should be used sparingly. Do not hesitate to use frozen vegetables and fruits, which have excellent taste and nutrition. The salad bar is another great resource: Pack salads for lunch and dinner right after shopping, but avoid the high-fat items (such as salad dressing and salads made with mayonnaise).

2. Choose carefully in the dairy section, with the following guidelines:
   - Select nonfat milk (or reduced-fat and fortified soy milk, although this may be in the canned milk aisle).
   - Reach for reduced-fat or low-fat yogurt—those with 150 calories or less per 8 ounces.
   - Choose nonfat cream cheese and nonfat sour cream.
   - Search for reduced-fat cheese. Check the label carefully for those that have 5 grams fat or less per ounce.

3. You do not have to avoid the bakery section: In fact, regard it as the place to purchase fresh whole-grain foods, such as 10-grain bread and rye bagels. Take advantage of the opportunity to buy one portion of dessert foods, which allows you to enjoy your favorite dessert once a week.

4. Spend more time at the fish case (either fresh or frozen) than at the meat case; also, pick up canned tuna and salmon (look for reduced-salt and packed-in-water cans). Purchase enough fish for two fish meals weekly, each a 3- to 5-ounce portion size per person (purchase 4 to 6 ounces per person to allow for shrinkage). When choosing meat, select the leanest cuts of each meat. While many of them are more expensive cuts, you will be buying smaller portions and having just one meat meal per week (see Lean Cuts of Meat, page 252).

5. Acquaint yourself with legumes and soy-based foods in your grocery store. The soybean has been used as a food source for 5,000 years. It has recently emerged from Chinese kitchens to Western ones, and its health benefits are equaled by the variety of forms in which it can be enjoyed.
   - Select either uncooked dried beans and peas and cook them yourself, or purchase the cooked versions, available in cans.
   - Find the soy products in your store: tofu is located in either the dairy section or the produce section (choose the reduced-fat version). Some supermarkets have tempeh, but a trip to the health food store may be necessary. Accumulate at least 25 grams of soy protein daily (see Soybean Products, page 253).

Lean Cuts of Meat*

Cut of Meat	Calories	Protein (grams)	Total Fat (grams)	Saturated Fat (grams)	Cholesterol (milligrams)
PORK					
Tenderloin	159	26	5	2	80
Canadian bacon	157	21	7	2	49
Sirloin	181	24	9	3	72
Center loin	199	22	12	4	68
Whole ham	125	19	5	2	44
BEEF					
Tenderloin	180	24	9	3	71
Top sirloin	166	26	6	2	76
Sirloin strip	176	24	8	3	65
Top round	153	27	4	1	72
Eye round	149	25	5	2	59
Round sirloin tip roast	157	24	6	2	69
Flank steak	176	23	9	4	57
VEAL					
Leg	128	24	3	1	88
LAMB					
Loin chop	184	26	8	3	81
Foreshank	159	26	5	2	89
Sirloin leg	174	24	8	3	78

*Each 3-oz serving of these meats, trimmed, provides 200 calories or less. All decimal values have been rounded.

■ Choose packaged and frozen convenience foods carefully. Many are extremely high in sodium and fat (especially saturated fat), while others can be a part of a heart-healthy diet (see Choosing Healthier Convenience Foods, page 254).

In the Kitchen

Planning healthier meals and shopping smarter covers two important steps to eating healthier. The last step is just as important: cooking leaner and lighter. To achieve this, acquire a few essential pieces of cooking equipment, considering them an investment in health. The items you cannot be without in the heart-healthy kitchen include

■ Nonstick sauté pans, in two sizes (8-inch and 12-inch)

■ Spoons and spatulas for nonstick pans

Soybean Products

Food	Serving Size	Grams Soy Protein
Miso: Fermented soybean paste made by injecting cooked soybeans with a mold cultivated in either barley, rice, or soybean base. Rich in B vitamins and protein, miso is used in soups, sauces, salad dressings, dips, and marinades.	¹/₂ cup	16
Soy flour, defatted: Fine, fat-free flour made by grinding defatted soybeans. Used in baking and for binding sauces; in baking, it should be combined with other flours to promote rising. One of the highest-protein flours.	¹/₂ cup	23.5
Soy flour, full fat: Same as above, but this version is made by grinding whole soybeans.	¹/₂ cup	14.5
Soybeans, cooked (boiled): Use the whole cooked soybean on salads or in soups and casseroles.	¹/₂ cup	14.3
Soy milk (reduced-fat, fortified): This nondairy product is made by pressing ground, cooked soybeans. Soy milk is higher in protein than cow's milk and can be used whenever a recipe calls for cow's milk. Choose the fortified version.	8 ounces (1 cup)	10
Soy nuts: Made by first boiling and then roasting the whole soybean.	1/4 cup	15
Tempeh: Made by fermenting soybeans then pressing them into a cake. Has a slightly yeasty, nutty flavor and can be used as a meat substitute in stir-fries.	¹/₂ cup	15
Tofu (reduced-fat, firm): Also called soybean curd and bean curd, tofu is made from curdled soy milk, an iron-rich liquid extracted from ground, cooked soybeans. The curds are then drained and pressed in a fashion similar to cheesemaking. Use tofu in soups, stir-fries, casseroles, salads, sandwiches, salad dressings, sauces, and cold fruit drinks.	6 ounces	12

Choosing Healthier Convenience Foods

Follow these guidelines to choose healthier convenience foods:

■ *Serving size:* Nutrition information is provided for 1 serving, with the serving size indicated on the Nutrition Facts label (see page 38). Even if a package seems like a 1-serving size, it may be 2 or even 3, according to the manufacturer. If you eat a whole package of a food as 2 servings, double the figures to tally what you have eaten.

■ *Calories:* Choose full meals with no more than 300 to 600 calories, depending on the number of calories you eat daily. A good rule of thumb is to limit a full meal to no more than one-third of a day's total calorie allotment.

■ *Fat:* Full meals should have no more than 15 fat grams, and meal accompaniments a maximum of 3 to 5 fat grams (depending on the fat content of the rest of the meal).

■ *Sodium:* Full meals should have a maximum of 750 grams sodium, except for people on very restricted sodium diets (whose meals should have no more than one-third of a day's allotment). Prepared convenience food is probably the highest sodium item for the day; look for low-sodium varieties and limit higher-sodium versions to no more than one convenience food meal each day.

■ *Protein:* Full meals should have at least 15 grams of protein.

■ *Dietary fiber:* Look for dinners with at least 5 grams of dietary fiber. The pictures on the labels provide a good clue: Those with more vegetables generally have more fiber.

■ Cutting board

■ One very sharp, high-quality chef's paring knife

■ Nonstick baking dish

■ Clay roaster

Optional equipment, but items that make life easier and healthier cooking faster, include

■ Food processor

■ Blender

■ Mini-food processor

■ Garlic press

Calorie- and Fat-Reducing Cooking Techniques

The following tips can turn your healthy purchases into the healthy food your heart needs:

- For cooking meat, fish, and poultry: steam, "stir-sizzle" (like stir-frying, but using broth instead of oil), roast, poach, braise, bake in parchment paper.

- Toast or roast herbs and nuts to intensify flavor. Place herbs or nuts in a dry nonstick sauté pan, toss over medium heat for 3 to 4 minutes until lightly toasted.

- Use a little butter or margarine—for example, as a topping for fish—but stick to one teaspoon. Intensify flavor by adding fresh herbs to melted butter.

- Extend butter or margarine by mixing it with juices or flavored vinegars.

- Use no-calorie extracts to replace high-calorie ingredients, such as coconut and rum extracts instead of the real thing.

- Replace high-fat ingredients with lower-fat alternatives. For example, use Canadian bacon or turkey bacon for regular bacon in recipes.

- Use smaller amounts of high-fat, high-calorie ingredients, but cut them up smaller to disperse them throughout the food. For example, instead of coarsely chopped nuts, chop them finely; the same is true for olives. Another example: when a recipe calls for chocolate chips, use mini-morsels, but cut the quantity in half.

- Use the most intense flavor of a food or ingredient. For example, choose extra virgin olive oil and dark sesame oil. Use Kosher salt or sea salt instead of regular table salt; these types of salt have more intense flavor, so you can use less.

- Grease pans and muffin tins with vegetable-oil spray instead of regular oil.

- Stir-fry with vegetable-oil spray and broth instead of oil; alternatively, use very small amounts of an intensely flavored oil, such as dark sesame oil.

- Choose the leanest cuts of meat.

- Use nonstick cookware and utensils so you can use less fat or no fat.

- When making soups and stocks, leave enough time to let them chill, and then skim the fat off the top. Or use a fat separator, a device similar to a measuring cup but with a spout at the bottom, so that you can pour off fat-free broth and leave the fat behind.

- Use reduced-fat and fat-free dairy products (milk, sour cream, cream cheese, yogurt, and cheese). Experiment and determine when you can use each and enjoy it; for example, sometimes nonfat cream cheese is acceptable in a recipe but not on a bagel. Similarly, reduced-fat cheese may melt on top of a casserole, but nonfat will not.

- Use strongly flavored cheeses, such as feta and goat, and use less of them.

- Marinate meats and vegetables in reduced-fat and fat-free marinades to intensify flavor.

- Make and use yogurt cheese from nonfat and reduced-fat yogurts as a substitute for cream cheese, butter, and sour cream.

- Replace fat with sweet. For example, use fruit salsas with pork, lamb, and fish and marmalades with poultry.

- Use a food processor to help you chop, cut, and grate vegetables for recipes: You are more likely to prepare those recipes if you have some help.

- If you do not like to prepare fresh whole vegetables, buy frozen or already-chopped fresh from the produce section.

- When baking, substitute applesauce or pureed prunes for up to half the oil; experiment with favorite recipes to find the right balance.

- Substitute textured vegetable protein (a soy food) for all or a part of ground beef in chili, spaghetti, lasagna, and sloppy joes. This cuts the fat and calories and increases the nutrition considerably.

- Double the vegetables in most recipes to increase the nutrition and decrease the fat and calories. For example if a chicken and broccoli casserole calls for 1 cup broccoli and $1/4$ cup chopped onions, double both.

Prioritizing Exercise for the Family

Exercise can be literally lifesaving for someone with heart disease, but it is also healthy for everyone in the family. Making it a family matter makes it much easier for the person with heart disease who must exercise to continue on an exercise plan. Even more important, exercise should become a priority in a family's busy schedule.

According to the 1995 National Institutes of Health Consensus Development Conference Statement on Physical Activity and Cardiovascular Health, you should engage in moderate-intensity exercise for at least 30 minutes most, and preferably all, days of the week. If you generally do not have 30 consecutive minutes on any day, you can gain the same benefits by accumulating the 30 minutes in 10-minute increments throughout the day.

Moderate-intensity exercise is commonly called aerobic exercise. It causes a person to break a sweat and to use the large muscle groups. This type of exercise includes walking, swimming, jogging, dancing, and hiking. More strenuous exercise, such as stair-climbing and running, is fine but not necessary to realize cardiac benefits.

When you exercise at moderate intensity the goal is to work at 60 to 70 percent of age-predicted maximal heart rate (the maximal heart rate is about 220 beats per minute minus your age). If you have not been exercising, start slowly—aiming for a heart rate lower than your target heart rate. This will avoid muscle injury and will not overtax your heart and lungs, since you have grown accustomed to a more sedentary lifestyle.

For example, begin with shorter bouts of exercise, such as 15 to 20 minutes of exercise every other day. Progress slowly, by 3- to 5-minute increments per week until you are exercising at the goal of 30 minutes each day.

You may have to modify this advice according to your diagnosis and the condition of your heart. This is why everyone, not just those with heart disease, should discuss the amount and type of exercise that is safe for them with their doctors.

In addition to a daily exercise routine, families can invigorate their lifestyles by rethinking social activities. Instead of going out for dinner every weekend, for example, families can plan enjoyable physical activities. Depending on your climate and where you live, this could include packing a picnic and bicycling to a local park or forest preserve, tobogganing, ice skating, roller skating, or exploring neighborhoods on foot. Even when dinner plans are on the agenda, consider walking to a favorite neighborhood restaurant.

Bicycling for 15 minutes to a favorite picnic spot and then back again counts as 1 day's exercise. Pulling a toboggan up a hill 5 to 6 times (5 minutes of uphill walking each time) also qualifies as 1 day's worth of exercise. The same is true for 30 minutes of ice skating or roller skating. It is very important to have fun when you exercise—adding the enjoyment component makes it easier to stick to a lifelong exercise plan.

Living with a Person with Heart Disease

When a person is diagnosed with heart disease, the whole family is affected. While it is essential for family members to provide support, it is also important that they realize the effect this diagnosis has on them. It has long been known that anxiety and depression are common among people with heart disease, especially among those who have undergone heart surgery. However, such feelings are also common among spouses of people with heart disease and might be even stronger among spouses, especially when their loved one begins cardiac rehabilitation. Parents of children with heart disease may be similarly affected.

Recuperation and Rehabilitation After Surgery

For information on postsurgery recuperation and rehabilitation, see Chapter 11.

Dealing with Angina, or Chest Pain.

Depending on what type of heart disease a person has, he may experience bouts of angina (see also page 85). Family members can be helpful in making sure their loved one always carries nitroglycerin, the medication that relieves angina by dilating the coronary arteries, and that it has not expired (nitroglycerin is ineffective past its expiration date). The family should also know what a person with angina should do when an attack begins:

- Stop activity and rest.
- Place one nitroglycerin tablet under the tongue or spray the nitroglycerin into the mouth, under the tongue. Wait 5 minutes.
- If the discomfort is not relieved, another nitroglycerin tablet or dose of spray can be used. Wait 5 minutes.
- If the discomfort is not relieved, another dose can be used. Wait 5 minutes.
- If the pain persists after 3 doses, call for emergency assistance (911) at once. It is very important to have chest pain evaluated quickly in order to prevent serious complications, such as a heart attack.

Psychological Support for the Affected Family Member

People with heart disease can feel many different emotions, including anger, anxiety, depression, frustration, lack of control, fear, and denial. It is common for people to be angry when heart disease is first diagnosed, and this anger can make them difficult to live with. Some people might be anxious that they will suffer angina or a heart attack, so they become fearful of engaging in any physical activity. Others may be frustrated that they have to change some aspect of their lifestyle, which could also make them irritable and difficult to live with.

Another possible reaction some people have is to feel not in control of their lives. This can lead to inertia, or an inability to carry on. Denial is also common: Some people who have been diagnosed with heart disease deny that they have it and continue living as if they do not. Some people may feel all these emotions, in some combination or in cycles. In some cases, they might not even understand what they are feeling or know how to express their feelings.

When family members understand this range of emotions, they can be appropriately supportive. Sometimes, giving the affected person space and time—especially if he is angry or particularly cranky—is the best strategy. In addition, family members can provide an opportunity to discuss feelings by making appropriate statements, such as, "It must be frightening to wonder whether you'll have chest pain when you exercise," or "Are you angry that you have to make so many changes in your diet?"

In some cases, it may be helpful for family members to suggest that a loved one seek assistance from a counselor or psychologist. A doctor is generally a good resource for seeking an appropriate mental-health professional.

With the guidance of a healthcare professional, family members may have to "push" the person with heart disease to return to some of his previous activities, especially after a heart attack or surgery. For example, he should be encouraged to return to hobbies and social activities.

When the person with heart disease is a child, it might be necessary to enlist the aid of a school psychologist to help the child deal with both having an illness and growing up. Preadolescents and adolescents, in particular, might have a difficult time facing everything before them, and the extra help is particularly valuable for the whole family. Some pediatric congenital heart centers employ a social worker and other mental health professionals for this purpose.

Another strategy to help the affected family member alleviate fear and anxiety is for everyone involved to learn about the condition's symptoms and then to continue to reinforce what these symptoms mean. For example, people with heart disease may have palpitations, bouts of angina, and fatigue, but if they are reminded that these symptoms are to be expected, rather than an ominous sign, the associated fear and anxiety may be relieved. The family and doctor can discuss the issue of when symptoms require consultation as well as when and how to deal with symptoms at home.

Assisting with Lifestyle Changes

It is sometimes difficult for family members to strike a balance between being appropriately supportive and helpful and not "nagging" or becoming too parental (when the person with heart disease is an adult). Understandably, spouses and children of people with heart disease want to make certain that their loved one takes all medications, exercises just enough but not too much, eats appropriately, and keeps all doctor appointments.

At the same time, if they take too much control of these responsibilities, the diagnosed family member can become angry, frustrated, or resentful. It is possible that, in turn, the person might respond by not following through with the actions that can protect and heal the heart. Some people with heart disease may respond by giving up all responsibility for the changes they need to make and become dependent on others to help them remember to take medications, exercise, and eat healthily.

The best way for family members to help yet avoid taking control is for them to discuss openly how to be of assistance in all these lifestyle changes. One method of helping with medications is to print up a medication schedule and post it inside the medicine cabinet. Giving the person with heart disease a membership to a health club can provide motivation to exercise without nagging.

Depending on their age, children with heart disease may need a little more help in taking medications and making the appropriate dietary changes, although they need to understand the importance of these measures and to take some responsibility as early as possible. Giving them some responsibility from an early age will help them carry through with lifestyle changes as they grow into adolescence and adulthood.

Another strategy to support lifestyle changes is for all family members to make some changes. Adopting healthier eating and exercise habits makes the change a positive—and even fun—family project, rather than a chore for the family member with heart disease.

Care for the Caregiver

Whether you are the spouse, child, or parent of someone with heart disease, you will also need support yourself. It is normal for you to have feelings of anxiety, fear, and frustration. Sometimes a good friend who is willing to serve as a sounding board may be all the support you need, but do not hesitate to consult a mental health professional if the changes and tasks at hand are overwhelming. Doing so will not only help you, but also the affected family member.

Travel Concerns

Whether you have been diagnosed with heart disease or have had a heart attack or heart surgery, planning ahead can make a trip safer and more enjoyable. Some of the issues that are important to consider include the following:

■ *Timing the trip:* Appropriate timing is essential if you have had a myocardial infarction (heart attack), congestive heart failure, arrhythmias, hypertension, or a blood clot. While your doctor should give the final guidance, travel experts suggest avoiding air travel for the following length of time after

- Myocardial infarction: 6 weeks
- Decompensated congestive heart failure: 2 weeks
- Uncontrolled arrhythmias: 2 weeks
- Uncontrolled severe hypertension: 2 weeks
- Deep venous thrombosis (a type of blood clot): 6 weeks

■ *Getting a doctor's clearance:* Whether traveling 2 hours away from home by car or halfway around the globe by air, a doctor's clearance is important if you have heart disease. The doctor may change or add medications or perhaps give guidance about how to make car or air travel safer. For example, if you are traveling by car, the doctor may advise you to stop every hour and walk. This will avoid the possibility of developing a thrombus (blot clot) because of being cramped too long in one position. The same advice may apply when traveling for an extended period by air.

■ *Carrying medications:* If you have heart disease (or any other condition requiring medications) pack all medications in a carry-on bag that you can keep with you at all times. This avoids the difficulties that ensue if luggage is lost or delayed.

■ *Carrying medical information and records:* If you have a pacemaker, carry copies of electrocardiograms (ECGs or EKGs) performed both with and without pacemaker activation. This is especially true if you are leaving the country, as electronic telephone checks of pacemaker function cannot be transmitted by international satellites.

■ *Hypertension at high altitudes:* If you have hypertension, be aware that hypertension may be difficult to control at high altitudes and you may have to take extra precautions or extra medications to control it. Decreasing salt intake more than usual and increasing rest during the first few days may be helpful. Some people may need different or increased doses of medications, an issue the doctor can help with before leaving.

■ *Identifying medical resources at the destination:* Consult with your doctor or a medical travel center (generally at large universities) about the medical resources available at your destination. You should carry the phone number and address of such resources with you and also know how payment is expected at such places—some may accept any medical insurance, others may require cash or credit card payment.

■ *Caring for diabetes:* If you have diabetes, all medications, syringes, and blood-testing supplies should be kept (including extra batteries for the glucose monitor) in a carry-on bag that is always accessible; so should extra snacks and meals. Carry a letter from your doctor stating why you must carry syringes with you; this is especially important for international travel. You should not count on being fed on time on airplanes, as turbulence may delay meals. When traveling east or west through more than six time zones, insulin dosage may have to be adjusted, an issue to discuss with your doctor before leaving.

■ *Carrying medical identification:* If you have a pacemaker, take certain medications (especially blood thinners and diabetes medications), or have medication allergies, wear a medical alert bracelet or necklace. For any type of heart disease carry a card or letter stating your diagnosis, medications, allergies, doctor's name and phone number, and a person to call in case of an emergency.

CHAPTER 13

Cardiac Research

Introduction

Cardiac research tackles the many types of heart disease, from the approaches of both prevention and treatment. Areas of research can overlap; for example, the discoveries made in the quest to halt the deterioration of a diseased heart muscle may offer insight into how to stop coronary artery disease (CAD) from leading to a weakened heart. Heart research occurs on many fronts: the search for the genesis of heart disease, the pursuit of new medications to prevent and treat heart disease, the quest for superior instrumentation to view the heart and its structures, and the development of better and safer surgical procedures.

While tests and treatments in humans is the ultimate goal of heart disease research, investigation begins many steps before that. Building up to human-subject research, as it is called, ensures the safety of the people participating in such research.

The Basics of Research

Any new treatment (drug or device) that is promising has already undergone extensive testing before it is evaluated in people. The prehuman testing involves rigorous basic science and experiments in animals. After initial testing in small numbers of people (phase I), a new therapy has to be assessed in much larger trials (phase II and III) before it is approved for widescale, routine use.

Research can be viewed as an excellent opportunity because it is cutting edge work, providing access to a potentially very important new therapy. All standard components of therapy are provided; most often the research is testing a new dimension or improvement of therapy.

In addition, if the new therapy "pans out," participation in a research project may help many future generations of people with the same disease.

Am I a Candidate for Heart Research?

The cardiac research team of doctors and scientists would not be complete without two sets of people: those who already have a diagnosis of heart disease and those with a significant family history of heart disease who are still healthy. It is by studying these two groups of people that heart researchers make advances in the knowledge about the causes and treatments of heart disease.

Whether you have a diseased heart valve, a genetic heart defect, or a family history of coronary artery disease, you may indeed have much to offer the future of heart disease treatment. As another step, however, in the safety of heart disease research, investigators carefully consider the types of people who can safely participate in any particular study. Two main lists of criteria are developed: inclusion criteria, or the criteria that would include a participant, and exclusion criteria, or the criteria that would exclude a participant. Each list describes how well a person's personal and medical characteristics match the study at hand. Among the factors included in the criteria are the following:

- Age

- Gender

- History of heart disease: Some studies may include only people with heart disease, while others may exclude those who are already diagnosed with heart disease

- Laboratory value parameters: For example, a study may require that participants have high cholesterol readings but excludes those with a low red-blood-cell count indicating anemia.

- Medication or supplement usage: This is often a very important determining factor regarding a person's eligibility to participate in a study, and it is imperative that you review the inclusion and exclusion criteria carefully in determining your own eligibility. Over-the-counter medication usage, including vitamin and mineral supplements, can be just as important as prescription medication usage in determining eligibility. Vitamin E supplements, for example, can significantly alter results in some cases.

If you decide to participate in a research trial, you have to make a commitment to the study design. In some studies, you might have to stop taking vitamin and mineral supplements for the duration of the study. Other investigations may require you to keep careful dietary records and to include, for example, a serving of soy foods daily. In yet other studies, you may have to commit to taking the study medication at a certain time of the day. Carefully following the study protocol is the only method of testing the hypothesis, or the study question. People who do not wish to make the commitment the study requires should not choose to participate, as they risk jeopardizing the results of the research. Any participants in clinic trials must receive complete disclosure on any potential risks of the trial.

There are several advantages to participation in a clinical trial: You may receive new drugs, devices, or procedures that will benefit you or your children, and you will be contributing to important scientific research.

If you are interested in participating in research trials, contact the academic institution nearest to you to determine the type of research being conducted there, and then speak with the study coordinator to assess your eligibility.

On the Horizon

Heart disease researchers are pursuing new treatments in a variety of areas, including the following:

- Coronary artery disease, including revascularization and restenosis prevention
- Heart failure
- Cardiovascular imaging
- Electrophysiology
- Valve disease
- Depression and heart disease

Coronary Artery Disease

CAD research is being approached from many different angles, which are reviewed below.

Revascularization and the Prevention of Restenosis

The advancement of procedures to revascularize the heart (reopen blocked passages in coronary arteries) has been incredibly important in saving lives. These interventional procedures, as they are called, are many and increasingly sophisticated. However, they have not yet eradicated the renarrowing problem. Restenosis, or the reclosing of arteries after they have been once opened, remains a continual problem. Patients undergoing these procedures have been treated with aspirin, heparin, or both as a means of preventing thrombosis (blood clots). Some of the recent developments and new avenues being explored in revascularization and the prevention of restenosis are described below.

Platelet Glycoprotein IIb-IIIa Inhibitors. The arsenal of antithrombotic (anti–blood clotting) agents has been augmented by the addition of a new class of drugs, glycoprotein IIb-IIIa inhibitors, which include abciximab, eptifibatide, and tirofiban. Unlike aspirin or heparin, which inhibit some but not all pathways leading to thrombosis, GP IIb-IIIa inhibitors block the final common pathway of platelet aggregation. Cardiologists continue to investigate the use of these new agents, alone or in conjunction with the traditional agents, to find the best treatment with the fewest side effects.

Percutaneous Myocardial Revascularization. Researchers are investigating whether catheter revascularization (angioplasty or atherectomy; see Chapter 5, Coronary Artery Disease) alone or in combination with the drilling of tiny holes in the heart muscle (transmyocardial revascularization; see page 106) produces superior results for people with severe blockages. Cardiologists are especially interested in how this combination of procedures might work in people at particularly high risk for restenosis.

Antirestenosis Agents. Investigators continue their quest for the best medications to use at the time of catheter revascularization in order to prevent future restenosis. They continue to study the effects of medications that stop cells from building up at the site of the damage, comparing those injected directly into the arteries at the time of the revascularization against medications given intravenously following the procedure.

Role of Platelet Function. Cardiologists are studying the association between the level of platelet function and the occurrence of death, myocardial infarction, and the need for repeat revascularization procedures following initial revascularization.

Inflammation and Plaque Instability. Even people with large amounts of plaque, or atherosclerotic damage in their blood vessels, may fare quite well without suffering an event such as a myocardial infarction. For some of these people, it is only when the plaque becomes unstable, or breaks off, that an infarction will occur. This is somewhat akin to a piece of rust flaking off of a rusting piece of metal. Research is aimed at understanding what makes plaque stable and unstable and how to make it more stable and prevent events. Some researchers are trying to determine what is responsible for changing the surface temperature of plaque, noting that higher temperatures and inflammation make plaque more likely to rupture. Other investigators are studying the effect of various substances, such as glycoprotein IIb-IIIa inhibitors, on platelets, and therefore on the stability of plaque. Central to this research is the use of imaging techniques that afford heart scientists a direct view of plaque and the factors that affect its stability. Answers may lead to clues about substances, such as foods or vitamins, that may act as antioxidants to stabilize plaque.

Genetics

Researchers are currently seeking to identify specific genes that may determine a person's risk for CAD. Evidence linking genetic variations and defects to predisposition to CAD is growing. Genes may play a role in obesity or high cholesterol levels or determine how a person metabolizes fats in the blood. Future treatments may involve the insertion of genetically altered cells to prevent blood clots from forming, for example, or to stimulate new blood vessel growth. Researchers are also working to identify the specific genes that cause each disease, including CAD.

Lipid Management

Heart disease experts have a good understanding of methods to lower total and low-density lipoprotein (LDL) cholesterol levels—both significant risk factors for the development of CAD. Two areas of study, however, are the roles of high-density lipoprotein (HDL) cholesterol and triglycerides in heart disease and how these levels are best managed. (See Understanding Cholesterol, page 23.) Current methods of raising HDL, the desirable cholesterol component, remain inadequate, and new methods must be developed to fully test the hypothesis that raising HDL will decrease atherosclerotic disease or cardiovascular events, such as myocardial infarction (heart attack). Similarly, while triglycerides are identified as a risk factor for the development of heart disease, researchers do not fully understand how best to lower them without adversely affecting other lipid levels.

Estrogen Therapy

Estrogen therapy for postmenopausal women who have had bypass surgery is a prime research area. The National Institutes of Health is sponsoring a study to investigate whether women who have had bypass surgery will have reduced recurrence of heart disease if they receive hormone therapy. Women will be divided into two groups following bypass surgery. Some will take estrogen, others will take a placebo, or a sugar pill, and then all will be followed for more than 3 years. Researchers will test to see if estrogen therapy decreases the chances that a woman will suffer blockages or atherosclerosis in their bypass grafts.

Combination Therapies for Lipid Lowering

While there are several excellent lipid-lowering therapies available, researchers are always seeking better alternatives. One alternative therapy being studied is the combination of different medications. In one line of research, investigators are studying a new medication in a class called bile-acid binders. Bile-acid binders are medications that bind to bile acids (chemicals formed from cholesterol in the liver) in the intestines, preventing the bile acids from re-entering the bloodstream and causing them to be eliminated instead. A reduction of bile acids in the body causes the liver to use more cholesterol to produce more bile acids, thus lowering cholesterol levels. Researchers are administering the new substance alone and in combination with a proven cholesterol-lowering medication called lovastatin (Mevacor), an inhibitor of HMG-CoA reductase (an enzyme essential to the production of cholesterol in the liver).

Cholesterol Testing

Early diagnosis of CAD remains essential in preventing possible consequences, such as myocardial infarction. Easy screening methods translate into more widespread testing, which identifies a greater number of people at risk. In one line of current research, investigators are determining the accuracy of skin testing for cholesterol levels. Such testing is performed simply by placing a drop of a chemical on the skin and observing the change in color—a much easier screening tool than drawing a blood sample. Approximately 11 percent of the body's cholesterol is contained in the skin, and preliminary research suggests that cholesterol levels in the skin correlate well with levels in the blood.

Treatment of Familial Hypercholesterolemia

One approach to high cholesterol levels is to aggressively treat children and adolescents who have a family history of high cholesterol levels (hypercholesterolemia). Atherosclerosis can begin as early as age 3, especially in familial, or genetically based, hypercholesterolemia. Questions remain about when and how aggressively to treat such children, especially when their cholesterol levels are elevated. Research is now addressing the safety and efficacy, for example, of treating children and adolescents with cholesterol-lowering medications originally developed for use in adults.

Intensive Cholesterol Lowering

Cardiologists around the country are currently striving to lower total and LDL cholesterol levels in order to decrease the risk of developing CAD. Some research, however, is investigating the results of lowering blood lipid levels even further by diet and medication. Researchers will track the number of coronary events (such as angina and myocardial infarction) as well as the need for revascularization (procedures that restore blood flow), to determine if more aggressive risk-factor lowering pays off.

Investigators are also studying the effects of aggressive cholesterol lowering in improving blood flow to the heart. The study hypothesizes that intensive lowering of cholesterol over a short period of time will lead to improvements in vascular function and blood cholesterol levels, and ultimately to improvements in blood flow to the heart muscle itself and to a decrease of cardiac symptoms.

Hypertension Treatment and Myocardial Infarction Prevention

Hypertension, or high blood pressure, is a well known risk factor for myocardial infarction. Researchers continually seek the best and safest treatments for hypertension and are currently comparing several drugs and their abilities to prevent myocardial infarction and death from heart disease.

Dietary Supplements and Cholesterol Lowering

Some high fiber foods, such as oats, have been proven to lower total and LDL cholesterol levels. Scientists continue to test the effectiveness of other fiber supplements, given as a medication twice daily, in achieving further cholesterol lowering.

Heart Failure

With an ever-aging population and an increased number of survivors of myocardial infarction, the incidence of heart failure in the population is increasing. (See Chapter 8, Heart Failure.) Researchers are searching for ways to prevent further damage to the heart muscle as well as ways to maximize heart function in such people. Some of the many avenues being investigated are described below.

Left Ventricular Assist Devices

Research continues on left ventricular assist devices (LVAD; see page 173) for people with severe heart failure. These devices help the heart pump more efficiently and are currently used as a bridge to heart transplantation; studies are ongoing to determine if they can be used on a long-term or permanent basis.

Medication Therapy to Improve Blood Flow in the Peripheral Arteries

When the heart muscle has failed to any degree, the heart cannot perform its function of distributing oxygen-rich blood to the rest of the body effectively. Researchers are testing the use of medications to improve the functioning of blood vessels in moving blood through the body. One such agent under investigation is endothelin, a vasoconstrictor, or medication used to stimulate blood vessel contraction. It is hoped that endothelin will slow the progression of congestive heart failure and also improve patients' quality of life.

Modulating Neurohormones in Heart Failure

Neurohormones (a type of body chemical) play an important role in heart function, especially in people with heart failure. Several lines of research are aimed at studying the effects of various medications on neurohormone function in people with heart failure. Medications are used alone and in combinations, and at varying dosages.

Tumor Necrosis Factor Receptor

In this genetically based research, investigators are studying the ability of various medications to modify the receptor of a body chemical called tumor necrosis factor (TNF) in people with chronic heart failure. TNF may cause left ventricular dysfunction, left ventricular remodeling (the reshaping of the left ventricle that occurs with heart failure), pulmonary edema (fluid in the lungs), and cardiomyopathy (disease of the heart muscle). It is hypothesized that blocking the effects of TNF may improve the condition of patients with heart failure. Researchers have identified and synthesized an agent capable of blocking TNF and are now studying it in class II to class IV heart failure patients (see page 160).

Cardiovascular Imaging Research: Looking Inside the Heart

Better imaging of the inside of the heart leads to more accurate diagnoses and treatments. While the advances in cardiac imaging have been astounding, imaging experts continue to push the frontiers forward at an incredible rate. Some of the investigations in imaging are discussed below.

Echocardiography in Valvular Heart Disease

Clinical trials are investigating the use of echocardiography (see page 71) to help doctors better understand the mechanism of valve disease and the secondary effects it has on the heart and blood vessels. The hope is that such an understanding will aid doctors in defining the best moment for intervention and will provide them with a better understanding of outcomes. In related research, echocardiographers are studying the effects of drugs given during various stages of valvular heart disease.

Three-Dimensional Echocardiography

Clinical trials are ongoing to develop 3-D echocardiography to better define cardiac function in heart failure, valvular disease, and CAD. It is hoped that the use of 3-D echocardiography will significantly shorten the exam and capture more precise data.

Echocardiography in Space

Heart researchers are collaborating with researchers from NASA and the International Space Station to study the use of echocardiography in space. With people spending longer periods of time in space, the need to image their hearts has become a real concern, especially in regard to the effects of long-term weightlessness on the heart. The Cleveland Clinic is working with NASA to develop methods that will enable astronauts to image the human heart in space and transmit digital images to earth via satellite for quick diagnosis.

Echocardiography Contrast Agents

Investigators are working on developing and testing the use of improved contrast agents, or dyes, that they think will help better define the areas of decreased blood flow to the heart muscle as a result of CAD. The contrast agents may increase image quality and thus enhance the interpretation process of echo images.

Echocardiography and Atrial Fibrillation

Echocardiographers are involved in tests using transesophageal echocardiography (TEE; see page 79) as part of a strategy for treating patients with atrial fibrillation (see page 151). By using TEE to screen for blood clots in the atria prior to cardioversion (shock treatment to stabilize heart rhythm) for atrial fibrillation, cardiologists may be able to prevent the strokes often associated with cardioversion. Such screening may improve symptoms and also shorten the period before restoration of normal rhythm. In related research, investigators are exploring the use of a new form of self-administered heparin, a natural substance resistant to blood clotting, to be taken prior to atrial cardioversion. Such therapy may eliminate the need for hospitalization and thus lower medical costs.

Intravascular Ultrasound

Angiography shows where arteries are narrowed but cannot show the interior of the artery. Intravascular ultrasound (IVUS) is performed in the catheterization laboratory in conjunction with angiography. The IVUS miniature transducer is placed into the coronary arteries through a catheter and, using sound waves, produces pictures of the interior of the arteries. Researchers are currently analyzing the IVUS procedure to determine how frequently and in which patients it should be used.

Cardiac Tagging

A special MRI technique called cardiac tagging provides physicians with a way to visually quantify heart function within the ventricles. It shows the difference between healthy heart muscle and tissue scarred by a myocardial infarction. Researchers hope that cardiac tagging will one day indicate which patients may benefit from TMR procedures (see page 106).

Electrophysiological Advances

Electrophysiologic studies involve understanding and modulating the electrical impulses of the heart in order to better diagnose and treat arrythmias (rhythm disorders). The research studies underway on electrophysiology are quite intricate and include a number of approaches. Areas of study include topics such as

- The effect on survival of controlling rate versus rhythm in people with atrial fibrillation (see page 151)

- The efficacy of medications to control heart rhythm anomalies in patients who have suffered a myocardial infarction and are at high risk of sudden death from arrhythmias

- The use of "overdrive pacing" in the prevention of paroxysmal atrial fibrillation (atrial fibrillation that occurs suddenly and without warning)

- The use of catheter ablation (a minimally invasive procedure involving a catheter, a long, thin tube, which is inserted into a vein and advanced to the heart; during the procedure, the malfunctioning tissues are ablated, or removed) in people with supraventricular tachycardia (see page 150) that is causing symptoms and is resistant to drug treatment

- The efficacy of implantable defibrillators (see page 141) to convert or stop spontaneous atrial fibrillation

- The use of dual-chamber pacemakers (see page 145) in patients with sick sinus syndrome (see page 146) to prevent cardiac events such as myocardial infarction and to improve quality of life. It is thought that this type of pacemaker is more effective and cost efficient than single-chamber pacemakers.

■ Identifying the genetic basis of arrhythmia. Electrophysiologists and geneticists are working together to map genes responsible for several inherited human diseases that affect rhythm, such as idiopathic cardiomyopathy (see page 164), congenital and acquired arrythmias, aortic coarctation (see page 218), and congenital atrioventricular block (see page148).

Valve Disease Research

Ongoing examinations of mechanical, biologic, and homograft valves (see page 122) is being conducted to determine the long-term effectiveness of replacement valves. Surgical tools and approaches to valve replacement and repair also undergo constant study and refinement.

Depression and Heart Disease

Although it is normal for people to feel depressed after having a heart attack, heart experts wonder about the effects of a prolonged depression. Could such depression increase the severity of underlying heart disease and precipitate another heart attack? Research is aimed at exploring this relationship, as well as the efficacy of treating depression with medications.

On the Cutting Edge

With the prevalence and costs of heart disease so high, millions of dollars and hours of human resources are dedicated annually to cardiac research. Consequently, new developments in the cardiac arena are announced every day. Many new study results and research findings are announced at large annual professional meetings like the American Heart Association Annual Scientific Sessions (generally held in November) and the American College of Cardiology Scientific Sessions (generally held in March). As we enter a new millennium, several important new findings have recently been announced.

Combination of Coronary Stents and a Blood-Thinning Medication Reduces Deaths and Heart Attacks

Ongoing result analysis of the EPISTENT trial, testing the use of abciximab (a platelet bocker) with stents (see page 97) versus angioplasty (see page 96) alone or with abciximab, shows that the combination of stenting plus abciximab reduces myocardial infarction and death in the short term—at 1-month, 6-month, and 1-year time frames.

Super Aspirins Reduce Heart Attacks and Save Lives

Three "super aspirins" including eptifibatide, tirofiban, and abciximab have now been proven to reduce heart attacks in people with unstable angina or those undergoing angioplasty and stenting. These powerful platelet blockers prevent clotting that can complicate cardiac interventional procedures such as angioplasty or even cause death. These medications are given intravenously on a short-term basis (12 hours to 3 days). Abciximab (ReoPro) has also been shown to save lives when used with stenting.

Simple Test Predicts Cardiac Risk

Heart rate recovery—a simple measurement taken during routine stress exercise tests—is a powerful predictor of mortality that can help cardiologists determine if a patient needs immediate and aggressive treatment for coronary artery disease. In a study of 2,428 adults suspected of having heart disease, researchers found that patients who had a slow heart rate recovery (less than 12 beats per minute during the first minute after exercise) were at more risk of death from coronary artery disease than those whose heart rate recovery was normal (15 to 25 beats per minute during the first minute after exercise).

Bioventricular Pacemakers for Heart Failure Patients

Biventricular pacing, the simultaneous electrical stimulation of both ventricles and the atrium, is showing promise for patients with heart failure. The device coordinates the contraction of both ventricles, producing a more efficient heartbeat, better blood flow, and less symptoms of heart failure. Today's pacemakers and defibrillators are being evaluated for a new approach to heart failure.

Ace Inhibitors Prevent Arterial Disease

New research on ACE inhibitors (see page 93)—and specifically ramipril—may serve a role in disease prevention as well as in heart failure and hypertension. The HOPE (Heart Outcomes Prevention Evaluation) study was stopped prematurely in 1999 because of overwhelming evidence that ramipril prevents all forms of cardiovascular events including heart attack, stroke, and the need for revascularization procedures.

How to Evaluate Study Results

Today's consumers are often overwhelmed by a plethora of information about cardiac research. Hardly a day passes without some new study result being announced by the media. Before taking action based on random studies, consider these basic guidelines:

- *How large was the study group?* The most reputable studies are conducted in large groups of people. Ideally, they should be conducted in many different locations.

- *What was the control group?* Every study should be conducted with some control group—a group of people who do not receive the treatment under investigation—so that all experimental results can be compared to them.

- *What was the endpoint?* Studies are designed to find out one or two things. A reputable study will answer the question related to its specific endpoint, although other related findings may be made.

- *Do the findings advocate a radical change in lifestyle?* In general, most doctors agree that moderation is the key to maintaining a healthy lifestyle and quality of life. If a new study advocates a radical departure from your normal activity, you should consult with your doctor.

Before undertaking any major changes in lifestyle, exercise, diet, or medication based on research findings, consult your doctor or seek a second opinion.

The Future

Doctors and researchers around the world are working to eliminate the devastating effects of heart disease. The Cleveland Clinic Heart Center encourages people to support cardiac research so that future generations will not have to combat diseases of the heart.

Emergency Response

Introduction

Having a medical emergency, and needing to act quickly and surely, is something that most of us dread, but that many of us will face at one time or another. A little common sense will go a long way if you happen to have a medical crisis, whether it involves you or someone you care about.

- First, try not to panic. Stay as calm as possible.

- If the emergency involves someone else, offer reassurance.

- If there is any possibility that touching or moving the person will cause further harm—don't.

- When in doubt, seek help. We all try to second-guess a situation, and no one wants to call for help when it is not needed. But, it is better to be more active rather than less, safe than sorry.

It is not always easy to tell how serious chest pain is—especially when you are worried that it could be a myocardial infarction (heart attack). Chest pain can be caused by a number of nonemergency conditions: indigestion, allergies or asthma, and stress and, while you should not ignore them, they are most likely not emergencies. Other conditions, such as unstable angina (see page 86), are serious but do not necessarily present an urgent crisis. Still other conditions—myocardial infarction, pulmonary embolism, pericarditis (infection), or stroke—require immediate emergency assistance. And some conditions, such as sudden cardiac arrest—when the heart stops—must be attended to *without delay.*

Which Conditions Require Emergency Medical Assistance

Each year, more than a quarter of a million people die of a myocardial infarction within 1 hour of the onset of the first symptom. These people never reach the hospital, and this number is certainly alarming. At the same time, if a person receives treatment soon after the first symptoms are noticed, much can be done to prevent serious damage or death. Therefore, call 911 or your local emergency medical service (EMS) number immediately if you experience any of the following symptoms:

■ Pain in the center of the chest that radiates to the left side of the neck, shoulder and back, and/or down the abdomen, coupled with breathlessness. This could be a symptom of pericarditis, infection of the pericardium, the sac surrounding the myocardium (heart muscle).

■ Sudden sharp pain coupled with difficulty swallowing and breathing, cough (especially coughing up blood), or sweating. This could be a symptom of pulmonary embolism, an embolus (blood clot) that has closed the pulmonary artery (the artery in which blood flows to the lungs to become oxygenated).

■ Dull chest pain coupled with breathlessness, dizziness, pale or bluish pallor, or cold clammy skin. This could be a symptom of a heart attack.

■ Sudden paralysis, numbness, or weakness in one side of the body or face; sudden blindness or double vision; speech difficulties; or sudden loss of coordination or balance. This could be a symptom of a stroke.

Calling EMS

When you dial 911 or your local emergency service, stay calm and try to speak clearly. The dispatcher will ask for your name and the name of the victim, your location, and the nature of the problem. Stay on the line until you are sure the dispatcher has all the information needed.

Emergency Warning Signs

Although the thought of having a heart attack or a stroke can be frightening, if you or someone close to you acts immediately in the face of an emergency, a life can be saved and serious damage or disability prevented.

New treatments, when administered quickly, offer great promise to people who have had a myocardial infarction or stroke. But unnecessary delays in seeking emergency can result in permanent damage, and perhaps death (see also Thirty Minutes to Treatment, page 279). If you or someone close to you experiences any of these classic warning signs, pay close attention to them, and seek immediate medical assistance.

Signs of a Heart Attack

■ Intense or persistent pressure, pain, or a tight, full squeezing sensation centered in the chest that lasts more than a few minutes

■ Discomfort that lasts at least 20 minutes that is not relieved by changing position

Thirty Minutes to Treatment

"Thirty minutes to treatment" is a simple phrase but one that could help you or someone you love survive a heart attack. Here's why.

A recent report by the National Institutes of Health determined that people have a better chance of surviving when they get to a hospital within 30 minutes of the onset of heart attack symptoms, and treatment begins within the next 30 minutes. How much better? About 40 percent. Plus, the study showed that treatment that begins within the first hour from the onset of symptoms helps lessen heart muscle damage (see also page 280).

- Pain that radiates out from the chest to the shoulders, neck, arms, teeth, or jaw
- Chest discomfort or a burning sensation in the upper abdomen or midsternum (breastbone) coupled with fainting, sweating, nausea, vomiting, or shortness of breath
- Chest pain accompanied by skin that turns ashen or blue, particularly around the mouth
- Cold sweat or clammy skin
- A sense of impending doom or anxiety or certainty that death is imminent

Signs of a Stroke

- Sudden paralysis, numbness, or weakness in one side of the face or body
- Sudden partial or complete blindness, double or blurred vision
- Inability to speak or make sense
- Sudden loss of physical coordination or balance
- Sudden intense headache

Emergency Care for a Heart Attack

It may not be possible to judge with certainty whether you are experiencing a heart attack. Although in some instances chest pains are so intense that they leave little doubt that you should seek immediate help, most often symptoms are subtle and uncertain, such as a nagging discomfort in the chest, pressure, or nausea. Symptoms can come on suddenly or may be vaguely present for some time.

Nevertheless, chest pain should never be taken lightly. If you or someone close to you has a family history of heart disease or any of the risk factors associated with heart disease, such as hypertension, high blood cholesterol, or smoking, you should become familiar with the warning signs of a heart attack. If there is any question that what you are feeling is heart pain, call your doctor.

If you think you are having a heart attack, it is important to get to the hospital emergency room as quickly as possible. Immediate and aggressive treatment is needed to restore blood flow and oxygen to the heart muscle in order to prevent large portions of tissue from dying. Most permanent damage to the heart occurs during the first hour of an attack. The sooner the blood supply is restored, the less permanent damage takes place and the greater the chance of full recovery. Rapid emergency room treatment can reduce mortality by as much as 40 percent.

What to Do If You Think You Are Having a Heart Attack

■ Remain as calm as possible.

■ Call 911, your local emergency number, or your doctor, or have someone do it for you.

■ Lie down and breathe deeply and slowly.

■ If you take nitroglycerin, use it and repeat every 3 minutes.

■ Chew an aspirin to inhibit blood clotting.

Do not attempt to drive yourself to a hospital emergency room because of the risk of having an accident. If you live near the hospital, though, someone else could drive—if you think it will be faster than waiting for an ambulance. On the other hand, bear in mind that if you call for an ambulance, an emergency medical technician will likely begin treatment en route to the hospital.

Treatment is most effective if administered within 3 hours of the start of a myocardial infarction. In most cases, the damage to the myocardium may be stopped and even reversed if caught within 2 to 3 hours of the event.

What to Do If Someone Else Is Having a Heart Attack

It is not always easy to know when another person is having a heart attack, and it may be tempting to discount the signs and therefore not to act. However, if someone seems to be experiencing significant or intense chest pains, do not second guess:

- Call 911 or your local emergency medical service number.
- If the person is unconscious, check for breathing and a pulse.
- If the person cannot be roused, perform cardiopulmonary resuscitation (CPR, see below).
- If he is conscious, help him sit in a relaxed position with his back supported and his knees raised up with a pillow.
- Reassure him that help is on the way.
- Loosen his collar or shirt, and perhaps his belt and waistband.
- Do not let him walk about.
- Ask if he is taking nitroglycerin for a heart condition. If so, help him take it according to instructions. Also, help him take an aspirin.

Cardiopulmonary Resuscitation

Cardiopulmonary resuscitation (CPR) is a relatively simple technique that can save lives. It can be used if a person is unconscious and cannot be aroused, has stopped breathing, and has no pulse. These signs usually indicate cardiac arrest—the heart has stopped. In cardiac arrest, the heart has stopped pumping blood, and the brain can be damaged within a short period of time without continuous blood flow. CPR is a technique designed to keep blood moving through the body until the heart can be restarted.

CPR combines chest compression with artificial (mouth-to-mouth) respiration. Even if CPR does not start the heart beating again, it can provide sufficient oxygen until more advanced techniques can be applied to restart the heart. As a result, the use of CPR can significantly increase the chances of survival.

What follows is a step-by-step guide for CPR for adults and children over 8 years of age. You would use a slightly different technique for 1- to 8-year-old children and for infants, and these variations are noted after the main CPR description. The best way to learn CPR as it applies to all ages is to take a course. CPR courses are offered by local hospitals, employers, the American Red Cross, and the American Heart Association.

The American Heart Association has devised a simple ABC way of remembering the steps in the CPR process:

- **A** for airway
- **B** for breathing
- **C** for circulation

Rescue Steps for Adults and Children Over 8 Years

Assess the Situation

1. To check if a person is in fact unconscious, ask loudly, "Are you okay?" Tap him on his shoulder.

2. If there is no response, call for help, either by calling 911 or your local emergency medical services (EMS) number. If there are others around, ask someone else to call for help as you continue to assist the victim.

3. If the victim is conscious and breathing, check his pulse (see point 9 on page 284), and continue to monitor his vital signs. If he loses consciousness or stops responding, begin the Airway, Breathing, and Circulation steps (ABCs) described below.

4. If the victim does not respond, begin the ABCs described below.

Airway

5. Position the victim on his back, arms at the side. That may mean rolling the person over onto his back. Squat on your knees at the victim's shoulders.

6. Lift the victim's chin and tilt his head by putting your hand on his forehead and pushing gently back. In most cases, this movement will open the mouth and airways.

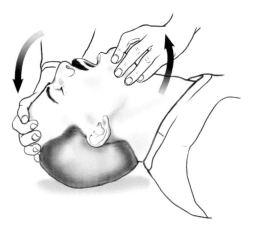

Lifting the victim's chin (text point 6).

Breathing

7. Listen for breathing by positioning your ear at the victim's mouth. Notice if his chest is rising and falling. If it is not, begin mouth-to-mouth resuscitation immediately.

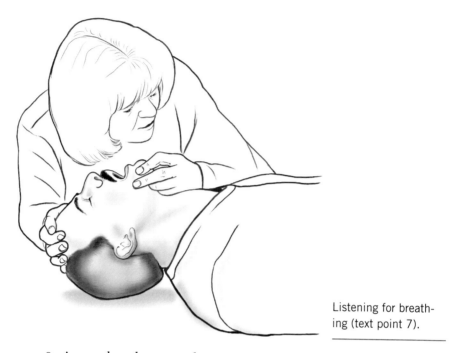

Listening for breath-
ing (text point 7).

8. As you kneel next to the victim, pinch his nose shut and inhale
deeply. Place your mouth over his so that there is no gap
through which air could escape. Exhale forcibly. Remove your

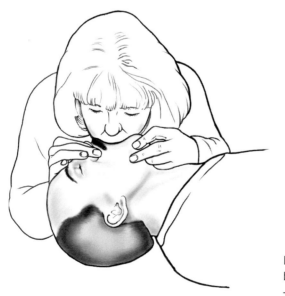

Delivering two powerful
breaths (text point 8).

mouth, inhale, and exhale again into the victim's mouth. That means delivering two powerful breaths. Notice if his chest rises, indicating that his lungs are expanding in response.

Circulation

9. Check for a pulse by placing two fingers on the carotid artery, on the side of the victim's neck, keeping your hand on the victim's forehead (not shown). When the heart is pumping, this artery will pulsate. *If there is a pulse, continue mouth-to-mouth resuscitation,* blowing a big breath into the victim every 5 seconds. Between breaths, watch for chest expansion and listen for the sound of breathing. Continue until breathing is restored or medical help arrives.

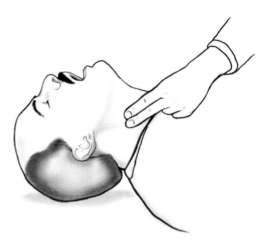

Checking for a pulse (text point 9).

10. *If there is no pulse, proceed to the next step—chest compressions—*which are alternated with mouth-to-mouth resuscitation. Also called closed heart massage, chest compressions work to restore blood flow to the brain. Mouth-to-mouth resuscitation delivers air to the lungs, while chest compressions pump oxygenated blood throughout the body.

11. Locate the base of the sternum (breastbone) by placing the index and middle fingers of one hand at the notch where the ribs meet in the center of the chest. Place the heel of the other hand just above your fingers (toward the victim's head). Then move the hand you used for the two-finger placement and place it on top of the other hand. Your hands should now be over the heart.

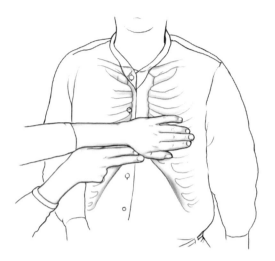

Locating the position for chest compressions (text point 11).

12. Straighten your arms. Your shoulders should be parallel directly above the victim.

13. Lean forward and compress the chest so that it falls by $1^1/_2$ to 2 inches. Ease up so that the chest rises beneath the heel of your hand after each compression, but do not remove your hands from the chest. Compress 15 times at the rate of 80 to 100 per minute, like a heartbeat. Count "one and, two and," up to "15 and." Do not rock.

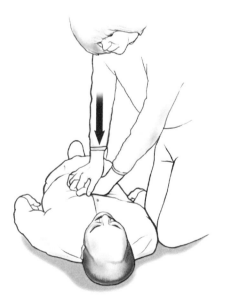

Performing chest compressions (text point 13).

14. After 15 chest compressions, perform mouth-to-mouth resuscitation again. Lift and tilt the victim's head, pinch his nose closed and exhale, with your mouth sealed over his, once, then again.

15. Repeat the 15 compressions, followed by the 2 breaths, until you have completed four complete cycles.

16. After the four cycles, check again for a pulse:
    - If there is still no pulse and the victim is not breathing, continue with the compression-breathing cycles until the victim starts to move, you are relieved by a medical professional, or you can no longer continue.
    - If there is a pulse and the victim is not breathing, continue giving breaths (1 breath every 5 seconds). Check the pulse after every 12 breaths.
    - If there is a pulse and the victim is breathing, stop CPR and attend to any other injuries.

Rescue Steps for Children 1 to 8 Years

The steps for CPR for children of this age are the same as those above with the following differences:

- When performing mouth-to-mouth resuscitation (after the initial 2 breaths), blow one breath every 4 seconds.

- Use only the heel of one hand—do not use both hands for compressions.

- Compress the chest only 1 to $1^1/_2$ inches.

- Do only 5 compressions, stop, and give just 1 breath, then repeat this cycle for a total of 10 times.

- After the first 10 cycles, recheck the pulse:

  - If there is no pulse and the child is still not breathing, continue with the compression-breathing cycles, until the child starts to move, you are relieved by a medical professional, or you cannot continue.

  - If there is a pulse but the child is not breathing, continue giving breaths: one breath every 4 seconds and check the pulse after every 15 breaths.

  - If there is a pulse and the child is breathing, stop CPR and attend to any other injuries.

Rescue Steps for Infants (Under 1 Year)

The steps for CPR for infants are the same as those for adults, with the following differences:

■ When performing mouth-to-mouth breathing, cover the infant's mouth and nose, and puff gently.

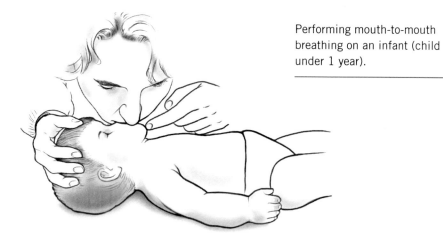

Performing mouth-to-mouth breathing on an infant (child under 1 year).

■ After the initial two breaths, blow one breath every 3 seconds.

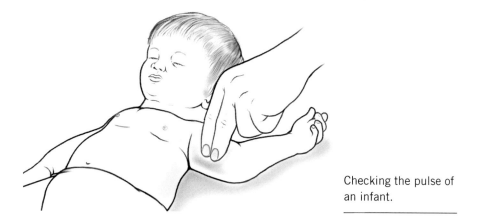

Checking the pulse of an infant.

■ When checking the infant's pulse, check the brachial artery in the upper arm. Keep your hand on the infant's forehead (not shown).

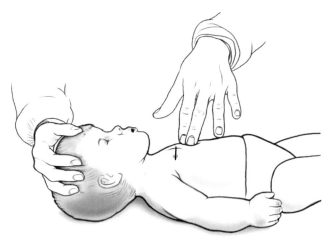

Locating the position for chest compressions on an infant: Place your index finger one finger width below the center of an imaginary line running between the baby's nipples. Use these two fingers for chest compression.

- To position for chest compressions, imagine a line connecting the baby's nipples. Place your index finger one finger width below the center of this line and your middle finger right next to your index finger. Use these two fingers for chest compression.

- Compress the chest only $1/2$ to 1 inch.

- Do only 5 compressions, stop and give just 1 breath, and then repeat this cycle for a total of 10 times. Compressions should be at the rate of 100 a minute (5 every 3 seconds).

- After the first 10 cycles, recheck the pulse:

  - If there is still no pulse and the child is not breathing, continue with the compression-breathing cycles, until the infant starts to move, you are relieved by a medical professional, or you can no longer continue.

  - If there is a pulse but the child is still not breathing, continue giving breaths (1 breath every 3 seconds). Check the pulse after every 20 breaths.

  - If there is a pulse and the child is breathing, stop CPR and attend to any other injuries.

EMS and Advanced Cardiac Life Support

Each year, at least 300,000 people in the United States experience cardiac arrest. When the heart ceases functioning, death can occur almost immediately. Thousands have other cardiac emergencies. However, resuscitation efforts can effectively restore heart function in approximately one-half of all cases. In addition, when resuscitative techniques are initiated early, long-term survival rates are greatly improved.

In the Emergency Room

If you experience signs of a heart attack (see page 89), go to an emergency room immediately. Do not dismiss the signs or put off going to the emergency room—a heart attack requires immediate attention. Once there, you will receive a full examination. The health care professionals will give you a painkiller, perhaps morphine, to kill the pain and to alleviate some of the anxiety that usually accompanies a heart attack. You will be given oxygen to help the blood circulate and an electrocardiogram (ECG or EKG) will be done. If there are signs of arrhythmias (disturbances in heart rhythm), medication or electric shock will be given to restore normal rhythm. If there are no abnormalities in the heart's pulsation, further tests will be run, including blood tests, to determine whether there was any cell death in the heart.

Most heart attacks are caused by clots of plaque that have broken off and lodged in a coronary artery, abruptly blocking the blood flow and oxygen supply to the heart. The extent of damage and complications caused by a heart attack is largely determined by where and for how long the obstruction has lodged. Thrombolytic agents are administered to dissolve the clot that is blocking blood flow. Early administration of these clot-dissolving drugs has greatly reduced mortality from heart attack. In some instances, emergency balloon angioplasty is performed to open the clogged artery. In rarer, more severe cases, emergency bypass surgery is performed to create a detour around the blockage and restore blood flow (see also Chapter 5, Coronary Artery Disease).

If the heart attack has been severe or you undergo emergency angioplasty or bypass surgery, you will stay in the cardiac intensive care unit (ICU) and be closely monitored for about 24 to 36 hours.

As most cardiac emergencies happen outside the hospital, it is likely that the initial response will be provided by emergency medical services (EMS). Typically, highly trained emergency medical technicians (EMTs) and paramedics are dispatched once 911 is notified. Most medical professionals who are called in to treat a cardiac emergency, whether it is at the emergency site, in the ambulance, or in the hospital emergency room, are trained to use a systematic procedure for resuscitation.

Basic Life Support

Basic life support is the term for the resuscitative technique outlined above under the cardiopulmonary resuscitation (CPR) section. The emergency team will do a quick assessment, checking for consciousness, a pulse, and respiration. If there is no sign of consciousness or major pulse, it is likely that there is cardiac arrest. When that is the case, a medical professional starts basic life support to keep the victim's blood oxygenated. Early CPR is used to maintain blood flow and oxygenation. In this way, the heart and central nervous system are supported until more definitive treatment can be brought in to restore normal function. For a short time, mouth-to-mouth breathing and chest compressions can substitute in part for normal heart-lung functions.

Advanced Cardiac Life Support

The next step in emergency response is to provide advanced cardiac life support (ACLS). Most medical emergency professionals in the United States are trained in this resuscitation protocol. Advanced cardiac life support concentrates on restarting the heart with defibrillators, drugs, and special techniques. The key for the medical staff involved in resuscitation is regular training, practice, and a calm approach.

The techniques of ACLS include the following:

- *Intravenous catheter:* An intravenous (IV) catheter is a tube inserted into a vein so that fluids and medications can be administered directly into the victim's blood.

- *Automatic chest compression:* Rescue teams can use machines to perform chest compressions, instead of compressing the chest by hand. Machines provide a strong, uniform compression, freeing rescuers to perform other lifesaving measures.

- *Defibrillators:* Automatic external defibrillators (AEDs) are devices that deliver an electric shock to the heart in order to correct a faulty heart rhythm. Newer models can also provide a quick reading of the heart's contractions, providing a diagnosis of the rhythm problem.

AEDs are used to reverse both ventricular fibrillation and ventricular tachycardia, two types of arrhythmias. Ventricular fibrillation is the most common cause of cardiac arrest and involves highly chaotic and unsynchronized contractions of the ventricular muscle fibers. Ventricular tachycardia is an abnormally rapid heart rate; when it occurs in a person who is also without a pulse, defibrillation is given to correct the rapid rhythm.

During defibrillation, paddles are placed over the heart, and three shocks are given, usually within 45 seconds. The high-energy electric shock is sent through the heart, stopping it momentarily. Often the electric current serves to restart the heart's own pacemaker, the sinoatrial node, prompting the myocardium to resume a coordinated rhythm. However, in some cases, ventricular fibrillation recurs, so multiple shocks are used routinely. As soon as the pulse returns, defibrillation is stopped and the patient's condition will be reassessed. Similarly, if the heart rhythm changes, another technique may be used.

- *Endotracheal intubation:* If ventricular fibrillation or pulseless ventricular tachycardia is still present after three shocks from an AED, oxygen is given, and the drug epinephrine is administered intravenously. Endotracheal intubation may also be performed. A flexible plastic tube is placed into the trachea (windpipe) to ventilate the lungs directly with oxygen. The tube is passed into the mouth and upper airway with the aid of a laryngoscope (an instrument used to view the inside of the throat). When the emergency involves asystole (complete ventricular standstill), endotracheal intubation is performed as soon as possible, and epinephrine is given intravenously to start the heart.

- *External pacemaker:* In some instances, an external pacemaker can help the heart establish and maintain a regular rhythm when its natural pacemaker, the sinoatrial node, is not working correctly. In the case of sudden cardiac arrest, this device is occasionally used in resuscitation efforts. Electrodes and monitor leads are placed on

Automated External Defibrillators (AED)

The development of automated external defibrillators (AEDs) has had an enormous impact on on-site emergency care. Because doctors cannot always be present at the site of a cardiac emergency, paramedics and emergency medicine technicians (EMTs) are trained to use external defibrillators (portable devices the size of a laptop computer), to provide life-saving treatment for a person suffering from sudden cardiac arrest. Cardiac arrest is most often prompted by a malfunction in the heart's electric current, usually ventricular fibrillation (see above). Defibrillation, which sends a pulse of electricity to the myocardium, is the best treatment to restart the heart and restore a healthy rhythm.

Because the chances of long-term survival are highest when the heart is restarted within 3 minutes of an arrest, the availability of automated external defibrillators at many local public centers can spell the difference between life and death. Therefore, not only do most ambulances and EMTs carry these devices, but many fire department personnel and police officers carry them as well. Increasingly, people are trained to use external defibrillators in the workplace and in public gathering places, such as stadiums, theaters, and airports and on public transportation, increasing the likelihood that a person experiencing sudden cardiac arrest will survive.

the patient's chest. The desired heart rate is programmed and an electric current is sent through to the heart. The current is increased until the heart echoes back the rhythm and assumes its pulsating activity.

After circulation has been restored and the victim has been stabilized, he is transported to the intensive care or coronary care unit, where a full diagnosis is conducted and a treatment plan developed.

Emergency Care for a Stroke

A stroke occurs when the blood flow to the brain is blocked, placing brain tissue at risk of damage (see also Chapter 9, Diseases of the Blood Vessels). Whenever symptoms of a stroke occur—sudden loss of the ability to speak, feel, stand, or see—immediate attention is crucial. Do not wait to see whether the symptoms will pass. Even if it is a transient ischemic attack (TIA or ministroke), and the symptoms subside or disappear relatively quickly, they must be taken seriously. More than one-third of people who have ministrokes go on to have full-blown strokes within a year or two.

A major stroke deprives brain cells of blood, and tissue begins to die within minutes. This damage can cause a permanent neurologic loss of control of body parts and functioning. Fortunately, prompt medical intervention can prevent death or disability from a stroke.

If you have a family history of stroke or any of the risk factors associated with stroke, such as hypertension, high blood cholesterol, or smoking, become familiar with the warning signs of stroke. Any related symptoms, however mild, should be taken seriously.

What to Do If You Think You Are Having A Stroke

- At the first sign of stroke, call 911 or your local emergency medical service (EMS).

- If you are not sure that you are having a stroke, call your doctor.

What to Do If Someone Else Is Having a Stroke

- If someone appears to be having a stroke, call 911 or your local EMS.

- If the victim is unconscious, check the victim's ABCs (airway, breathing, and circulation). If you are unable to rouse him, administer cardiopulmonary resuscitation (CPR; see page 281).

■ If the victim is unconscious but breathing and you can feel a pulse, roll him to his left side to allow fluids to drain from the mouth.

■ If the victim is conscious, reassure and calm him, and place him in a comfortable position. Turn his face to the side to prevent choking. If there are signs of paralysis, turn his head so that the paralyzed side faces up.

■ Do not let the victim have anything to eat or drink.

Guidelines for Safe Medication Use

1. Become familiar with the name of each medication you take and why you take it.

2. Take the medication at the same easy-to-remember time each day.

3. Do not take a double dose of medication to make up for a missed one. If you miss a dose, contact your doctor or pharmacist for advice.

4. Consult your doctor or pharmacist before taking any over-the-counter drugs, such as aspirin, vitamins, laxatives, or antacids, which can interact with other medications.

5. Medications—especially heart medications—are only for the patient to whom they have been prescribed. Do not offer another person your medications or prescriptions, and do not take anyone else's.

6. Keep medications in their original containers with their original information.

7. If you have any questions about a medication, consult your doctor or pharmacist before taking it.

8. Store medications at room temperature, away from moisture, and out of direct sunlight.

9. Contact your doctor or pharmacist to determine if a medication more than 6 months old should be discontinued or replaced.

10. Many medications may initially cause side effects, such as dizziness, headache, or nausea, which often disappear after several days and do not usually require stopping the medication. Inform your doctor if unusual or severe side effects occur or persist.

11. A medication can cause an allergic or unanticipated reaction. Report any unusual signs or symptoms to your doctor.

12. Some medications may interact or interfere with each other. Make sure that all doctors (including the dentist) know exactly which medications you are taking.

13. Some foods may interfere with the optimal results of certain medications by interfering with absorption as well as by other mechanisms. Consult your doctor or pharmacist if you have questions regarding a food-drug interaction.

14. Always have an adequate supply of medication, especially when taking a trip, expecting visitors, or doing anything different from your normal routine. Carry a several-day supply of medications when traveling.

15. Keep all medications away from children and in bottles with childproof caps.

16. When seeing your doctor, bring the medications you are taking or a list of them.

17. With most cardiac medications, the brand-name drug is preferable to the generic version. Your doctor and pharmacist can help you make the determination. Whichever you choose, use the same product consistently.

18. If a medication has LA, SR, XL, or CR (abbreviations for "long acting," "sustained release," and "controlled release") after its name, swallow it whole; do not crush it.

19. Avoid alcohol-containing drinks, which interfere with many cardiovascular drugs.

Types of Cardiac Drugs

Alpha Blockers

What They're For

Alpha blockers lower blood pressure.

How They Work

Alpha blockers relax small blood vessels throughout the body, which reduces blood pressure.

Possible Side Effects

Common: dizziness, drowsiness, edema (fluid retention). Less common: nasal congestion, nausea, irregular heartbeat, blurred vision.

Precautions and Special Information

Change positions from lying to standing slowly to avoid dizziness. The first dose and any increases in dosage should be taken before going to sleep; potentially hazardous activities should not be undertaken for the following 12 hours.

Generic Name	Brand Name
Doxazosin	Cardura
Prazosin	Minipress
Terazosin	Hytrin

Angiotensin-Converting Enzyme (ACE) Inhibitors

What They're For

Angiotensin-converting enzyme (ACE) inhibitors lower blood pressure.

How They Work

ACE inhibitors affect the process in which kidneys regulate blood pressure. The kidneys release renin, a hormone that causes small arteries to contract, thus raising blood pressure. ACE inhibitors interfere with this process, and thereby lower blood pressure.

Since they reduce the heart's workload by widening the arteries, some ACE inhibitors are used to treat congestive heart failure.

Possible Side Effects

Common: dry, tickling cough. Less common: altered sense of taste, fatigue, headache. Rare: swelling of the face and throat.

Precautions and Special Information

Because ACE inhibitors cause the kidneys to retain potassium, diuretics—drugs that cause the kidneys to secrete potassium in the urine—are often used with ACE inhibitors. Salt substitutes that contain potassium should not be used without a doctor's approval.

Generic Name	Brand Name
Benazepril	Lotensin
Captopril	Capoten
Enalapril	Vasotec
Fosinopril	Monopril
Lisinopril	Prinivil, Zestril
Moexipril	Univasc
Quinapril	Accupril
Ramipril	Altace
Trandolapril	Mavik

Angiotensin II Receptor Blockers (ARBs)

What They're For

Angiotensin II receptor blockers lower blood pressure.

How They Work

These drugs block the action of angiotensin II, a powerful vasoconstrictive hormone. As a result, blood pressure is decreased.

Possible Side Effects

Common: upper respiratory tract infection. Less common: dizziness, diarrhea, cough, headache, fatigue, upset stomach.

Precautions and Special Information

Angiotensin II receptor blockers should not be administered to pregnant women. A lower dose should be considered for people with impaired liver function.

Generic Name	Brand Name
Candesartan	Atacand
Irbesartan	Avapro
Losartan	Cozaar
Valsartan	Diovan

Antiarrhythmics

What They're For

Antiarrhythmics treat heart rhythm disorders.

How They Work

Irregular heartbeats can develop when part of the myocardium (heart muscle) is damaged or when its electrical system is disrupted. Antiarrhythmics make the myocardium less sensitive to disruptions so it can resume a regular beat.

Possible Side Effects

Common: Dizziness, drowsiness, headache, insomnia, weakness, increased blood sugar.

Precautions and Special Information

Antiarrythmics should not be stopped without a doctor's approval. Stopping suddenly may cause a serious disruption in heart rhythm.

Generic Name	Brand Name
Amiodarone	Cordarone, Pacerone
Disopyramide	Norpace
Flecainide	Tambocor
Mexiletine	Mexitil
Moricizine	Ethmozine
Procainamide	Procanbid, Pronestyl
Propafenone	Rythmol
Quinidine gluconate	Quinaglute
Quinidine sulfate	Quinidex
Sotalol	Betapace
Tocainide	Tonocard

Anticoagulants

What They're For

Anticoagulants reduce the blood's ability to clot and lower the risk of stroke in conditions such as atrial fibrillation.

How They Work

Anticoagulants diminish the blood's ability to clot by reducing the proteins involved in coagulation or interfering with their functioning.

Possible Side Effects

Common: bleeding (with warfarin); contact your doctor in all cases of abnormal bleeding. Less common: cramps, nausea, vomiting, diarrhea, itching, rash.

Precautions and Special Information

Use of anticoagulants may be suspended before surgery or dental procedures. These drugs can lead to anemia or cause a pre-existing bleeding disorder to become manifest.

Generic Name	Brand Names
Aspirin	Bayer, Bufferin, Ecotrin, Empirin (many brand names available)

Clopidogrel	Plavix
Dipyridamole	Persantine
Pentoxifylline	Trental
Ticlopidine	Ticlid
Warfarin	Coumadin

Beta Blockers

What They're For

Beta blockers lower blood pressure and reduce the heart's need for oxygen.

How They Work

Beta blockers block the hormone epinephrine (which makes the heart beat faster) from attaching to its receptors. As a result, the heart beats slower and less forcefully, which lowers blood pressure and enables the myocardium (heart muscle) to use less oxygen.

Possible Side Effects

Common: excessive slowing of the heartbeat, fatigue, vivid dreams, depression, increased blood sugar and cholesterol levels.

Precautions and Special Information

People with asthma should not take beta blockers; they narrow the small air passages in the lungs. In people with diabetes, beta blockers may hide the warning symptoms of an insulin reaction.

Generic Name	**Brand Name**
Acebutolol	Sectral
Atenolol	Tenormin
Betaxolol	Kerlone
Bisoprolol	Zebeta
Carteolol	Cartrol
Carvedilol	Coreg
Labetalol	Normodyne, Trandate
Metoprolol	Lopressor, Toprol XL
Nadolol	Corgard
Penbutolol	Levatol
Pindolol	Visken
Propranolol	Inderal
Sotalol	Betapace
Timolol	Blocadren

Calcium-Channel Blockers

What They're For

Calcium-channel blockers lower high blood pressure and control angina (chest pain caused by reduced blood flow to the coronary arteries).

How They Work

Calcium-channel blockers interrupt the flow of calcium through coronary arteries, which inhibits their contraction.

Possible Side Effects

Common: headaches and swelling of the ankles. Verapamil can cause constipation and excessive slowing of the heartbeat.

Precautions and Special Information

Because calcium-channel blockers tend to slow the heart rate in the same way as beta blockers, the two drugs should not be taken together.

Generic Name	Brand Name
Amlodipine	Norvasc
Bepridil	Vascor
Diltiazem	Cardizem, Dilacor, Tiazac
Felodipine	Plendil
Isradipine	DynaCirc
Nicardipine	Cardene
Nifedipine	Adalat, Procardia
Nisoldipine	Sular
Verapamil	Calan, Covera-HS, Isoptin, Verelan

Cardiac Glycosides (Digitalis)

What They're For

Digitalis, the active ingredient of the purple foxglove plant, has been used for centuries to treat heart failure.

How They Work

Cardiac glycosides cause the heart to beat slower and more forcefully, increasing the amount of blood the heart can pump and thus improving circulation.

Possible Side Effects

Stomach upset and loss of appetite.

Precautions and Special Information

A daily pulse reading may be necessary prior to taking the medication, and a doctor should be notified if the pulse falls below 60 when taking digitalis. Low potassium levels can increase sensitivity to side effects; diuretics may affect potassium levels. Daily monitoring of weight may be necessary; rapid weight gain may mean that water is being retained, in which case a low-salt diet may be recommended.

Generic Name	Brand Name
Digoxin	Lanoxin

Central Alpha Agonists

What They're For

Central alpha agonists lower blood pressure.

How They Work

Central alpha agonists affect control centers in the brain that regulate blood pressure.

Possible Side Effects

Common: dizziness, dry mouth, drowsiness.

Precautions and Special Information

To avoid dizziness, stand slowly from a lying position to prevent a sudden drop in blood pressure that can occur while taking central alpha agonists. To avoid drowsiness, take medication at bedtime. Do not stop taking the medication abruptly; blood pressure can "rebound" higher than it was previous to taking the medication.

Generic Name	Brand Name
Clonidine	Catapres
Guanabenz	Wytensin
Guanfacine	Tenex
Methyldopa	Aldomet

Cholesterol-Lowering Drugs

What They're For

Cholesterol-lowering drugs lower blood cholesterol levels in people with a genetic predisposition to high cholesterol who cannot lower cholesterol solely through diet modifications.

Cholesterol-lowering drugs are more effective when used together with a low-cholesterol diet.

Fibrates

How They Work

Fibrates lower the level of triglycerides in the blood by blocking production of triglycerides in the liver, and also moderately reduce cholesterol levels.

Possible Side Effects

Clofibrate: most common—nausea; less common—diarrhea, drowsiness, weakness, headache; rare—rash, muscle cramps, stiffness.
Fenofibrate: upset stomach, headache, rash, flulike symptoms, muscle aches.
Gemfibrozil: most common—stomach upset, abdominal pain, nausea, diarrhea, vomiting, gas; less common—rash, itching, muscle pain, dizziness, blurred vision, headache.

Generic Name	Brand Name
Clofibrate	Atromid-S
Fenobirate	Tricor
Gemfibrozil	Lopid

Niacin

How It Works

Niacin, a B-complex vitamin, reduces the body's ability to manufacture very-low-density lipoprotein (VLDL) cholesterol.

Possible Side Effects

Common: flushing, itching, tingling sensation, headache.

Generic Name	Brand Name
Niacin	Niaspan

Bile-Acid Binders

How They Work

Bile-acid binders deplete the body's supply of cholesterol. Bile acids, made from cholesterol in the liver, aid in digesting dietary fats. After bile acids are used, they are normally reabsorbed. Bile-acid binders prevent this reabsorption, causing the liver to use its reserved cholesterol to make more bile acids.

Possible Side Effects

Common: constipation, gas, stomach upset.

Generic Name	Brand Name
Cholestyramine	Prevalite, Questran
Colestipol	Colestid

HMG-CoA Reductase Inhibitors

How They Work

HMG-CoA reductase inhibitors block production of cholesterol in the liver.

Possible Side Effects

Common: stomach upset, liver function problems; rarely: muscle tenderness.

Generic Name	Brand Name
Atorvastatin	Lipitor
Cerivastatin	Baycol
Fluvastatin	Lescol
Lovastatin	Mevacor
Pravastatin	Pravachol
Simvastatin	Zocor

Diuretics

What They're For

Diuretics lower blood pressure. In people with congestive heart failure, diuretics reduce swelling and the accumulation of fluid.

There are three types of diuretics: *Thiazide diuretics* are mainly used to treat hypertension. The more powerful *loop diuretics* are used in heart and kidney failure. *Potassium-sparing diuretics* are mild diuretics mainly used with thiazides to prevent the loss of potassium that thiazides cause.

How They Work

Diuretics induce the kidneys to remove sodium. High blood sodium levels cause water retention and elevate blood pressure.

Possible Side Effects

Thiazide and loop diuretics: lowered potassium levels (which can cause nausea, numbness, confusion, drowsiness, and weakness), increased blood cholesterol and sugar levels, lowered calcium, sensitivity to sunburn, rash.

Potassium-sparing diuretics: increased level of potassium in the blood (which can cause weakness, numbness, confusion, and heaviness in the legs).

Precautions and Special Information

Because thiazide and loop diuretics make the kidneys excrete more potassium, a doctor or dietitian may recommend a diet of foods high in potassium, like fresh fruits and vegetables. Do not use a salt substitute that contains potassium, except under a doctor's supervision. Since these diuretics can increase the levels of uric acid in the blood, people with gout should have their levels of uric acid measured by a doctor.

Thiazide Diuretics

Generic Name	Brand Name
Chlorthalidone	Hygroton, Thalitone
Chlorothiazide	Diurigen, Diuril
Hydrochlorothiazide	Esidrix, Ezide, HydroDiuril, Hydro-Par, Oretic
Metolazone	Mykrox, Zaroxolyn

Loop Diuretics

Generic Name	Brand Name
Bumetanide	Bumex
Ethacrynic acid	Edecrin
Furosemide	Lasix
Torsemide	Demadex

Potassium-Sparing Diuretics

Generic Name	Brand Name
Amiloride	Midamor
Spironolactone	Aldactone
Triamterene	Dyrenium

Combinations

Generic Name	Brand Name
Amiloride/hydrochlorothiazide	Moduretic
Hydralazine/hydrochlorothiazide	Apresazide
Methyldopa/hydrochlorothiazide	Aldoril
Spironolactone/hydrochlorothiazide	Aldactazide
Triamterene/hydrochlorothiazide	Dyazide, Maxzide

Immunosuppressants

What They're For

Immunosuppressants are prescribed in heart transplantation to fight organ rejection.

How They Work

Immunosuppressants inhibit the production of T-lymphocytes, cells that are essential to the body's immune response.

Possible Side Effects

Common: kidney and liver toxicity, increased susceptibility to infections. Rare: tremors, cramps, acne.

Precautions and Special Information

Only doctors experienced in the management of immunosupressive therapy should prescribe these medications.

Generic Name	Brand Name
Azathiaprine	Imuran
Cyclosporine	Neoral, Sandimmune

Nitrates

What They're For

Nitrates prevent and treat attacks of angina, chest pain that occurs when the heart muscle does not receive enough blood.

How They Work

Nitrates dilate blood vessels throughout the body, decreasing stress on the heart's workload and increasing the blood flow through partially blocked coronary arteries.

Possible Side Effects

Common: headache, rapid pulse, flushing, sweating.

Precautions and Special Information

Avoid alcohol, which exacerbates nitrates' side effects. The anti-impotence medication Viagra cannot be taken while taking nitrates. Avoid physically stressful activities, which can bring on an angina attack. If one begins, stop all activity, sit or lie down, and take the medication immediately.

Generic Name	Brand Name
Isosorbide mononitrate	Monoket, Imdur, ISMO
Isosorbide dinitrate	Isordil, Sorbitrate
Nitroglycerin	Minitran, Nitro-Bid, Nitrodisc, Nitrogard, Nitrolingual, Nitrostat, Transderm-Nitro (many brand names available)
Pentaerythritol tetranitrate	Peritrate

Vasodilators

What They're For

Vasodilators lower blood pressure.

How They Work

Vasodilators cause blood vessels to dilate, thus reducing blood pressure. Vasodilators are often used in combination with other blood-pressure-lowering drugs such as diuretics and beta blockers. Many kinds of vasodilators are available, including alpha blockers and nitrates.

Possible Side Effects

Common: headache, rapid heart rate, flushing, sweating. In people with coronary artery disease, vasodilators can cause symptoms of angina. Loniten (minoxidil) causes hair growth.

Precautions and Special Information

To avoid dizziness, stand slowly from a lying position to prevent a sudden drop in blood pressure that can occur while taking vasodilators. At high doses, hydralazine (Apresoline) can cause symptoms of lupus—fever, joint pain, a general feeling of being unwell. Contact your doctor immediately if this occurs.

Generic Name	Brand Name
Hydralazine	Apresoline
Minoxidil	Loniten
Prazosin	Minipress
Terazosin	Hytrin

Glossary

Ablation The surgical removal or destruction of tissue.

Aerobic exercise Activity that conditions the heart and lungs and increases endurance by enhancing the body's ability to use oxygen. Regular aerobic exercise, such as jogging or swimming, can reduce the risk of coronary artery disease and improve cardiovascular health.

Alveolus One of the tiny air sacs at the ends of the bronchioles, the air passages in the lungs. During respiration, the alveoli release fresh oxygen into the bloodstream and absorb gaseous waste products such as carbon dioxide.

Amino acid An organic compound composed of carbon, oxygen, hydrogen, and nitrogen. All proteins, including such important cardiac proteins as hemoglobin, are built out of amino acids.

Amyloidosis A rare autoimmune disorder characterized by the buildup of abnormal protein in tissues. Amyloidosis can be a cause of heart valve disorders and heart failure.

Anemia A condition characterized by a deficiency of erythrocytes (red blood cells). Anemia, which reduces the amount of oxygen available to the body, can cause an irregular heartbeat.

Aneurysm A sac formed by the bulging of a blood vessel wall or section of heart tissue. An aneurysm, which is filled with fluid or clotted blood, can occur in any artery and is associated with atherosclerosis and hypertension.

Angina pectoris Chest pain or pressure, lasting a matter of minutes, that may radiate into the neck or arm. A common symptom of coronary artery disease, angina occurs during periods of physical or emotional stress and is relieved by rest.

Angiogenesis The spontaneous or drug-induced growth of new blood vessels. The growth of these vessels may help to alleviate coronary artery disease by rerouting blood flow around clogged arteries.

Angiography An invasive imaging procedure that usually involves inserting a catheter into an artery leading to the heart muscle or brain and injecting a radioactive tracer into the bloodstream via the catheter. Coronary angiography is particularly helpful in evaluating coronary artery disease, heart valve function, and the strength of the heart muscle.

Angioplasty   An invasive procedure in which a catheter is inserted into a narrowed artery. A tiny balloon may be placed at the tip of the catheter; it is inflated in order to widen the vessel. Or, a laser may be used to improve blood flow.

Angiotensin-converting enzyme (ACE) inhibitor   A type of medication that dilates blood vessels by slowing the body's production of angiotensin, a chemical that causes vessels to constrict. These medications, lower blood pressure.

Angiotensin II receptor blockers (ARBs)   A new class of medication that lowers blood pressure by blocking the action of angiotensin II, a chemical that causes blood vessels to constrict. These medications can be used to treat hypertension and congestive heart failure.

Annulus   A ring of fibrous tissue attached to the leaflets of a heart valve. The annulus helps to maintain the valve's structural integrity.

Antiarrhythmic   A medication used to treat irregular heartbeat.

Anticoagulant   A medication or body chemical that prevents blood clotting. Anticoagulant medications can be used to prevent myocardial infarction or stroke in people at high risk. Also called blood thinners.

Antihypertensive   A medication used to lower blood pressure.

Antioxidant   One of a group of vitamins—including A, B, C, and E—that may help to limit the cellular damage caused by free radicals. Studies suggest that certain antioxidants may help to prevent cardiovascular disease.

Aorta   The largest artery in the body. All blood pumped out of the left ventricle travels through the aorta on its way to other parts of the body.

Aortic valve   The strong valve that regulates blood flow between the left ventricle and the aorta. The heart's ability to pump blood may be affected if this valve is partially closed due to disease or a congenital defect.

Arrhythmia   An irregular heartbeat. While occasional episodes of irregular heartbeat are common, a persistent arrhythmia can be a symptom of heart disease.

Arterial pressure line   A catheter placed in an artery in the arm that is used to monitor blood pressure during recuperation from cardiac surgery.

Arteriole   A small artery. Arterioles are the vessels that connect arteries to capillaries.

Arteriosclerosis   A general term describing the thickening and hardening of the arteries. Atherosclerosis is considered a form of arteriosclerosis.

Artery   A vessel that transports oxygen-rich blood away from the heart. When an artery supplying blood to the heart muscle or brain is obstructed, the result may be a myocardial infarction or stroke.

Aspirin   A pain reliever, anti-inflammatory, and anticoagulant that is used to help prevent myocardial infarction.

Atherectomy   An invasive surgical procedure designed to clear clogged arteries by ablating the obstruction. In atherectomy, plaque deposits are removed through the use of a small razor-like device or a diamond-tipped drill.

Atherosclerosis   Narrowing and hardening of the arteries. Atherosclerosis, which occurs as a result of calcification and plaque buildup, can lead to the development of coronary artery disease and other cardiovascular problems.

Atresia   The abnormal closure or absence of an opening or passage. Atresia affecting the aorta can lead to the development of valvular disease in the form of aortic stenosis.

Atrial fibrillation   A rhythm disorder in which the upper heart chambers twitch chaotically, and fail to fully empty their contents into the ventricles. As blood pools in the atria, the risk of thrombosis increases.

Atrioventricular (AV) node   A group of cells located near the center of the heart that regulates the electrical current that travels through the heart with each beat, slowing and distributing the current once it reaches the ventricles.

Atrium   The filling chamber of the heart located above each ventricle. The heart has two atria—the left and the right. The blood that fills the left atrium is newly oxygenated blood returning from the lungs. The blood that fills the right atrium is deoxygenated blood returning from all parts of the body.

Batista procedure   See Ventriculectomy.

Beta-adrenergic blockers   See Beta-blockers.

Beta-blockers   A type of medication that reduces the amount of blood pressure required by the heart for proper functioning. Beta-blockers, which work by inhibiting the stimulating effects of epinephrine on the heart, are used to treat hypertension, slow the progression of congestive heart failure, lower heart rate, and in some cases dilate blood vessels. Also called beta-adrenergic blockers.

Bicuspid valve   A heart valve with two cusps. See Mitral valve.

Biofeedback   A relaxation technique that involves conscious control of involuntary body functions such as heart rate and blood pressure. Biofeedback can be useful in the management of stress.

Biopsy   Removal and analysis of a tissue sample. Biopsies of the myocardium are performed periodically after cardiac transplantation in order to determine if the body is rejecting the donor organ.

Blood pressure   The pressure of blood on the arterial walls, produced by the contractions of the heart and dependent on the elasticity of the arterial walls and the volume of blood. It is expressed in two numbers—diastolic and systolic. Normal blood pressure for an adult is 120/80.

Blood vessel   A flexible tube that transports blood throughout the body. Arteries, veins, and capillaries are the body's blood vessels.

Body mass index   The number, derived by dividing body weight by height squared, used to determine the degree of cardiovascular disease risk created by excess body weight.

Bradyarrhythmia   See Bradycardia.

Bradycardia   An abnormally slow heart rate. Also called bradyarrhythmia.

Bronchi   A pair of breathing tubes that connect the trachea to the lungs. Oxygen and carbon dioxide travel in opposite directions through the bronchi.

Bundle of His A network of specialized muscle fibers in the ventricles of the heart. The bundle of His triggers the contractions of the ventricles by slowing and distributing the electrical impulses originating in the sinoatrial node during heartbeat.

Bypass surgery See Coronary artery bypass graft surgery.

Calcification A process in which tissue becomes hardened due to deposits of calcium salts. Calcification of blood vessels plays a role in the development of atherosclerosis.

Calcium A mineral found mainly in dairy products that is used by the body as a building block of bone and for the proper functioning of organs and muscles. It is needed in many phases of blood clotting. Calcium is also an ingredient of artery-clogging plaque.

Calcium channel blocker A type of medication used to dilate blood vessels and slow heart rate. Calcium channel blockers are used to treat hypertension and certain arrhythmias, as well as angina pectoris.

Capillary A tiny blood vessel connecting arteries to veins. In the capillaries, the body's smallest blood vessels, oxygen and nutrients in the blood are exchanged for carbon dioxide.

Carbohydrate An organic compound composed of carbon, hydrogen, and oxygen. Found in sugars, cereals, fruits, and vegetables, carbohydrates provide fuel for the body and assist in the metabolism of other nutrients.

Carbon dioxide A gaseous by-product created during metabolism, when cells use oxygen to burn fat and release energy. Carbon dioxide is transported by erythrocytes to the lungs, where it is expelled.

Carbon monoxide A gas found in cigarette smoke. Carbon monoxide significantly increases the risk of coronary artery disease and other cardiovascular problems by damaging artery walls and reducing the ability of blood to carry oxygen.

Cardiac arrest Sudden cessation of heartbeat and breathing. Most people who suffer cardiac arrest have an underlying heart condition such as coronary artery disease, hypertension, or congestive heart failure.

Cardiac auscultation The use of a stethoscope to listen to the sounds the heart makes as it contracts and relaxes. Cardiac auscultation can be used to evaluate heart rate and rhythm.

Cardiac catheterization   An invasive procedure in which a catheter is inserted into an artery or heart chamber, via an incision in the arm or groin, in order to examine the artery for blockage and assess blood flow or valve leakage. It can also be used to open blocked arteries.

Cardiac output   The amount of blood pumped by the left ventricle per minute. The cardiac output of an average adult is about 5 quarts.

Cardiac muscle   See Myocardium.

Cardiac transplantation   An operation in which a defective heart is replaced with a healthy donor organ. Cardiac transplantation may be recommended in cases of heart failure that do not respond to medication or alternate surgical procedures. Also called heart transplant surgery.

Cardiologist   A doctor who specializes in the study or treatment of the heart and its diseases.

Cardiomyopathy   A condition in which the myocardium deteriorates and fails to pump blood with sufficient force. Cardiomyopathy, which increases the risk of myocardial infarction and heart failure, can be caused by hypertension, coronary artery disease, heart valve disease, or congenital heart defects.

Cardiomyoplasty   An experimental, invasive procedure designed to increase the efficiency of the heart's pumping power; it involves transplanting muscle tissue from other parts of the body to the heart, and may be used in cases of heart failure.

Cardiopulmonary resuscitation (CPR)   A noninvasive technique designed to temporarily circulate oxygenated blood through the body of a person whose heart has stopped. CPR, which involves breathing for the victim and applying pressure to the chest, can often prevent death if it is performed during the first few minutes of a cardiac arrest.

Cardiovascular   Relating to the system composed of the heart and blood vessels. The cardiovascular system is responsible for circulating oxygen- and nutrient-rich blood throughout the body and removing waste products such as carbon dioxide.

Cardioversion   The process of reestablishing a normal heart rhythm by applying electric shock. Cardioversion may be accomplished using medications or a defibrillator.

Carotid artery The vessel that supplies the brain with oxygenated blood. A stroke can occur if the carotid artery or its branches become obstructed by an emboli or thrombus.

Carotid artery disease A progressive condition in which the carotid artery is damaged by atherosclerosis. Carotid artery disease can lead to stroke.

Carotid endarterectomy A surgical procedure used to treat carotid artery disease, wherein an incision is made in the neck, the carotid artery is opened, and the atherosclerotic plaque is removed.

Catecholamine A group of hormones, including epinephrine and norepinephrine, involved in the body's fight-or-flight response. An overproduction of catecholamines, such as that associated with chronic stress, can increase the risk of coronary artery disease.

Catheter A slender, flexible tube.

Catheterization See Cardiac catheterization.

Cell receptor A protein located on the surfaces of cells that binds with hormones and other chemicals in the bloodstream, including certain medications. Cell receptors are the means by which estrogen helps maintain cardiovascular health in premenopausal women.

Central nervous system The system composed of the brain and spinal cord. Besides governing higher functions such as thought, speech, and memory, the central nervous system helps to maintain cardiovascular health by regulating breathing rate and heartbeat and by making corrections in heart rhythm.

Cerebral embolism A common cause of stroke—an embolus that has moved through the bloodstream and obstructs an artery leading to the brain.

Cerebral hemorrhage The rupturing of an artery that supplies blood to the brain. Cerebral hemorrhage is a relatively uncommon cause of stroke.

Cholesterol A waxy substance produced by the body and found in foods that come from animals. Technically classified as a steroid, cholesterol is the main ingredient of atherosclerotic plaque.

Chordae tendinae The thin, fibrous cords that contribute structural support to the tricuspid and mitral valves. These two valves require the extra aid of chordae tendinae because they are large and fragile.

Clotting factors A group of chemicals in the blood, including fibrinogen, prothrombin, and calcium, that combine to form thrombi.

Coarctation of the aorta A severe constriction of the aorta, which becomes so narrowed that it fails to deliver sufficient blood flow to the lower part of the body. The result is an increase in blood pressure.

Collateral blood vessels Tiny, latent vessels that may spontaneously enlarge and become functional in people with coronary artery disease. Collateral vessels help to detour blood flow around plaque deposits in arteries.

Computed tomography (CT) An imaging procedure, which can be invasive or noninvasive, that uses x-rays and computers to create three-dimensional pictures of the inside of the body. Computed tomography can be used to gather information about the anatomy and functioning of the heart and the efficiency of blood flow through arteries.

Congenital Present at birth. Congenital heart defects are usually of unknown cause, but they may be hereditary or the result of disease contracted by the mother during pregnancy.

Congestive heart failure See Heart failure.

Coronary artery One of the vessels that supply the myocardium with oxygenated blood. A myocardial infarction can occur when one or more coronary arteries are obstructed by a thrombus.

Coronary artery bypass graft (CABG) surgery An invasive procedure that reroutes blood flow around an arterial obstruction by creating a shunt. The new passage bypasses the site of the blockage, allowing sufficient blood flow to nourish the myocardium.

Coronary artery disease A chronic, progressive condition in which a clogged coronary artery prevents the myocardium from receiving a sufficient supply of blood. When the arterial plaque ruptures and a thrombus forms at the site, the result is a myocardial infarction. Also called coronary heart disease or ischemic heart disease.

Coronary circulation The circulatory system that supplies the heart with blood. In coronary circulation, a portion of newly oxygenated blood pumped by the heart is sent directly to the myocardium via the coronary arteries.

Coronary heart disease See Coronary artery disease.

Coronary spasm An involuntary contraction of a coronary artery that temporarily obstructs blood flow to the myocardium. Coronary spasm, which tends to affect young men who smoke heavily, is associated with atherosclerosis and can trigger a myocardial infarction.

Cortisol A hormone produced in the adrenal glands and associated with the body's fight-or-flight response. Excessive production of cortisol can elevate blood pressure.

Cryotherapy An invasive procedure that involves freezing tissue in order to destroy it. Cryotherapy can be used to ablate abnormal tissue associated with cardiovascular disease.

Cyanosis A condition characterized by blue-tinted fingernails or skin, due to a lack of oxygen. It may occur in a newborn because of a heart defect.

Deep-vein thrombosis A thrombus (blood clot) in the deep veins of the legs or thighs. These clots, which can cause leg pain or swelling, may break off and become lodged in a smaller artery in the lungs—a potentially fatal complication.

Defibrillator A machine capable of re-establishing normal heart rhythm by administering an electric shock to the heart. Defibrillation can be administered externally or internally, via a device implanted under the skin.

Diabetes A disease in which the body either cannot produce enough insulin or properly metabolize the hormone, resulting in an excess amount of sugar in the blood. Even with treatment, diabetes significantly increases the risk of developing cardiovascular disease.

Diaphragm A muscle located below the sternum (breastbone) that aids in breathing.

Diastole The part of the heart cycle during which the myocardium relaxes and expands. During diastole, blood fills the heart chambers.

Dilated cardiomyopathy A degenerative, inflammatory disease of the myocardium that causes the heart cavity to become stretched and enlarged.

Diuretics A type of medication that helps the body eliminate excess fluids and sodium. They are used to treat hypertension, congestive heart failure, and certain types of irregular heartbeat.

Dyspnea Shortness of breath. Cardiac dyspnea is distressed breathing caused by heart disease.

Ebstein's anomaly A congenital malformation of the tricuspid valve. It usually occurs together with a septal defect.

Echocardiography An imaging procedure, which can be invasive or noninvasive, that creates a graphic outline of the heart's movement using high-frequency sound waves. Echocardiography is used to evaluate the heart's pumping action and detect valve abnormalities.

Ectopic Out of place. An ectopic heartbeat, for example, originates in an abnormal location of the heart.

Edema An abnormal swelling of tissue due to fluid buildup. Edema may be a complication of congestive heart failure, which may cause swelling in the legs, liver, and lungs.

Eisenmenger's complex A disease characterized by thickening of the pulmonary arteries, elevated blood pressure in the lungs, and heart failure. Eisenmenger's syndrome develops as a complication of ventricular septal defect, a congenital disorder.

Ejection fraction The amount of blood pumped out of a ventricle during heartbeat. The ejection fraction evaluates how well the heart is functioning. A healthy heart pumps out about 67 percent of the blood in each ventricle.

Electrocardiography Diagnostic testing, usually noninvasive, that produces a graph—an electrocardiogram (ECG or EKG)—representing the heart's electrical impulses.

Electrolyte One of the substances in the blood that helps to regulate the proper balance of body fluids. Electrolytes such as sodium and potassium are removed by the kidneys as needed in order to control the volume of fluid in the blood, which in turn helps to regulate blood pressure.

Electrophysiology study An invasive procedure that involves inserting a catheter into the myocardium, via an incision in the arm or groin, and stimulating the heart with a mild electrical charge in order to identify the origin of an abnormal heart rhythm.

Embolus A blood clot that moves through the bloodstream. When forced into a smaller blood vessel, it can create an obstruction. Embolism is the blocking of an artery by an embolus.

Endarterectomy A surgical procedure wherein an artery is opened and atherosclerotic plaque is removed. Often performed on the carotid artery to prevent stroke.

Endocarditis An infection of the inner lining of the heart or its valves. Endocarditis, which is caused by bacteria, is more likely to occur in people who have heart valve disorders or prosthetic valves.

Endocardium The smooth, inner lining of the heart chambers.

Endoscopy An invasive procedure in which an endoscope, a slender tube fitted with a miniature camera and light source, is used to produce images of the inside of the body on a monitor. These images can be used to provide a view of the interior of the heart during surgery to repair the organ or its valves.

Endothelium The interior surfaces of blood vessels. The endothelium, which is the site of atherosclerosis in arteries, is composed of specialized cells called epithelial cells.

Enzyme A protein in cells that stimulates chemical reactions in the body. Some enzymes, such as renin, help to regulate blood pressure and other aspects of cardiovascular health.

Epicardium The thin membrane surrounding the myocardium. Also called the visceral pericardium.

Epidemiology The study of large populations to determine the frequency, distribution, and risk factors associated with a particular disease. The data from epidemiologic studies, for example, suggest that moderate amounts of alcohol may help prevent cardiovascular disease.

Epinephrine A hormone produced by the adrenal glands that also acts as a neurotransmitter for nerve cells. As part of the fight-or-flight response, epinephrine signals the heart to pump harder, increases blood pressure, and has other effects on the cardiovascular system. Also called adrenaline.

Erythrocyte One of millions of red blood cells that deliver oxygen to tissues and removes carbon dioxide and other waste products. Also called red blood cells, red cells, or red corpuscles.

Esophagus The tube that connects the mouth to the stomach. Echocardiography is sometimes performed by placing the transducer, the instrument that bounces sound waves off the myocardium, inside the esophagus.

Essential fatty acid   A type of fatty acid that the body cannot produce and which must be obtained from food. Essential fatty acids, which are especially important when the body is recuperating from cardiac or other surgery, play a role in the making of cell membranes and also help prevent infection by strengthening the immune system.

Estrogen   The primary female sex hormone, which is thought to play a major role in maintaining cardiovascular health in women.

Exercise stress test   A test that provides information about the way the heart responds to physical exertion or emotional stress. An exercise stress test usually involves walking or jogging on a treadmill or pedaling a stationary bike while heart rate and blood pressure are monitored.

Fatty acid   A building block of fat. A fatty acid is classified as saturated, monounsaturated, or polyunsaturated depending on how much of the element hydrogen it contains.

Fiber   An indigestible carbohydrate found in fruits and vegetables that aids in digestion and may help to prevent heart disease. Studies suggest that one type of fiber, called soluble fiber, can lower total and low-density lipoprotein cholesterol.

Fibrillation   Abnormally rapid, inefficient contractions of the atria or ventricles. Fibrillation, which originates in tiny sections of myocardial fibers, can prevent the heart from pumping sufficient amounts of blood.

Fibrin   A protein that helps blood to clot and aids in the healing of wounds. Fibrin is also a component of artery-clogging plaque.

Flutter   A type of rapid heartbeat. Atrial flutter, which usually does not have serious health consequences, may occur after open-heart surgery or as a response to stimulants such as caffeine or nicotine.

Foley catheter   A catheter that connects the bladder to a urine collection bag via the urethra. A Foley catheter, which may be used during the first few days of recuperation from cardiac surgery, allows patients who are confined to bed to urinate.

Foramen ovale   An opening between the atria of the heart that normally closes shortly after birth. An atrial septal defect may develop if the foramen ovale fails to close properly.

Free radical A destructive fragment of oxygen produced as a by-product when cells use oxygen to burn fat. Free radicals can damage cells and the genes that regulate how cells grow.

Gangrene The death of tissue due to inadequate blood supply. Gangrene, which usually affects the extremities, is more likely to occur in people with atherosclerosis, vascular disease, or other conditions associated with poor blood circulation.

Glucose Blood sugar. Manufactured by the body from carbohydrates, protein, and fat, glucose is the main source of energy for all living organisms.

Great vessels The large blood vessels that enter the heart: the aorta, the pulmonary artery and vein, and the venae cavae.

Greater saphenous vein A long vein extending from the ankle to the groin that may be used to create a shunt during bypass surgery.

Heart attack See Myocardial infarction.

Heart block A condition in which the electrical current that triggers heartbeat is obstructed between the atria and ventricles. Heart block, which can cause dangerously slow heartbeat, may be a result of a myocardial infarction, thickening of the atrioventricular node, endocarditis, or calcification of the aortic or mitral valves.

Heart failure A chronic, progressive disease in which the myocardium becomes weakened and elongated. In congestive heart failure, the heart fails to pump with enough force to supply oxygenated blood to all parts of the body, and fluid collects throughout the body.

Heart-lung machine A machine that detours blood flow around the heart and lungs during surgery to replace the organs. A heart-lung machine, which removes carbon dioxide from the blood and replaces it with oxygen, is used during a heart or lung transplant.

Heart monitor An electrocardiography machine designed to monitor heart function continuously during rehabilitation from cardiac surgery. If the heart monitor detects an abnormality in heart rate or rhythm, it alerts nearby nurses by sounding an alarm.

Heart transplant surgery See Cardiac transplantation.

Hemoglobin A protein in erythrocytes that attracts oxygen and carbon dioxide and gives blood its red color. When blood passes through capillaries, the oxygen in hemoglobin is released into tissues and replaced with carbon dioxide.

Hemorrhaging Heavy bleeding. A cerebral hemorrhage can lead to a stroke.

Hepatitis Inflammation of the liver. Liver damage caused by hepatitis can affect the organ's ability to remove waste products from blood.

High blood pressure See Hypertension.

High-density lipoprotein A particle of protein, cholesterol, and triglyceride. It deposits its cargo of cholesterol in the liver, where it is excreted or used to make other substances needed by the body.

His-Purkinje system See Bundle of His.

Holter monitor A small and portable electrocardiography machine, worn on a shoulder sling for 12 to 48 hours, that records the heart's rhythm and can detect such abnormalities as flutters and skipped beats.

Homocysteine An amino acid. While necessary for good health, high levels of homocysteine can raise cholesterol levels and contribute to the development of atherosclerosis.

Hormone A chemical produced by the body that travels the bloodstream delivering messages between organs and glands. Hormones are used by the central nervous system to regulate heartbeat and blood pressure and to help the cardiovascular system to respond to changes in the internal and external environments.

Hydrogenation An industrial process used by food manufacturers that involves adding hydrogen to polyunsaturated fatty acids in order to increase the shelf-life of a product or make it thicker in consistency. The special breed of fatty acids created by this process, called transfatty acids, can raise total cholesterol levels and lower high-density lipoprotein cholesterol.

Hyperlipidemia Elevated blood levels of fatty substances, including cholesterol and triglycerides.

Hypertension High blood pressure. Elevated blood pressure can increase the heart's workload and contribute to the development of cardiovascular disease and kidney failure.

Hyperthyroidism A condition caused by excessive production of thyroid hormones. Hyperthyroidism can cause irregular heartbeat.

Hypertrophy An abnormal enlargement of an organ or thickening of its tissue. An enlarged left ventricle, called left ventricular hypertrophy, can lead to cardiac arrest.

Hypoplasia The incomplete development of an organ or tissue. In hypoplastic left heart syndrome, the left side of the heart does not develop normally during gestation and fails to pump sufficient amounts of blood.

Hypotension Low blood pressure.

Hysterectomy The surgical removal of the uterus and ovaries. The risk of heart disease rises when menopause is induced through a hysterectomy.

Idiopathic Of unknown origin. Some cardiovascular diseases, such as aortic stenosis, often occur idiopathically.

Iliac veins The two principal veins returning blood from the lower part of the body. The iliac veins eventually join to form the inferior vena cava.

Immunosuppression Lowering of the body's immune system response with the use of radiation or medication. Immunosuppressive drugs are used before and after heart transplant surgery to prevent the immune system from attacking and damaging the donor organ.

Infarction Tissue death caused by oxygen deprivation. The death of heart tissue occurs when the organ's blood supply is obstructed or severely reduced.

Innominate veins The two principal veins returning blood from the upper part of the body. The innominate veins eventually join to form the superior vena cava.

Inotropic medication A class of medications that strengthens heart muscle contractions and improves blood circulation. Inotropic drugs are often used in the treatment of congestive heart failure.

Insomnia Difficulty sleeping. Insomnia is a common problem during recuperation from cardiac surgery due to the lingering effects of anesthesia, the discomfort associated with healing, and recovery-related anxiety or stress.

Insulin   A hormone produced by the pancreas that helps the body to metabolize sugar.

Intermittent claudication   Reduced oxygen supply to the leg muscles due to a narrowed artery. Intermittent claudication, which causes lower leg pain during walking or exercise, can be caused by atherosclerosis or a spasm or occlusion in an artery.

Intima   The inner layer of the arterial wall. Atherosclerosis originates in the intima.

Intravascular   Within a blood vessel. Intravascular ultrasound, for example, involves inserting a catheter directly into the wall of a coronary blood vessel to examine it using a miniaturized ultrasound probe.

Invasive   Penetrating. Invasive tests or procedures, such as angiography, are those that penetrate the body or puncture the skin. They are generally associated with more risk and discomfort than are noninvasive tests.

Ischemia   Reduced blood flow to an area of the body due to an obstructed vessel. Ischemia usually occurs when a coronary artery becomes narrowed due to atherosclerosis.

Ischemic heart disease   See Coronary artery disease.

Leukocyte   One of millions of cells in the blood that seeks and destroys disease-causing microorganisms. Leukocytes play a role in the development of atherosclerosis by trapping particles of low-density lipoprotein cholesterol in artery walls. Also called white blood cells, white cells, or white corpuscles.

Linolenic acid   See Omega 3.

Lipid   Fat circulating in the blood, including particles of cholesterol or triglycerides. A lipid profile measures these fats.

Lipoprotein   A fat-protein combination that transports lipids in the blood. Lipoproteins are the means by which cholesterol and triglycerides travel through the bloodstream.

Low-density lipoprotein   A particle of protein, cholesterol, and triglyceride. Low-density lipoprotein is responsible for depositing cholesterol onto artery linings, where it can accumulate and form plaque.

Lumen   The hollow cavity of a blood vessel or other tubular organ.

Lupus See Systemic lupus erythematosus.

Magnetic resonance imaging (MRI) An imaging procedure, which can be invasive or noninvasive, that creates three-dimensional pictures of the inside of the body. MRI can be used to evaluate the functioning of the heart's chambers and reveal the presence of congenital defects.

Menopause The cessation of estrogen production by the ovaries. Several years after women complete menopause, they experience myocardial infarctions at about the same rate as men do.

Metabolism The sum of all processes involved in converting nutrients into energy for use by the body.

Mineral An inorganic compound needed by the body for good health, proper metabolic functioning, and disease prevention. Examples are calcium, magnesium, and iron.

Mini-stroke See Transient ischemic attack.

Mitral valve The high-pressure valve that regulates blood flow between the left atrium and ventricle. The heart's ability to pump blood may be affected if this valve is partially closed due to disease or a congenital defect. Also called the bicuspid valve.

Mitral valve prolapse See Prolapse.

mm Hg An abbreviation that stands for "millimeters of mercury." Blood pressure is measured in mm Hg.

Monounsaturated fat A fat composed mostly of monounsaturated fatty acids. Monounsaturated fat may help reduce the amount of low-density lipoprotein cholesterol in the blood.

Morbidity rate The percentage of people who have complications after a procedure or treatment.

Mortality rate The percentage of deaths associated with a disease or medical treatment.

Murmur An abnormal sound caused by the flow of blood through a defective heart valve or narrowed chamber. Murmurs, which can occur during the systolic or diastolic phases of heartbeat, are usually detected during cardiac auscultation.

Myocardial infarction A sudden obstruction of blood flow through a coronary artery that results in the death of heart tissue. The immediate cause of a myocardial infarction is usually a thrombus that forms near the site of ruptured plaque. Also called a heart attack.

Myocarditis An inflammation of the myocardium. Myocarditis can cause irregular heartbeat.

Myocardium The heart muscle; the muscular, middle layer of heart tissue that contracts rhythmically during heartbeat. When the myocardium becomes damaged or weakened due to reduced blood supply, the result may be heart failure or myocardial infarction.

Neurotransmitter A hormone that delivers messages between the brain and the cardiovascular system. Some neurotransmitters provide the brain with information regarding blood pressure and electrolyte levels in the blood, while others help regulate the breathing rate and the amount of oxygen supplied to tissues.

Nitroglycerin A coronary vasodilator which begins to work in less than a minute. It is the drug most frequently used to treat acute attacks of angina.

Noninvasive Nonpenetrating. Noninvasive tests or procedures, such as a blood pressure reading, do not penetrate the body and are usually considered low-risk and painless.

Norepinephrine A hormone produced by the adrenal glands that also acts as a neurotransmitter for nerve cells. As part of the fight-or-flight response, norepinephrine signals the heart to pump harder, increases blood pressure, and has other effects on the cardiovascular system.

Nuclear scan A general term for an imaging procedure that involves the injection or ingestion of a low-dose radioactive tracer before images are taken. Positron emission tomography (PET) is a nuclear scan used to help diagnose cardiovascular disease.

Obesity An excess of body fat that is 20 percent or more over a person's ideal weight. Obesity strains the cardiovascular system and increases the risk of diabetes, hypertension, and elevated lipid levels.

Occlusion Blockage. Most myocardial infarctions occur when a coronary artery becomes occluded due to a thrombus.

Omega 3 An essential fatty acid. Omega 3, which is found in fish and certain plants, may reduce the risk of cardiovascular disease and myocardial infarction by lowering triglyceride levels and blood pressure and preventing the formation of life-threatening thrombi. Also called linolenic acid.

Open-heart surgery   Any of a number of invasive cardiac surgical procedures. Open-heart surgery, which has been traditionally performed with the aid of a heart-lung machine, includes valve replacement, bypass, heart transplant, and other surgeries.

Oral contraceptives   Medications that use estrogen or progesterone to prevent conception. Women who take oral contraceptives with high levels of these hormones are at increased risk of developing cardiovascular problems.

Osteoporosis   A severe weakening of bone. Osteoporosis may occur as a long-term side effect of immunosuppressive medications, which are taken to prevent the rejection of a donor organ after heart transplant surgery.

Oxidation   A process in which free radicals released during metabolism damage cells and the DNA that control cell growth. Oxidation can accelerate the process of atherosclerosis by damaging particles of low-density lipoprotein cholesterol, making them more potent as plaque-builders.

Pacemaker   A small device capable of re-establishing normal heart rhythm by administering an electric shock to the heart. Pacemakers may be implanted under the skin or worn externally.

Palpitation   The sensation of rapid heartbeat or a missed beat. Palpitations are characterized by an increase in the frequency or force of heartbeat and are often accompanied by irregular heart rhythm.

Parietal pericardium   The fibrous outer layer of the pericardium.

Patency rate   The likelihood that a vessel will remain open. In coronary artery bypass surgery, a portion of the internal mammary artery is often used as a shunt because it has a high patency rate.

Pericardial cavity   The space between the epicardium and the outer layer of the pericardium. The cavity is normally filled with a small amount of clear fluid that reduces friction between the two membranes.

Pericarditis   An inflammation of the membrane surrounding the heart, usually accompanied by fluid buildup. Pericarditis can cause irregular heartbeat.

Pericardium   The translucent sac that encloses the heart. The pericardium protects the heart from infections originating in other parts of the body, such as the lungs.

Perimenopause   The several years preceding menopause, during which women may experience fluctuating hormone levels, irregular periods, occasional hot flashes, and fatigue. The symptoms of myocardial infarction in women may be confused with those of perimenopause.

Phytochemical   An organic compound found in plants that is believed to play a role in preventing cardiovascular or other diseases.

Plaque   Deposits of cholesterol, calcium salts, cellular waste, and fibrin on the inner linings of blood vessels. Plaque is the reason that arteries become thickened and hardened during the process of atherosclerosis.

Plasma   A translucent, watery liquid that accounts for about half of blood volume. Plasma transports most of the substances and gases found in blood, such as vitamins, minerals, oxygen, and fat.

Platelet   See Thrombocyte.

Platelet antagonist   A type of anticoagulant medication that prevents blood clotting by interfering with the activity of platelets. Aspirin is a platelet antagonist.

Pleura   The thin membrane that surrounds and cushions each lung. The pleura is composed of two layers with fluid between them.

Polyunsaturated fat   A fat composed mostly of polyunsaturated fatty acids. Polyunsaturated fat can lower blood cholesterol level.

Portal vein   The principal vein leading to the liver. Veins from the stomach, spleen, pancreas, and intestine are connected to the portal vein, which delivers blood into the liver for filtering.

Positron emission tomography (PET)   An invasive imaging procedure that creates three-dimensional pictures of the inside of the body and can monitor metabolic processes. This procedure, which involves an injection of a low-dose radioactive tracer before images are taken, is effective at detecting areas of oxygen deprivation in the myocardium.

Prinzmetal's angina   See Variant angina.

Prolapse   A condition in which an organ or other part of the body is not in its correct position. In mitral valve prolapse, for example, the leaflets of the valve enter the left atrium of the heart as the valve closes, allowing blood to flow backward into the left atrium.

Prophylaxis   The prevention of disease. Anticoagulant therapy may be used as a prophylactic measure to help prevent myocardial infarctions.

Protein   A group of organic compounds composed of amino acids and rich in nitrogen. Protein, which is required for the growth and repair of tissue and the formation of hormones and enzymes, is also used by the body to transport fat and cholesterol through the bloodstream.

Pulmonary artery   The vessel through which blood exits the right ventricle on its way to the lungs, where it receives oxygen. The pulmonary artery is the body's only artery that carries deoxygenated blood.

Pulmonary circulation   The circulation of blood from the right side of the heart, to the lungs, then to the left side of the heart. During pulmonary circulation, deoxygenated blood pumped through the lungs exchanges carbon dioxide for oxygen.

Pulmonary edema   An abnormal swelling of tissue in the lungs due to fluid buildup. Left-sided heart failure is a common cause of pulmonary edema.

Pulmonary valve   See Pulmonic valve.

Pulmonic valve   The valve that regulates blood flow between the right ventricle and the pulmonary artery. The pulmonic valve is less likely to be a cause of cardiovascular problems than the aortic or mitral valves. Also called the pulmonary valve.

Pulmonologist   A doctor who specializes in the study and treatment of the lungs and their diseases.

Pulse rate   The number of heartbeats per minute. The resting pulse rate of an average adult is between 60 and 100 beats per minute.

Radioactive tracer   A low-dose radioactive dye or contrast medium injected into a blood vessel as part of an imaging procedure. Radioactive tracers are used to enhance the quality of x-ray images.

Radiofrequency   An invasive procedure that involves heating tissue in order to destroy it. Radiofrequency can be used to ablate abnormal tissue associated with cardiovascular disease.

Radionuclide scan An invasive imaging procedure that involves an injection of a low-dose radioactive tracer that can highlight the interior of an organ such as the heart. A radionuclide scan can be used to evaluate blood flow to the heart and the functioning of its chambers and can also detect areas of heart muscle damage.

Red blood cell See Erythrocyte.

Red corpuscle See Erythrocyte.

Regurgitation A backward flow. Blood may be regurgitated into the heart or between its chambers due to the improper functioning of a heart valve.

Renin An enzyme produced by the kidneys. Renin is released into the bloodstream by the kidneys in order to regulate blood pressure.

Restenosis The closing or narrowing of an artery that was previously widened by a cardiac procedure such as angioplasty.

Rheumatic fever A systemic disease characterized by inflammation of the joints and muscles. Untreated rheumatic fever can cause damage to the mitral and aortic valves.

Rupture Break. A rupture of plaque in an artery is often the immediate cause of a myocardial infarction or stroke, because the rupture triggers the formation of a thrombus.

Saturated fat A fat composed mostly of saturated fatty acids. Saturated fat is the most important dietary factor in raising cholesterol levels.

Sepsis A serious infection in the bloodstream. Sepsis can lead to irregular heartbeat.

Septostomy An invasive procedure that temporarily redirects blood flow to ensure that sufficient amounts reach the lungs. Septostomy, which is often performed in infants with transposition of the great vessels, increases the amount of oxygen available to the body.

Septum The muscular wall separating the right and left sides of the heart. The septum prevents oxygenated blood in the left side of the heart from mixing with deoxygenated blood in the right side.

Shunt A surgically created passage between blood vessels that is designed to reroute blood flow.

Sinoatrial (SA) node A natural pacemaker located within a small bundle of specialized cells in the right atrium of the heart. Considered the starting point of the heartbeat, the sinoatrial node generates rhythmic electrical impulses that guide the contractions of the heart chambers. Also called sinus node.

Sinus node   See Sinoatrial Node.

Sphygmomanometer   Blood pressure cuff. The sphygmomanometer is wrapped around the arm and inflated with air during a typical blood pressure reading.

Spirometry   Noninvasive diagnostic testing used to evaluate the functioning of the lungs. Spirometry involves breathing forcefully into a machine (spirometer) that measures the volume and flow rate of air entering and exiting the lungs. Also called a ventilation test.

Stenosis   A condition in which a blood vessel or other passage in the body becomes abnormally narrow. Stenosis can restrict blood flow by narrowing arteries or heart valves.

Stent   A wire-mesh tube inserted after balloon angioplasty that functions to support the arterial wall and keeps the vessel dilated. A stent, which remains in the artery permanently, is effective at preventing restenosis and subsequent bypass surgery.

Stroke   A sudden obstruction or rupturing of an artery leading to the brain. During a stroke, brain cells in the affected area are starved for oxygen and subsequently die.

Syncope   A condition characterized by faintness or dizziness. Syncope can be a symptom of heart valve disease or other cardiovascular problems.

Systemic circulation   The circulation of blood from the left ventricle, through an extensive network of vessels that penetrate every part of the body, to the right side of the heart.

Systemic lupus erythematosus   A chronic autoimmune disorder in which a person's natural antibodies, which normally fight infection, damage parts of the central nervous system, connective tissue, or internal organs such as the lungs or kidneys. Lupus can cause heart valve disorders, including regurgitation and stenosis.

Systolic   Relating to the beating phase of the heart cycle, during which parts of the organ contract. It is during the systole phase that blood is propelled out of the heart through the left and right ventricles.

Tachyarrhythmia   See Tachycardia.

Tachycardia   An abnormally rapid heartbeat. Certain tachycardias, such as those originating in the ventricles, can trigger cardiac arrest if left untreated. Also called tachyarrhythmia.

Thrombocyte   One of the irregularly shaped cells in the blood that congregates at the site of internal or external wounds in order to seal off the injured area and stop the bleeding. While necessary for good health, thrombocytes also contribute to the formation of life-threatening blood clots in arteries. Also called platelet.

Thrombogenesis   The process of blood-clot formation.

Thrombolytics   A type of medication designed to dissolve clots that form in blood vessels. Administering a thrombolytic within a few hours after a heart attack can reduce the extent of heart muscle damage.

Thrombus   A blood clot. A thrombus, which is attached to the artery in which it forms, can obstruct blood flow and result in a heart attack or stroke. It may also break free to become an embolus and lodge elsewhere.

Tissue-plasminogen activator (t-PA)   A clot-dissolving agent that is injected directly into a clogged artery to break up a blood clot. If used within 3 hours after the start of a stroke, brain damage may be avoided.

Total cholesterol   The total amount of cholesterol in the blood. This measurement accounts for cholesterol carried by both high-density and low-density lipoprotein.

Transesophageal echocardiography   An invasive type of echocardiography in which the transducer, the instrument that bounces sound waves off the myocardium, is placed inside the esophagus. Transesophageal echocardiography provides clearer images of the heart's movement because the transducer's location in the esophagus is closer to the heart and limits interference.

Transient ischemic attack   A stroke-like event lasting several minutes that occurs when the brain is temporarily deprived of sufficient blood flow. A transient ischemic attack may increase the risk of stroke. Also called a mini-stroke.

Tricuspid valve   The valve that regulates blood flow between the right atrium and ventricle. The tricuspid valve is less likely to be a cause of cardiovascular problems than the aortic or mitral valves.

Triglyceride   A molecule composed of three fatty acids attached to a base of glycerol. Most dietary and body fat exists in the form of triglycerides.

Valvuloplasty   An invasive procedure in which a catheter is inserted into a narrowed heart valve and a tiny balloon at the tip of the catheter is inflated in order to widen the valve. Valvuloplasty can be used to improve blood flow in cases of aortic stenosis and other heart valve problems.

Variant angina   A type of angina that occurs at rest, usually during sleep, due to coronary artery spasm.

Vascular   Relating to the network of arteries, veins, and smaller vessels.

Vasodilator   A type of medication that increases blood flow to the heart by dilating blood vessels. Coronary vasodilators enlarge the arteries serving the heart and allow more oxygen and nutrients to reach the myocardium.

Vein   A vessel that transports blood from other parts of the body back to the heart. Unlike arteries, veins have tiny valves that prevent blood from flowing in the wrong direction.

Vena cava   The two large veins that collect blood returning from all parts of the body. Blood returning from the upper part of the body enters the right atrium through the superior vena cava, while blood from the lower extremities enters this filling chamber via the inferior vena cava inferior.

Venous thrombosis   A blockage in a vein caused by a thrombus. Blood cannot return to the heart; as a result, swelling and tenderness in the affected area may occur.

Ventilation test   See Spirometry.

Ventricle   The heart's pumping chambers. The heart has two atria—the left and the right—located below each atrium. The blood that fills the left atrium is newly oxygenated blood returning from the lungs. The stronger of the heart's two pumps, the left ventricle is responsible for pumping oxygenated blood to all parts of the body. The weaker of the heart's two pumps, the right ventricle is responsible for pumping blood into the nearby lungs, where it exchanges carbon dioxide for oxygen.

Ventriculectomy   An invasive procedure that increases the heart's pumping power by reducing the size of the left ventricle. Ventriculectomy, which involves removing small sections of the myocardium, may be used in cases of heart failure. Also called the Batista procedure.

Visceral pericardium   See Epicardium.

Vitamin   One of the organic compounds needed by the body for good health, proper metabolic functioning, and disease prevention.

White blood cell   See Leukocyte.

White corpuscle   See Leukocyte.

Index

A

Abciximab, combined with stents, 273
Ablation. *See also* Radiofrequency ablation
  defined, 309
ACE inhibitors
  defined, 310
  for heart disease prevention, 274
  for heart failure, 171
  pharmacology and types of, 297
  for promotion of new blood vessel growth, 93–94
Activity. *See* Exercise
Aerobic exercise. *See also* Exercise
  characteristics of, 257
  defined, 309
  examples of, 40
African Americans
  atherosclerosis risk in, 21
  vascular disease and stroke risk in, 188
Age and aging
  cardiac effects of, 161–62
  as contraindication to heart transplantation, 175
  dissecting aneurysm associated with, 200
  mitral valve stenosis severity related to, 117–18
  as risk factor
    for arteriosclerosis, 188
    for coronary artery disease, 20
    for stroke, 188
Alcohol consumption, 32–33
  avoiding, with platelet blockers, 94
  benefits of, 32
  guidelines for, 33
Aldactone (spironolactone), for heart failure, 170
Alpha agonists, central, 302
Alpha blockers, 296–97

Ambulation, after heart surgery, 233–34
American Heart Association
  recommendation for cholesterol screening, 63
  as source of information, 61
Amiodarone, for ventricular tachycardia, 143
Aneurysm, 198–202
  causes of, 48, 199–200
  with coarctation of aorta, 220
  defined, 48, 309
  degenerative, 198
  diagnosis and detection of, 200–201
  dissecting, 198, 200
  surgical therapy of, 201–2
    complications of, 202
  symptoms of, 199
  ventricular, surgical repair of, 174
Anger
  after diagnosis of heart disease, 258
  as risk factor for coronary artery disease, 26
Angina pectoris, 85–87
  in aortic valve regurgitation, 128
  in aortic valve stenosis, 117
  in coronary artery disease, 48
  defined, 309
  disorders with pains similar to, 66
  family information about, 258
  radiation of pain in, 86
  as signal for impending myocardial infarction, 87, 89
  signs and symptoms of, 64–65, 85–86
  unstable, 86
  variant (Prinzmetal's)
    calcium-channel blockers for, 92
    characteristics of, 85
    defined, 333
  vasospastic, 66
Angiogenesis
  ACE inhibitors for promoting, 93–94
  defined, 309